Advanced
EXERCISES IN DIAGNOSTIC RADIOLOGY

9

DIAGNOSTIC RADIOLOGY OF THE BRAIN: CT, DSA, NMR

Second Edition

RUTH G. RAMSEY, M.D.

Associate Professor of Radiology
Section of Neuroradiology
Rush-Presbyterian-St. Luke's Medical Center
Chicago, Illinois

W. B. SAUNDERS COMPANY • 1984
PHILADELPHIA • LONDON • TORONTO • MEXICO CITY • RIO DE JANEIRO • SYDNEY • TOKYO

W. B. Saunders Company: West Washington Square
Philadelphia, PA 19105

1 St. Anne's Road
Eastbourne, East Sussex BN21 3UN, England

1 Goldthorne Avenue
Toronto, Ontario M8Z 5T9, Canada

Apartado 26370—Cedro 512
Mexico 4, D.F., Mexico

Rua Coronel Cabrita, 8
Sao Cristovao Caixa Postal 21176
Rio de Janeiro, Brazil

9 Waltham Street
Artarmon, N.S.W. 2064, Australia

Ichibancho, Central Bldg., 22-1 Ichibancho
Chiyoda-Ku, Tokyo 102, Japan

Library of Congress Cataloging in Publication Data

Ramsey, Ruth G.

Diagnostic radiology of the brain.

(Advanced exercises in diagnostic radiology ; 9)

Rev. ed. of: Computed tomography of the brain. 1977.

Includes index.

1. Brain—Radiography. 2. Brain—Diseases—Diagnosis. 3. Diagnosis, Radioscopic. I. Title. II. Ramsey, Ruth G. Computed tomography of the brain. III. Series. [DNLM: 1. Brain—Radiography. 2. Tomography, X-ray computed. W1 AD402E v. 9 / WL 141 R183c]

RC78.E89 vol. 9, 1984 [RC386.6.R3] 616.07′57s
83–18946 [616.8′047572]

ISBN 0–7216–1177–X

Computed Tomography of the Brain ISBN 0-7216-1177-X

Last digit is the print number: 9 8 7 6 5 4 3 2 1

Dedicated to
M.M.R., J.J.F., M.S.H.

PREFACE
to the Second Edition

Since the first edition of this book, there have been a number of advances in the field of computed tomography. However, it is worthwhile to reiterate the virtues of this technique before discussing these new developments. It is not an exaggeration to say that computed tomography has revolutionized our approach to the diagnosis of intracranial abnormalities. The technique is essentially noninvasive, provides more and better definition of the intracranial structures than any other method, and is particularly useful in defining midline lesions of the brain and abnormalities of the posterior fossa. Computed tomography outlines the exact pathologic condition better than any other method and makes anatomic abnormalities readily apparent. The examination is easily performed with essentially no discomfort to the patient, usually as an out-patient procedure. In addition to its importance in diagnosis, the method has proved of great value in treatment planning and in follow-up care.

Newer scanners provide even more precise anatomic definition and sensitivity than the earlier models. The new scanners are also much more rapid and versatile than the older models.

In addition to the chapters on computed tomography of the brain and orbit in this edition, new chapters have been added that provide an introduction to the newer techniques of ultrasonography of the neonatal brain, digital subtraction angiography, and nuclear magnetic resonance imaging.

This book is not meant to be a comprehensive textbook on any of these topics but rather a basic "handbook" or readily available information source about these techniques. In the case of computed tomography of the brain and orbits, the newer method of study is compared with the older, more established methods in the hope of correlating the CT scans with the type of studies with which many are already familiar. Medical students and residents in radiology, neurology, neurosurgery, internal medicine, and other medical specialties as well as technologists will find this book especially helpful. The practicing physician will also find this book useful as a day-to-day reference.

ACKNOWLEDGMENTS

Many of the case examples contained in the first edition have been retained in this edition because they display a certain unique feature or because of their excellent correlation with the nuclear medicine scans. (In the age of computed tomography, radionuclide brain scanning has become almost extinct.) However, many new cases have also been added, and I wish to extend my thanks to many individuals who helped me with this second edition. Charles Havel, Robert Walker, Elissa Ray, and the entire photography staff of the Rush-Presbyterian–St. Luke's Hospital and Medical Center deserve special thanks, as does my secretary, Vanessa Baker.

I would also like to thank Mr. John Dyson of the W. B. Saunders Company for his able assistance.

PREFACE
to the First Edition

To extol the virtues of the technique of computed tomography of the brain one has only to list the clinical uses it serves. The technique is noninvasive, provides more and better definition of the intracranial structures than any other method and is particularly useful in detecting midline lesions. It outlines the exact anatomy better than other techniques, and makes defects visibly appreciable. The examination is easily performed, with essentially no discomfort to the patient, who need not be hospitalized. In addition to diagnosis, the method has proved of great value in treatment planning and treatment follow-up. It would not be an overstatement to say that computed tomography has revolutionized our approach to the diagnosis of intracranial abnormalities.

The main deficiencies of the technique are the long waiting list for nonemergency scans and the possibility of an allergic reaction to the infusion of iodinated contrast material. At present the scanning time of 4½ minutes is a problem, but with the new generation of scanners this time will be significantly shortened.

This book is not meant to be a comprehensive textbook on computed tomography, but rather a basic "handbook" to serve as an introduction to the technique and provide an elementary knowledge of computed tomography. The technique is compared to the older, more established methods, in the hope of correlating the computed tomograms (CT scans) with the methods with which everyone is already familiar. Because of the introductory nature of the material, I have felt it appropriate to dispense with the exercises format used in other books in this series.

All the scans were done using the EMI head scanner, and all the tissue absorption densities are expressed in EMI numbers (u).

These cases were all studied at the University of Chicago Billings Hospital.

RUTH G. RAMSEY, M.D.

TABLE OF CONTENTS

Chapter 1
INTRODUCTION AND NORMAL ANATOMY 1
Normal Postinfusion Anatomy 12
Normal Anatomy 13
Postinfusion Normal Anatomy 18
Postsurgical Changes 20

Chapter 2
PRIMARY BRAIN TUMORS 25
Gliomas 25
Pituitary Tumors 63
Meningiomas 77
Acoustic Neurinomas 98
Posterior Fossa Tumors 108

Chapter 3
METASTASES 125

Chapter 4
VASCULAR DISEASES 153
Infarcts 153
Spontaneous Intracerebral Hematomas 172
Aneurysms 191
Arteriovenous Malformations 201
Superior Sagittal Sinus Thrombosis 207

Chapter 5
POST-TRAUMATIC ABNORMALITIES 211

Chapter 6
ACQUIRED ABNORMALITIES 229
Atrophy 229
Other Acquired Abnormalities 232
Multiple Sclerosis 234

Chapter 7
CONGENITAL ABNORMALITIES 237
Porencephalic Cysts 240
Other Congenital Abnormalities 246

Chapter 8
ORBITAL SCANNING 253

Chapter 9
NEONATAL ULTRASOUND 267
Normal Examination and Method 267
Hemorrhage 269
Hydrocephalus 272
Subdural Extracerebral Collections 275
Intraoperative Ultrasound 275

Chapter 10
DIGITAL INTRAVENOUS SUBTRACTION ANGIOGRAPHY (DISA) 277

Chapter 11
NUCLEAR MAGNETIC RESONANCE 285

INDEX 289

CHAPTER 1

INTRODUCTION AND NORMAL ANATOMY

The technique of computed tomography (CT) was the concept of Geoffrey N. Hounsfield, scientist, EMI Ltd., Middlesex, England. The computed tomogram represents a mathematical reconstruction of computer-assisted absorption density measurements of tomographic cuts of the brain obtained in the axial projection. It should be emphasized that this is not a direct x-ray of the brain itself but rather a mathematical reconstruction of the brain. Hounsfield's original description is recommended to those readers who are interested in a more thorough description of the workings of the instrument.

Simply stated, the x-ray tube traverses back and forth on a rail at the side of the patient's head (Figure 1–1). Two hundred and forty

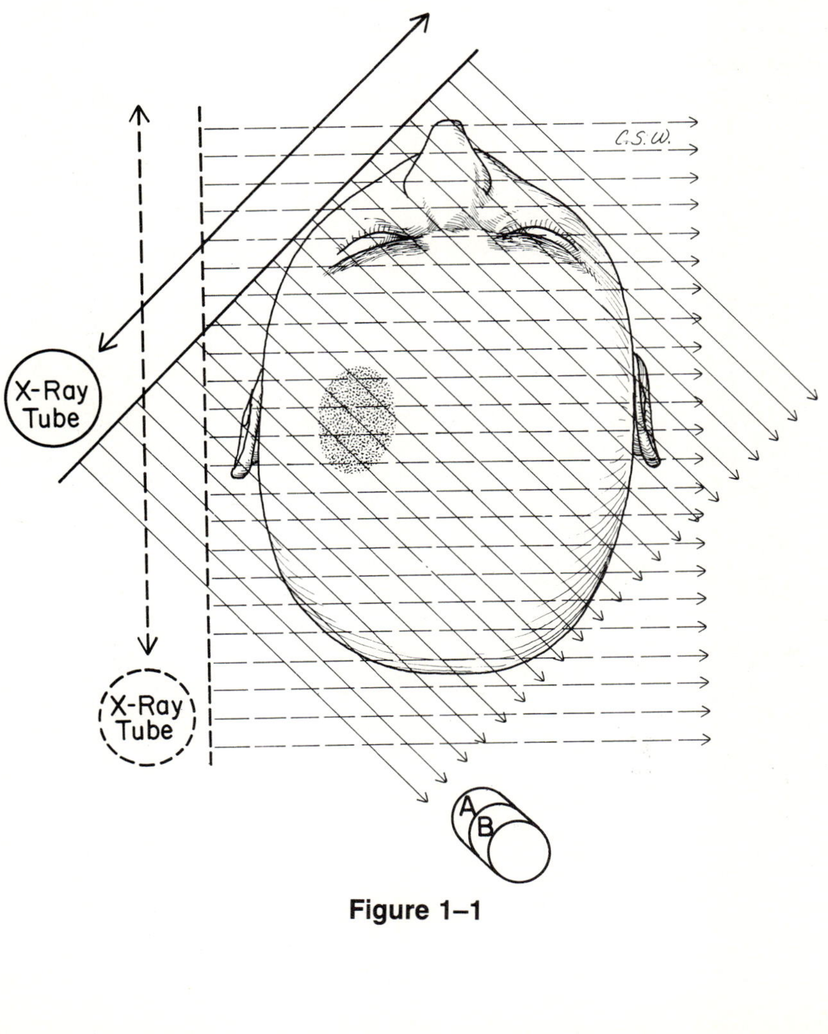

Figure 1–1

density measurements are made per traverse of the tube by detectors at the other side of the patient's head. In this example a "mass lesion" has been placed in the left hemisphere. Two sodium iodide crystal detectors, which are closely aligned with the x-ray tube, simultaneously record the finely collimated beam, resulting in two cuts per scan with a thickness of 1.3 cm per cut. After each traverse the scanning device rotates 1° until the unit has rotated 180°; at the completion of 180° of rotation the unit pauses, and in 30 seconds the computer simultaneously solves 43,200 equations of the tissue density measurements. The scan itself takes 4½ minutes. The result is a 160 × 160 dot matrix of tissue absorption density measurements of the brain, the skull, and the surrounding water bag. The A and B cuts of each level are obtained simultaneously with each 180° rotation of the unit. The dot matrix is made up of 25,600 points, each of which represents a column of tissue 13 mm tall and 1.5 × 1.5 mm square. The information is presented in three different ways—on the cathode-ray tube, where density measurements can be made; on the Polaroid picture, which can be used for permanent storage; or on the number printout sheet.

All of our scans are done initially with a standard technique. We attempt to position the patient in such a way that the cuts are obtained at an angle of 20 to 25° to the base of the skull. Cut 1A includes the fourth ventricle as well as the frontal lobes (Figure 1–2). The remainder of the cuts are above this level; each cut is right above the other, and each is 13 mm thick. We include all the brain tissue, even the high convexities; this is particularly important when a convexity meningioma is suspected. The completed scan consists of six or occasionally eight slices of the brain. The number of cuts necessarily varies with the size of the patient's head. If necessary, we perform an intravenous infusion of contrast material and repeat the initial cuts. For adults we use 300

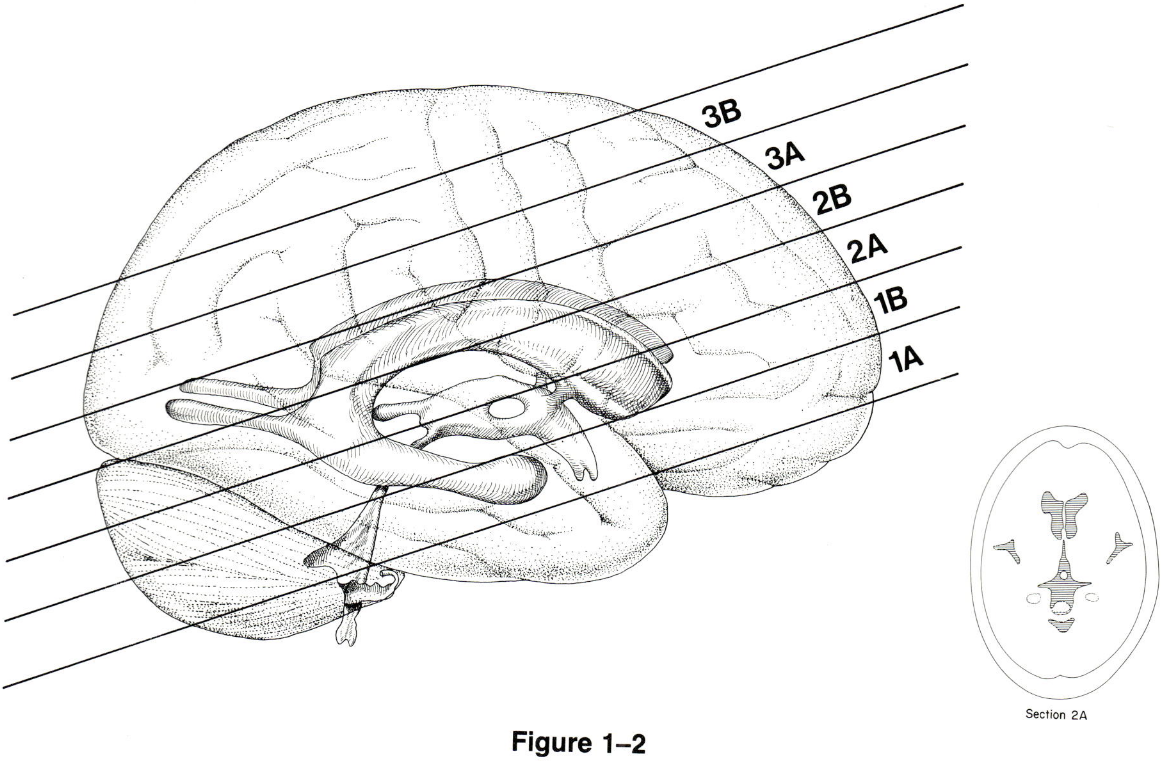

Figure 1–2

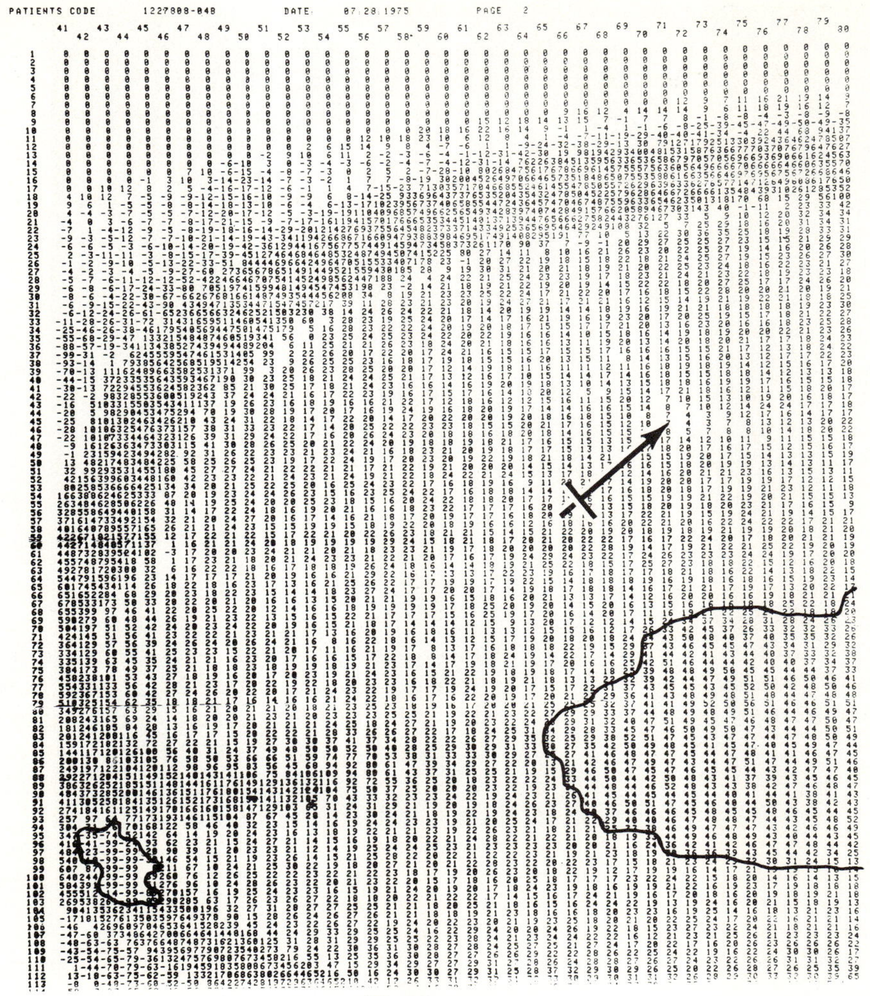

Figure 1–3

ml of methylglucamine diatrizoate 30 per cent contrast material. The first 150 ml is infused prior to beginning the scan; the remainder is infused slowly throughout the duration of the scan. For pediatric patients we use 4.4 ml/kg (2 ml/lb).

The number printout sheet requires eight large sheets of paper per cut and is a 160 × 160 dot matrix of the density values. The number printout sheet is useful for research and as a permanent data storage sheet of the numerical absorption density values. Figure 1–3 is a sample of a portion of a number printout sheet. The corresponding CT scan cut is adjacent to the printout sheet (Figure 1–4). Because the 3-digit number columns mechanically require a certain amount of space, the number printout sheet is distorted in such a way that the head appears shorter and wider than on the Polaroid picture. The area of the tumor has been outlined on the printout sheet (in this case, a tentorial meningioma). The small irregular circle of the left-hand side of the printout sheet represents the mastoid air cells that can be seen in the left petrous bone on the Polaroid picture (arrow). The dense petrous bone can also be visualized on the printout sheet as a roughly triangular density, extending medially from the mastoid air cells and pointing approximately toward the tumor. The low density of the left frontal horn can

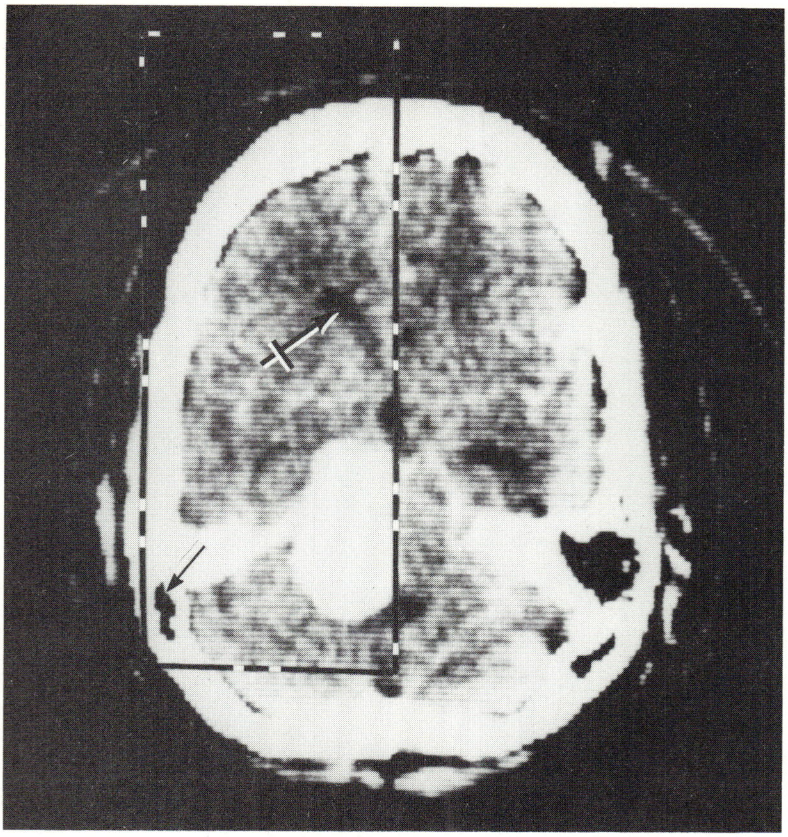

Figure 1–4

be readily identified both in the Polaroid picture and on the printout sheet (crossed arrow).

The following section is devoted to a review of normal computed tomographic anatomy as compared to normal pathologic neuroanatomy (Figures 1–5 to 1–11). The orientation is such that the right side of the Polaroid picture represents the right side of the patient—as if one were looking down at the patient's head. The important structures are labeled both on the pathologic specimen and on the corresponding tomographic cut. Throughout this book the preinfusion scans are labeled with a single digit number, and the postinfusion scans are labeled with a double digit number. The photos of those scans bearing the label *electronic enhancement* were taken with the control unit on the "measure" mode. This measure mode is used to obtain the density measurements and can also be used to bring out or enhance an abnormal area of increased or decreased density to better advantage. Our routine scans are photographed at a window width of 75 and a density of about 34 or 36.

Text continued on page 12

EMI COEFFICIENTS OF ABSORPTION IN HOUNSFIELD UNITS

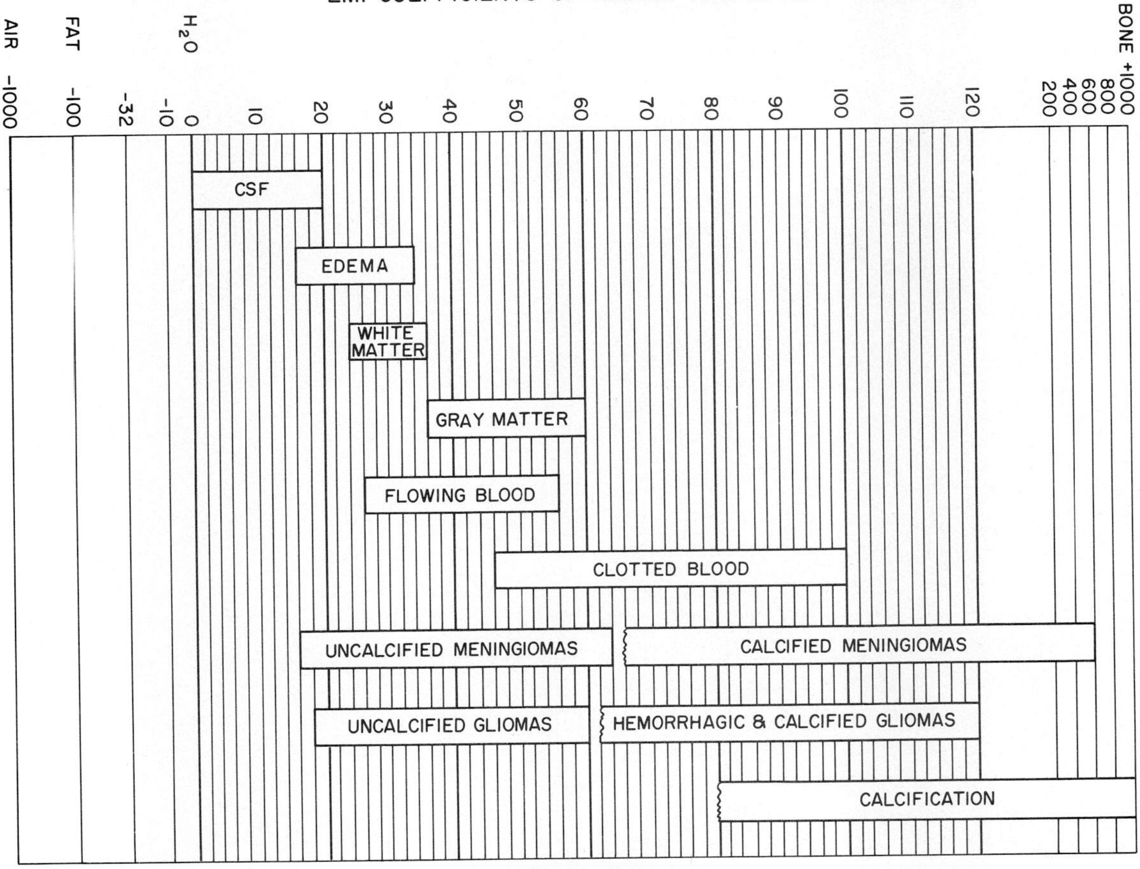

Figure 1–5

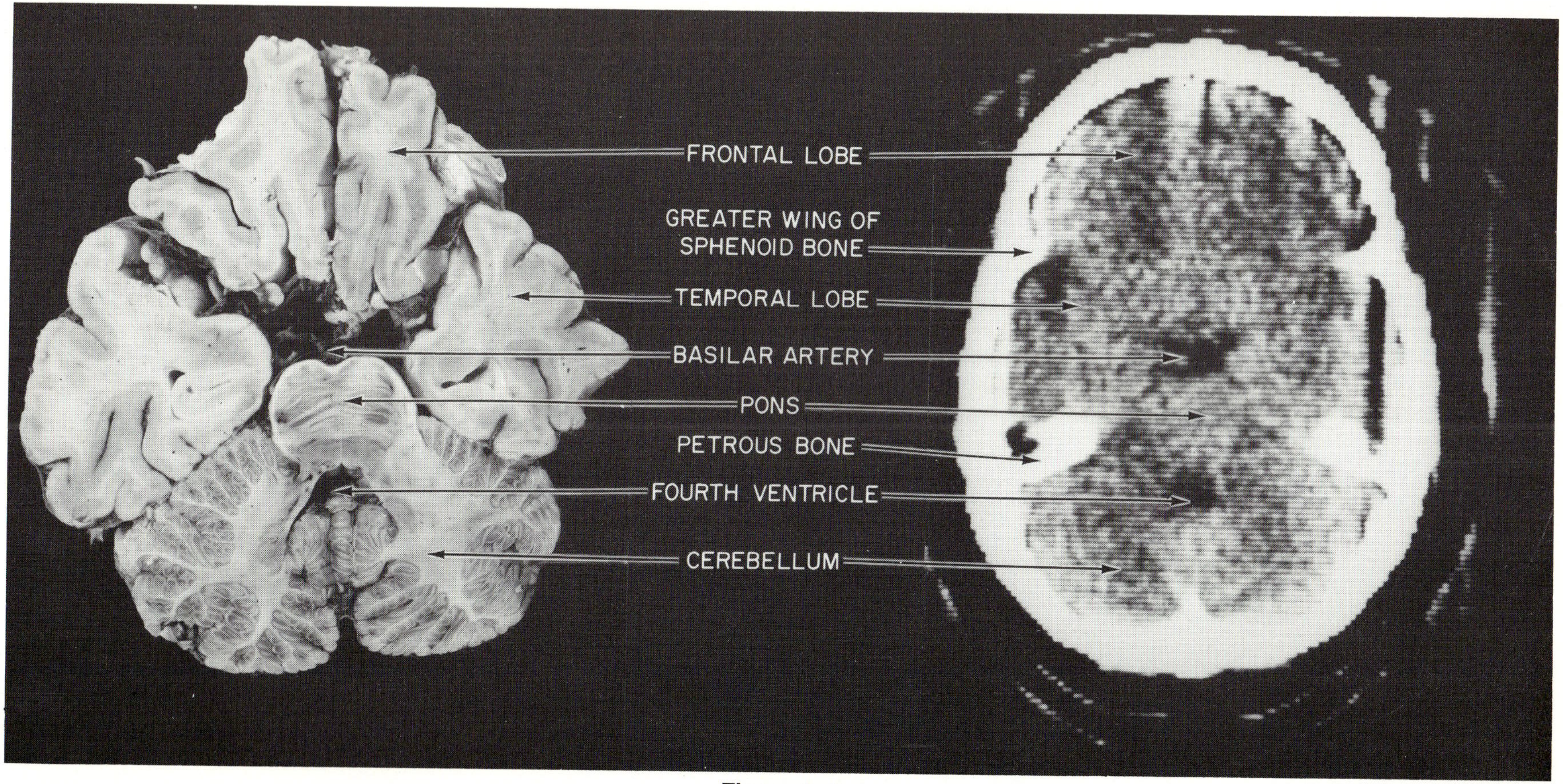
FRONTAL LOBE
GREATER WING OF SPHENOID BONE
TEMPORAL LOBE
BASILAR ARTERY
PONS
PETROUS BONE
FOURTH VENTRICLE
CEREBELLUM

Figure 1–6 **1A**

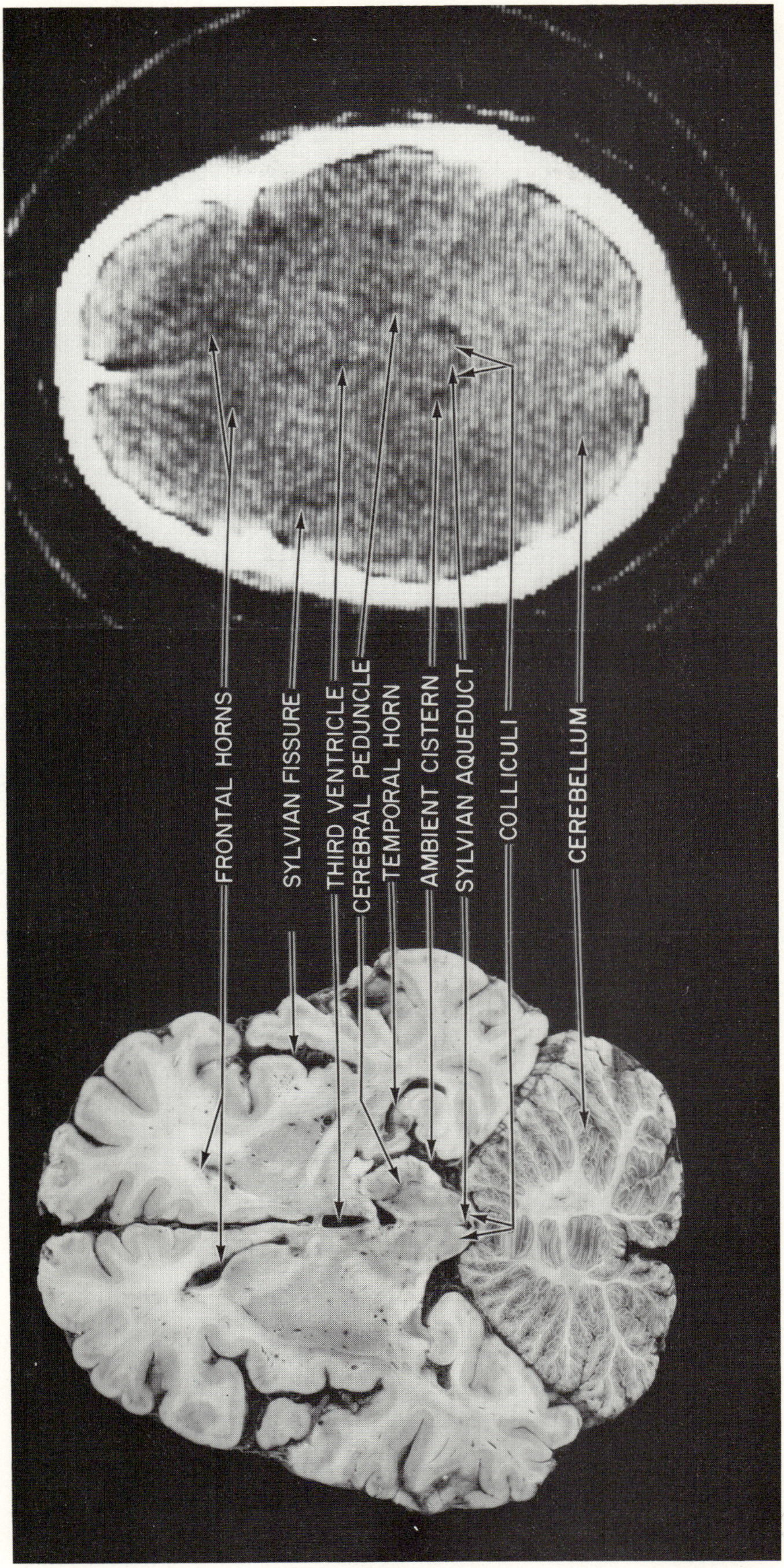
FRONTAL HORNS
SYLVIAN FISSURE
THIRD VENTRICLE
CEREBRAL PEDUNCLE
TEMPORAL HORN
AMBIENT CISTERN
SYLVIAN AQUEDUCT
COLLICULI
CEREBELLUM

Figure 1–7

1B

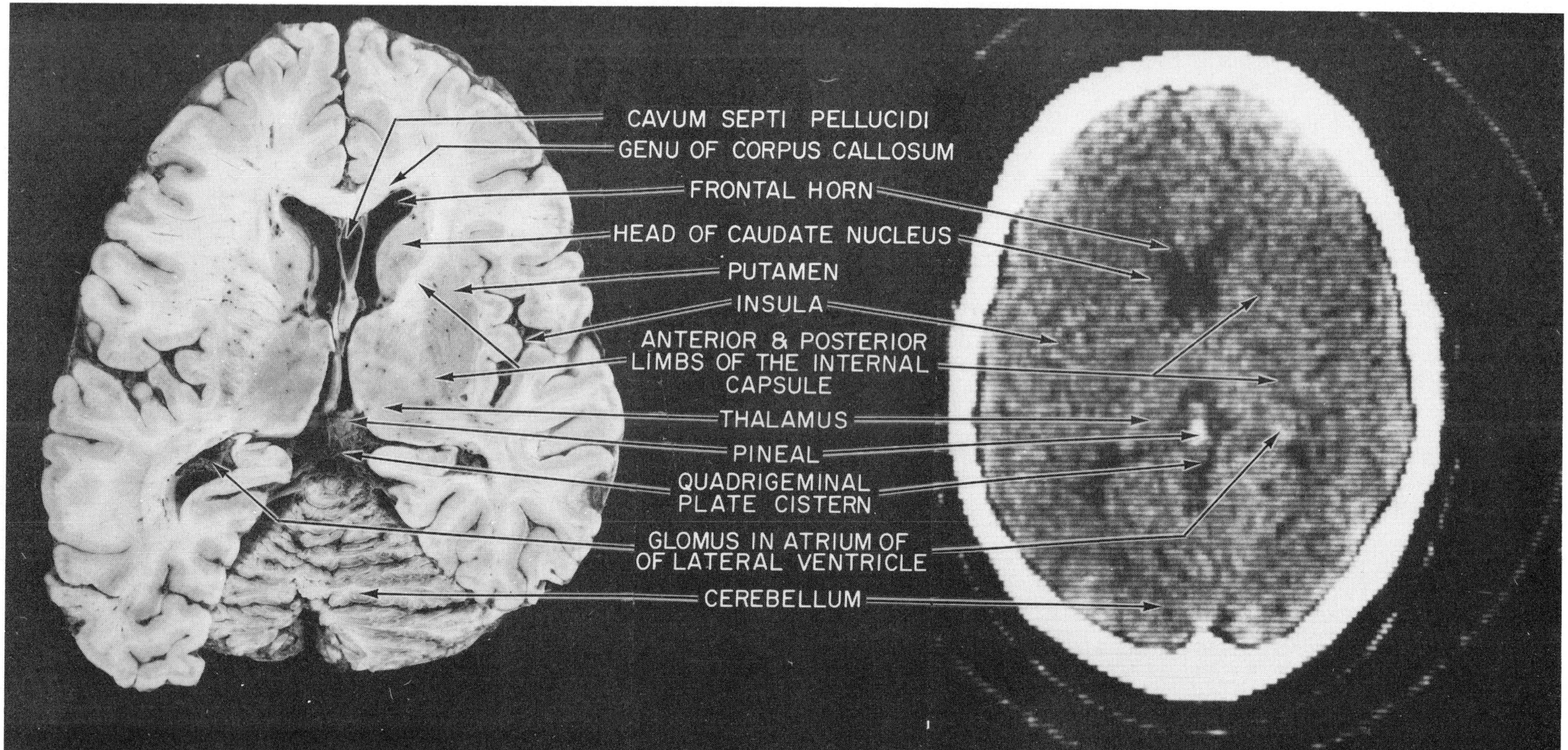
CAVUM SEPTI PELLUCIDI
GENU OF CORPUS CALLOSUM
FRONTAL HORN
HEAD OF CAUDATE NUCLEUS
PUTAMEN
INSULA
ANTERIOR & POSTERIOR LIMBS OF THE INTERNAL CAPSULE
THALAMUS
PINEAL
QUADRIGEMINAL PLATE CISTERN
GLOMUS IN ATRIUM OF OF LATERAL VENTRICLE
CEREBELLUM

Figure 1–8

2A

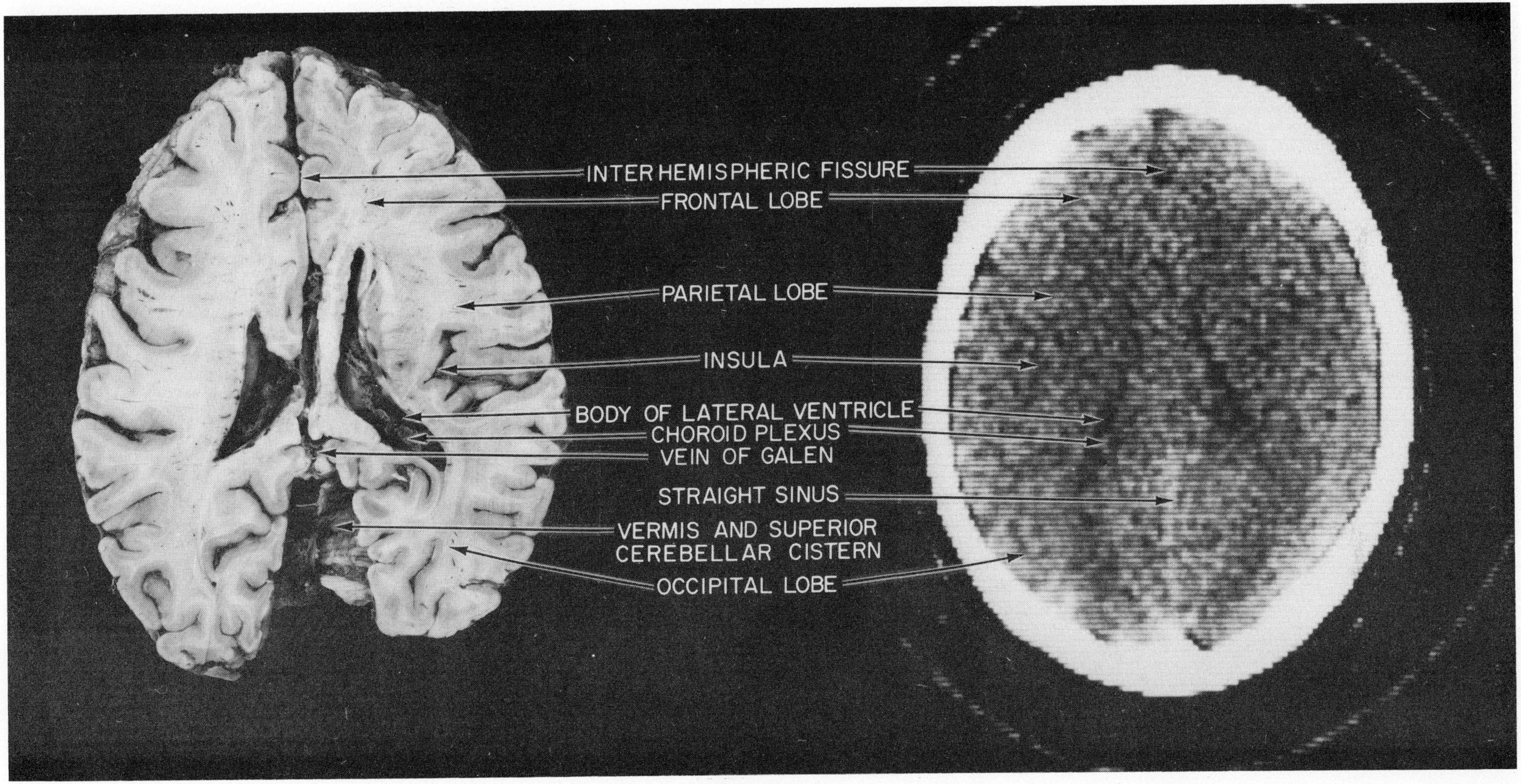
INTERHEMISPHERIC FISSURE
FRONTAL LOBE
PARIETAL LOBE
INSULA
BODY OF LATERAL VENTRICLE
CHOROID PLEXUS
VEIN OF GALEN
STRAIGHT SINUS
VERMIS AND SUPERIOR
CEREBELLAR CISTERN
OCCIPITAL LOBE

Figure 1–9 **2B**

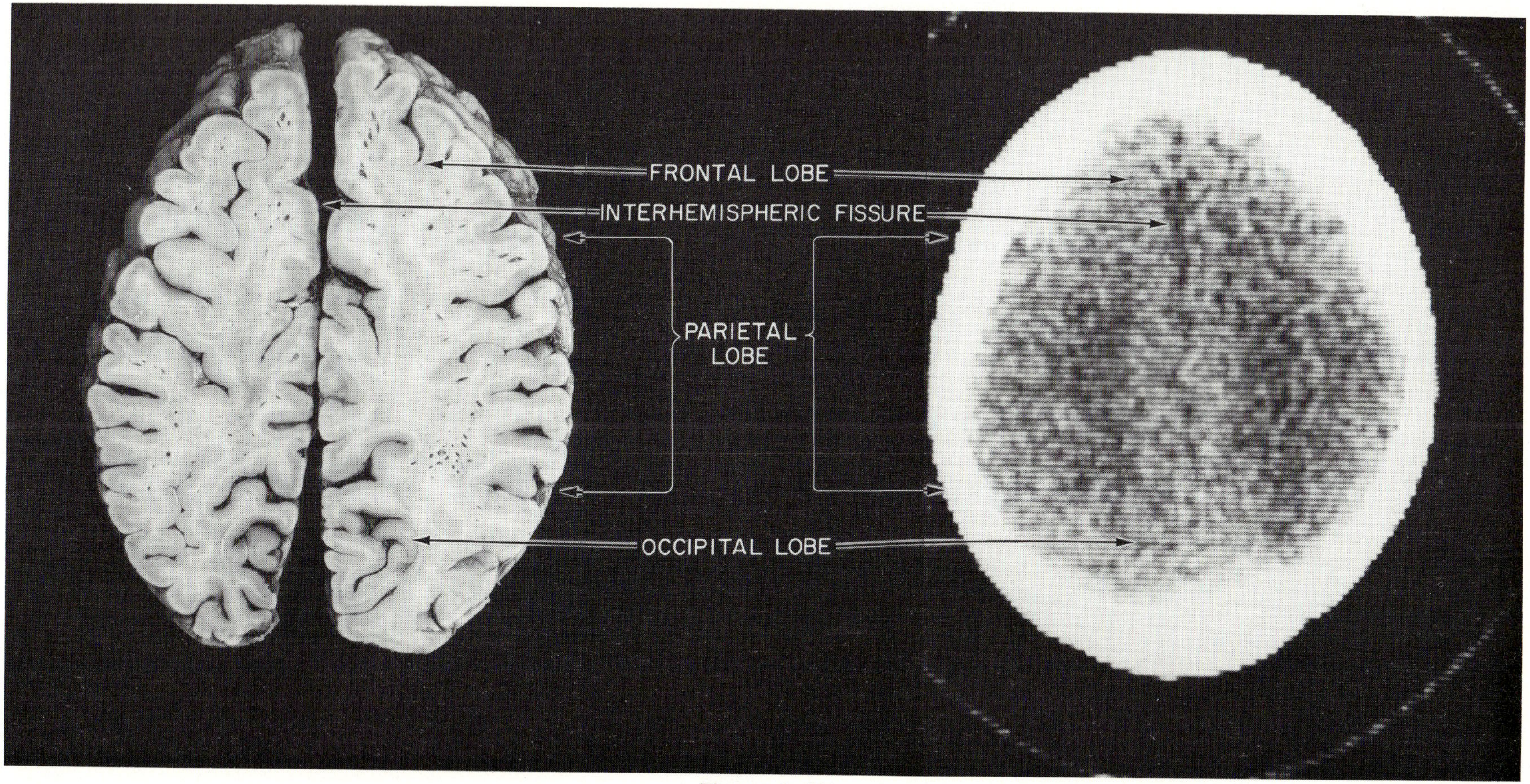

Figure 1–10

3A

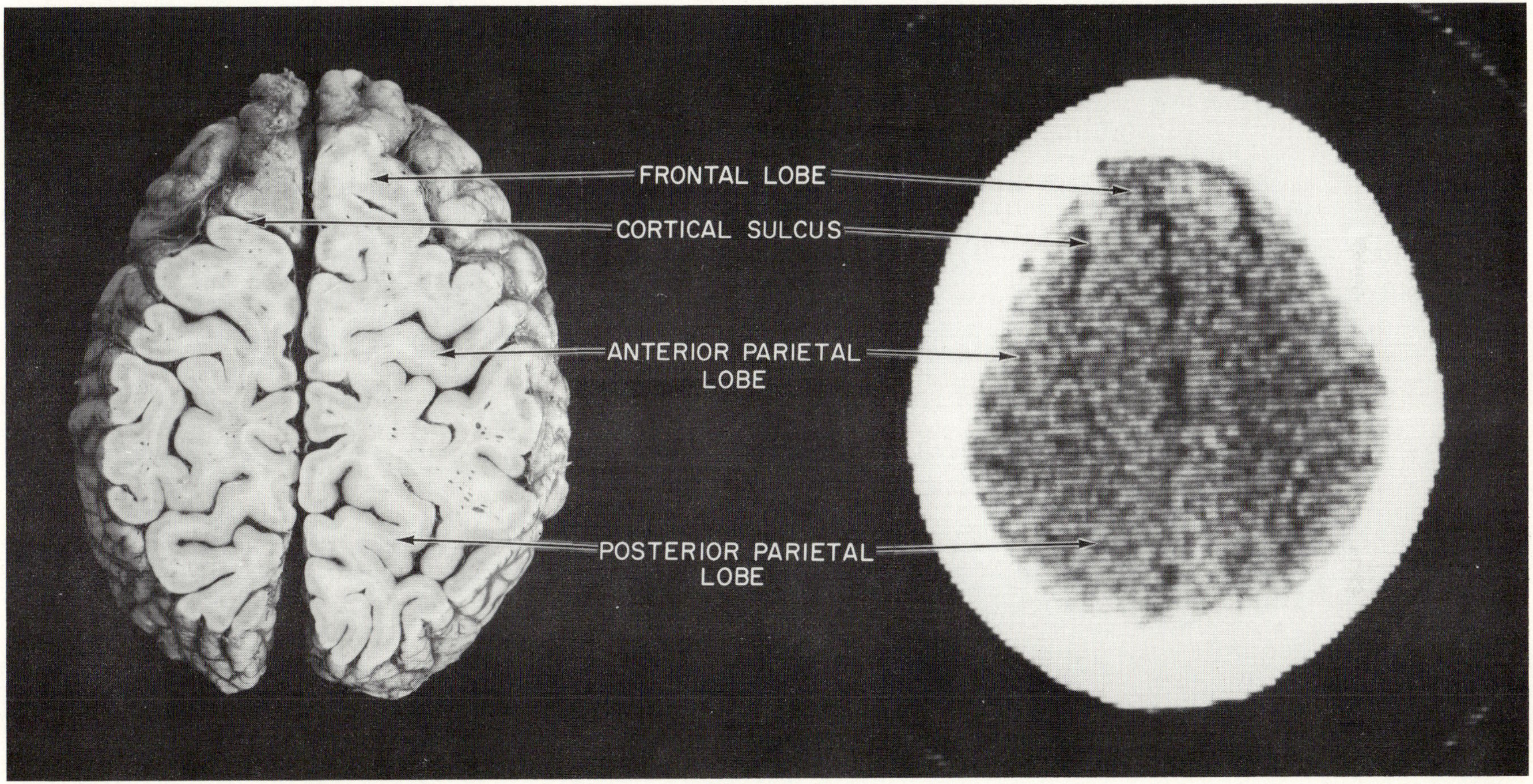

Figure 1–11

3B

Since the first edition of this book (1977), there have been marked advances in the technology of scanners. Initial rapid developments led to the appearance of the *second generation scanner*. This scanner was based on the same principles as the first generation translate-retake scanner, but could scan, process data, and solve equations much faster because it used newer, more advanced computers. Faster scanning of individual patients resulted in less interference from patient motion artifact.

The *third generation scanner* represented a new approach to CT. It introduced a rotating x-ray tube and an array of detectors. Again, new technology allowed for much more rapid scanning. In some cases individual scan slices could be performed in less than five seconds. Not only was this a great advantage for performing CT studies of the brain but it also permitted easier examination of the chest and abdomen. In addition, there was a trend toward increasing the dot matrix size in the new scanners. This increased resolution, making it possible to identify lesions as small as 1 cm. Of course, the increased size of the dot matrix also increased the number of equations to be solved with each scan slice, requiring a more sophisticated computer to handle the mathematical problems.

Fourth generation scanners also were introduced. These scanners have a rotating tube and an array of detectors fixed in a ring around the patient. In terms of diagnostic potential, there is no real difference between the third and fourth generation scanners.

Besides increased scanning speed, the greatest advantage of the newer scanners is their versatility. Many of the newer scanners are equipped with a gantry (entry aperture for the patient) that can tilt in a forward (positive) or reverse (negative) direction. This allows for easier patient positioning and examination of certain body parts—especially the orbits, the sella, and the internal auditory canals. By tilting the gantry and flexing or extending the patient's head, direct coronal examination of the region around the sella is possible. This is particularly helpful in detecting microadenomas of the pituitary gland or determining the suprasellar extension of a pituitary tumor. This new technology and the addition of metrizamide cisternography have essentially eliminated any need for pneumoencephalography.

Other advances in computer technology allow the manipulation of data in such a way that images can be converted from the axial plane to the coronal plane with the push of a button. In fact, any combination of scan planes can be performed if the appropriate computer capabilities are available.

Normal Postinfusion Anatomy

On the preinfusion scan the blood vessels and the flowing blood cannot be distinguished as such. However, after the infusion of contrast material, the circle of Willis can often be visualized. Figure 1–12 is an example of the normal anatomy that can be seen on the lowest postinfusion cut. In addition, one sees opacification of the falx cerebri, tentorium, straight sinus, lateral sinuses, sigmoid sinuses, and choroid plexus at various levels and positions. Examples of these will be given later.

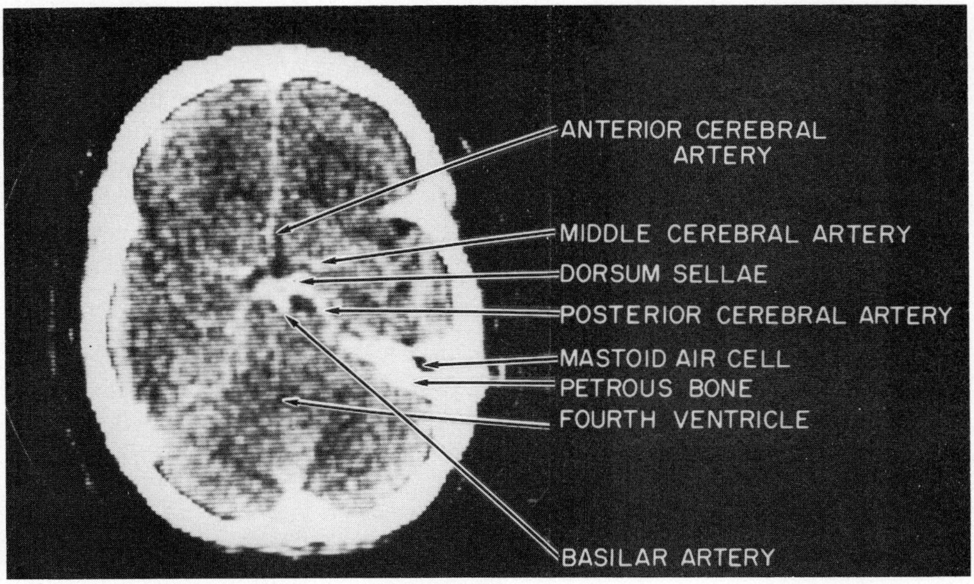

Figure 1–12

1A 2A 3A

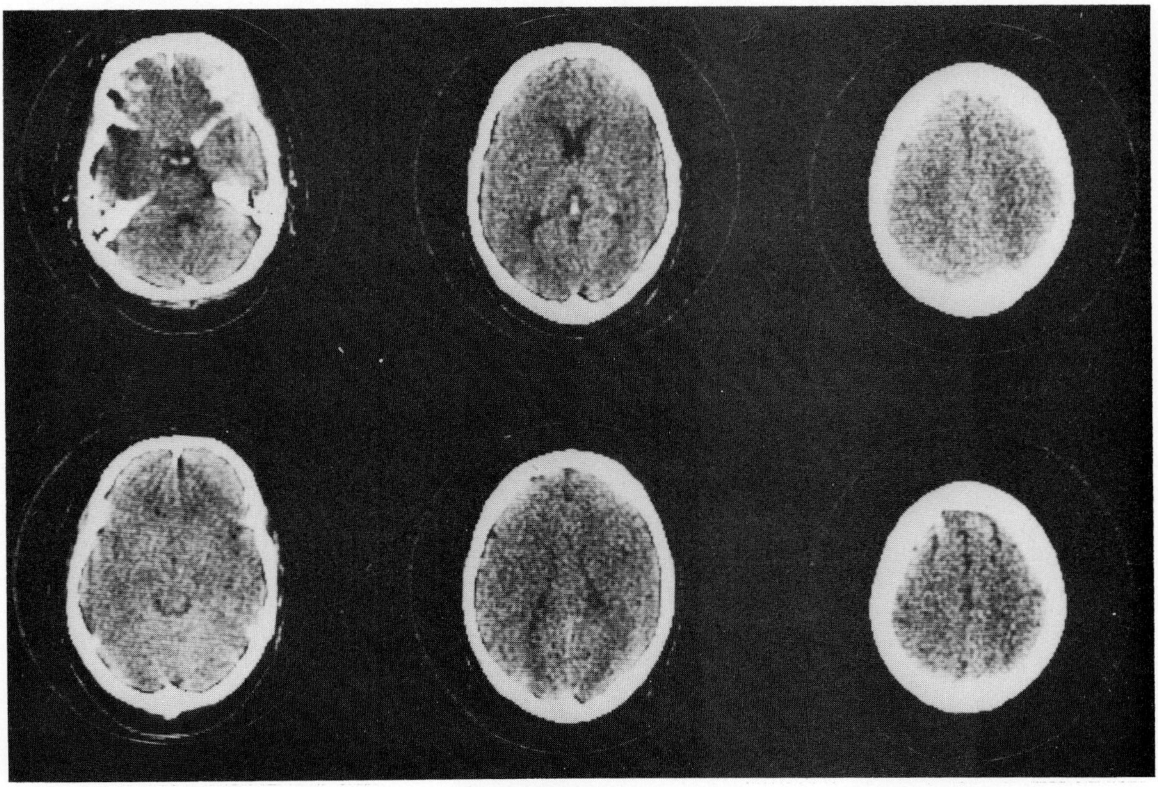

Figure 1–13

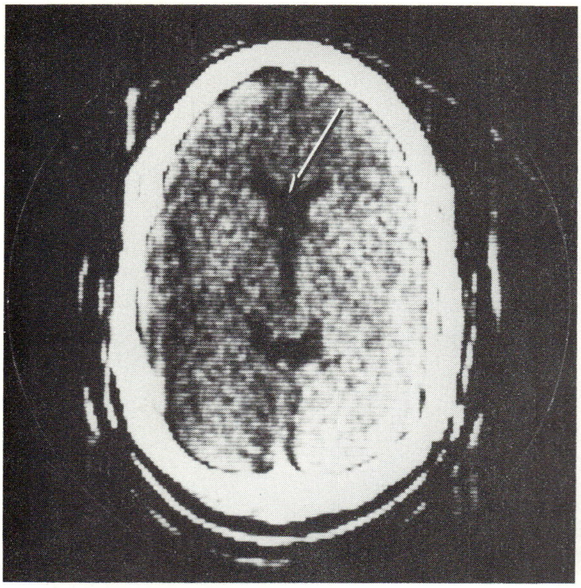

Figure 1–14

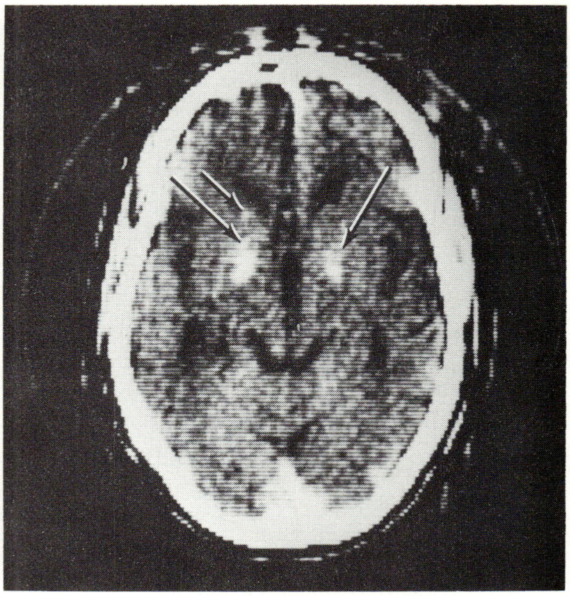

Figure 1–15

Normal Anatomy

A normal adult scan is shown in Figure 1–13. As in any biologic system, the normal scan has a good deal of variation. In addition to learning the normal anatomy, it is also necessary to become accustomed to the normal variations.

Figure 1–14 demonstrates cavum septum pellucidum (arrow), a normal variation.

Idiopathic basal ganglia calcification is shown in Figure 1–15. This may also be seen with hypoparathyroidism and pseudohypoparathyroidism.

In Figure 1–16 the calcified pineal gland can be seen in the quadrigeminal plate cistern. Posterior to this is the superior cerebellar cistern. The upper portion of the vermis of the cerebellum (arrow) is surrounded by the cistern. This should not be mistaken for a cystic tumor of the posterior fossa.

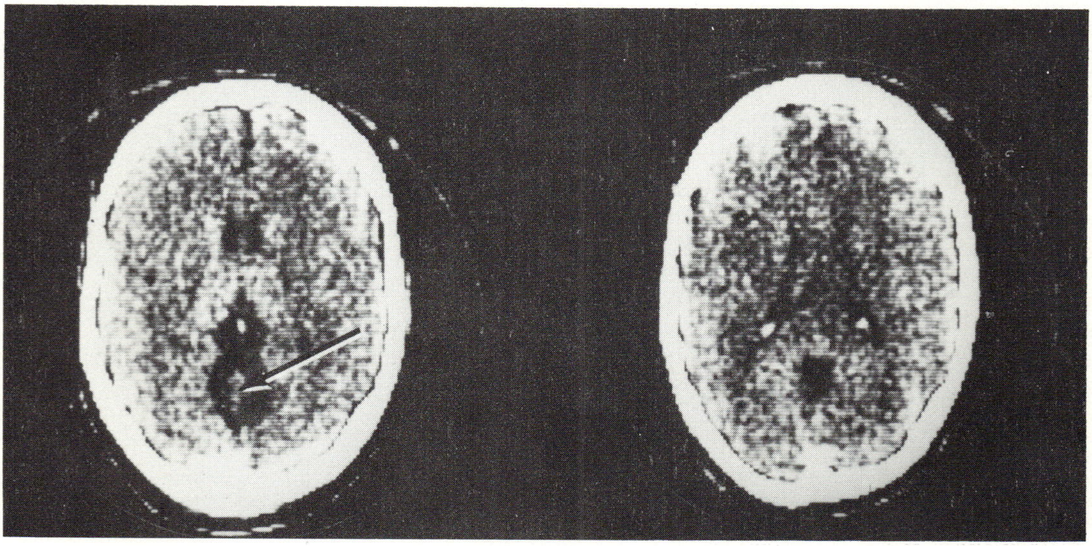

Figure 1–16

Figure 1–17, a low base cut, shows the anterior clinoids (upper arrow), the posterior clinoids and the dorsum sellae (crossed arrow), and the occipital condyles where the atlas articulates with the occipital bone. Also well seen are the petrous bones with the mastoid air cells.

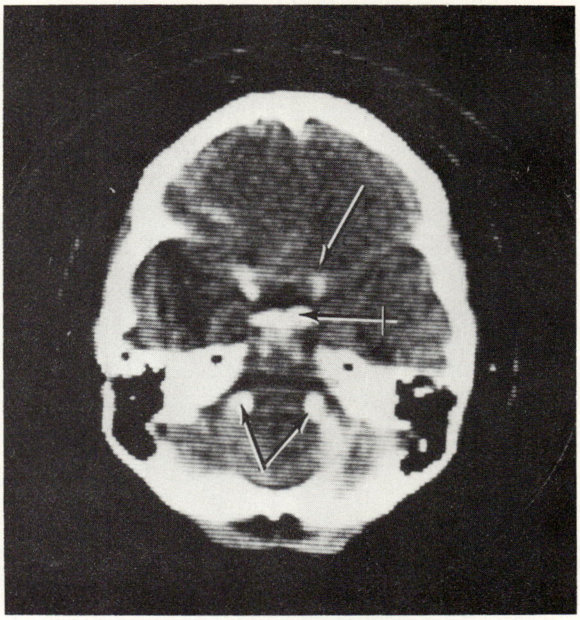

Figure 1–17

The two photographs in Figure 1–18 are identical except for the density level at which they were photographed. The sphenoid sinus (upper arrows) and external auditory canals can be readily identified (short arrows). The foramen magnum (crossed arrow) is best seen on the higher density photo.

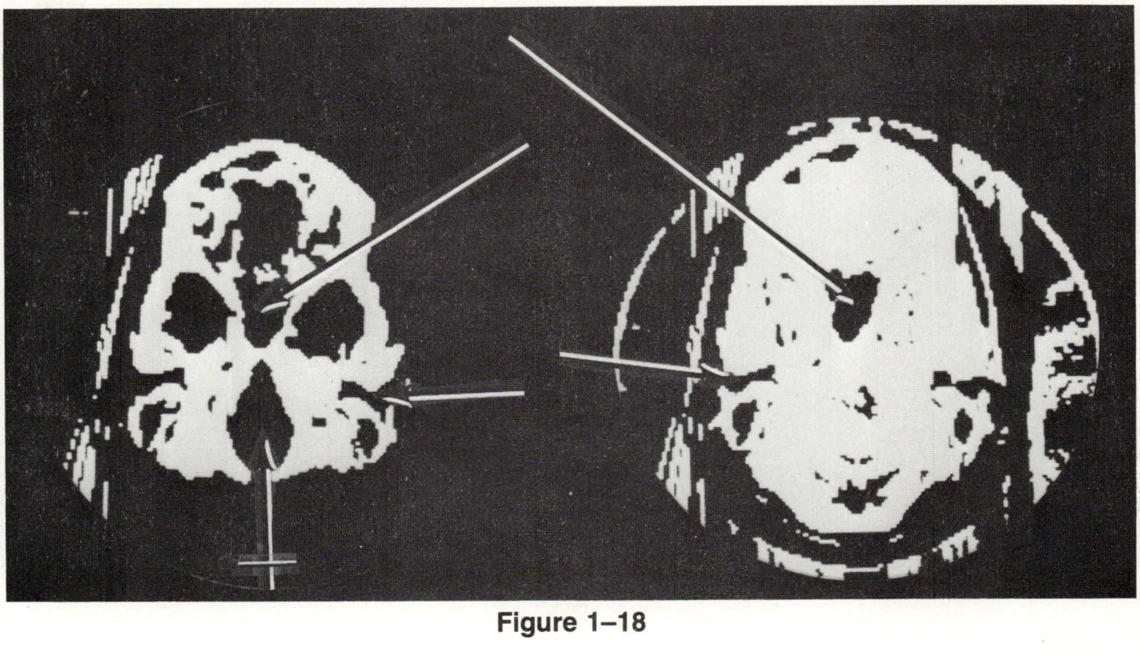

Figure 1–18

Figure 1–19 shows a normal pediatric scan on a 3 year old child. In addition to the smaller head, the lateral ventricles tend to be more delicate in size, although again it must be noted that there is also a variety of normals among pediatric patients.

The series of scans in Figure 1–20 is from a routine pediatric study that was performed both with and without the infusion of contrast material. The child was sedated prior to the study; with each succeeding scan one can see the increase in motion artifact as the sedation becomes ineffective. The scan is initially quite adequate, but eventually it becomes so degraded by motion artifact that it is virtually unreadable.

The dosage schedule in Table 1–1 has proved effective for children requiring neuroradiologic procedures. The same doses used for patients who required angiography or pneumoencephalography have proved to be safe and effective with computed tomography.

TABLE 1–1. Sedation Dosages for Children

Age (yrs)	Secobarbital (mg/kg)	Meperidine (mg/kg)	Atropine, Total Dose (mg)	Chlorpromazine (mg/kg)
1-4	8–10	1-1.5	0.1–0.2	1.5
5-8	5–7	1-1.5	0.3	1.0
9–12	3–4	1.0	0.4	0.75

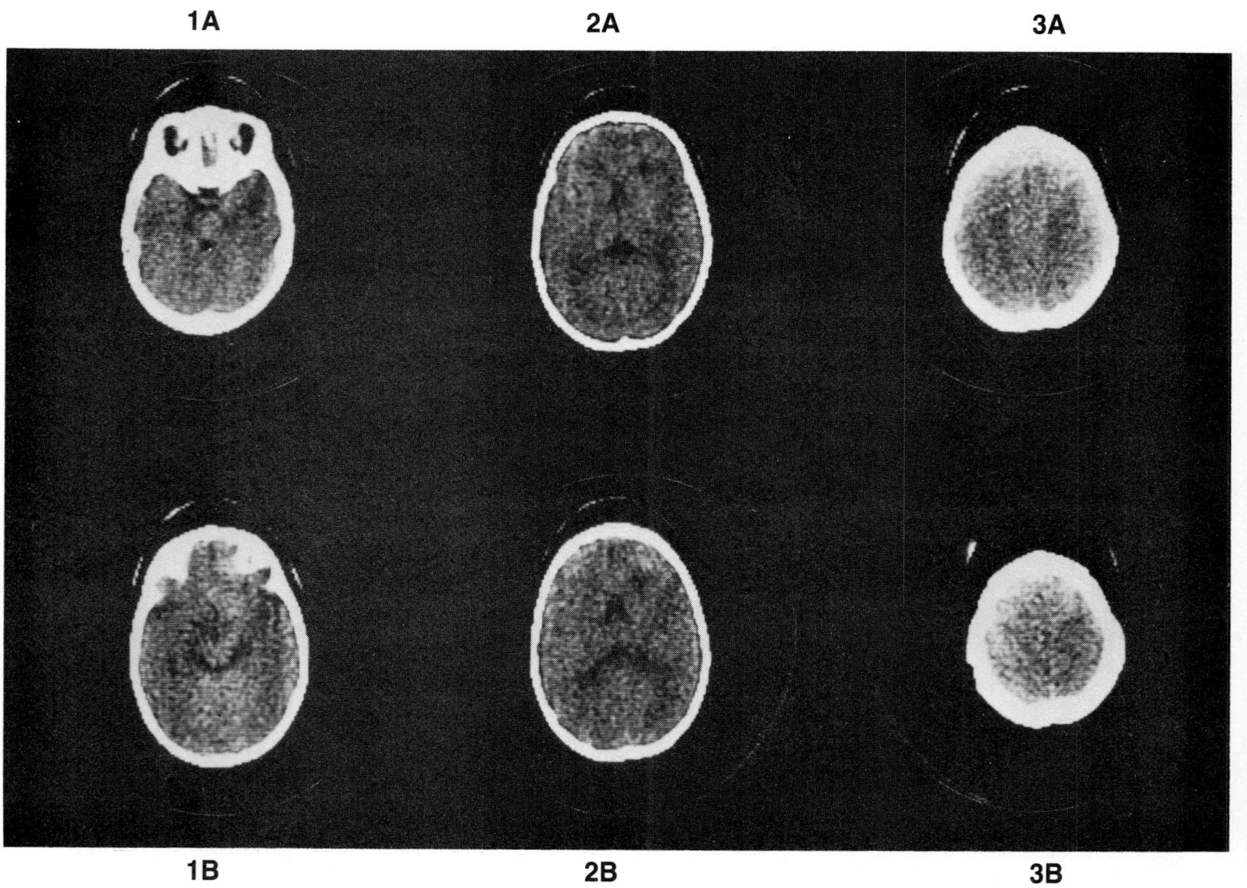

Figure 1–19

This sedation is administered intramuscularly 45 to 60 minutes before the procedure. In arteriography a lesser dose of secobarbital and a greater dose of meperidine are used. In pneumoencephalography a greater dose of secobarbital is used, and either less meperidine or none. Chlorpromazine should not be used in hypothalamic or brain stem lesions. For computed tomography I use the lower end of the dosage scale. These patients must be observed closely; if there is any depression of consciousness or of the vital signs, the sedation dose should be scaled down accordingly. Occasionally it will be necessary to perform the scan under general anesthesia for either a child or adult patient.

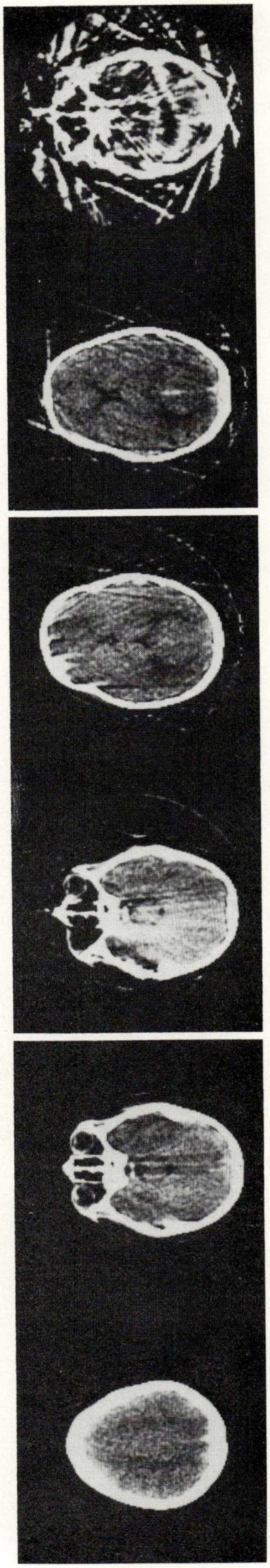

Figure 1–20

Postinfusion Normal Anatomy

Figure 1–21 demonstrates normal enhancement of the choroid plexus in the floor of the lateral ventricles (upper arrows) and opacification of the straight sinus.

Enhancement of the tentorial notch (upper arrows), the straight sinus (lower arrow), and the transverse sinus (crossed arrow) is shown in Figure 1–22.

Figure 1–23 shows opacification of the tentorium (the lower two photos are postinfusion) as it is cut in a parallel plane.

Choroid plexus enhancement in the roof of the temporal horns (arrows) is seen on the postinfusion cut (Figure 1–24).

Figure 1–25 represents opacification of the falx cerebri.

2B 12B

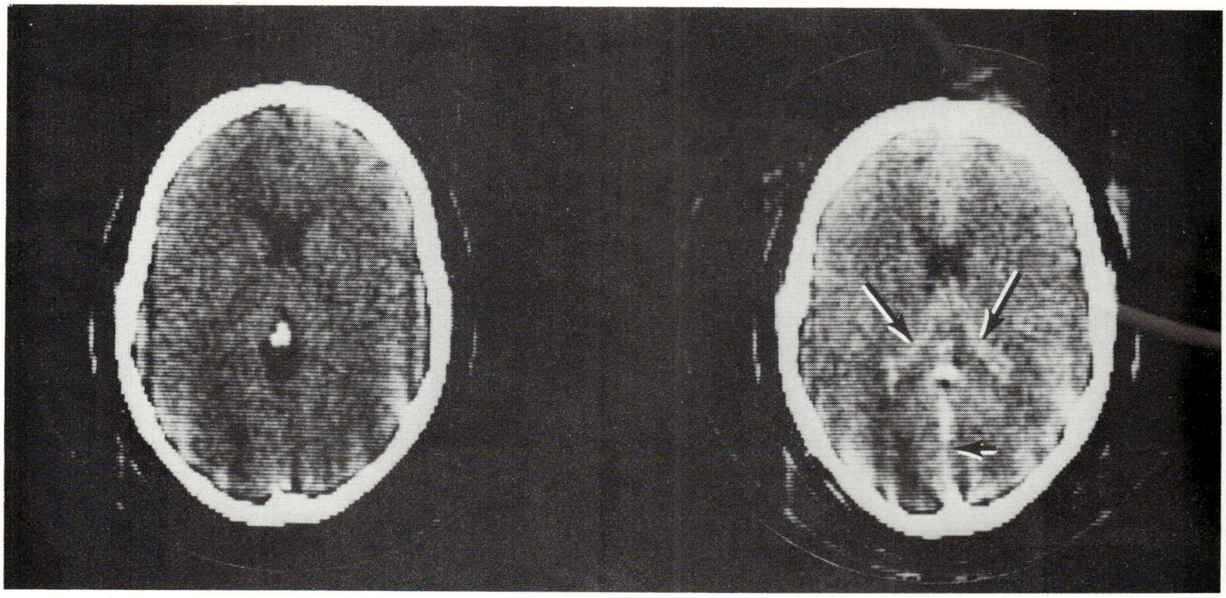

Figure 1–21

12B

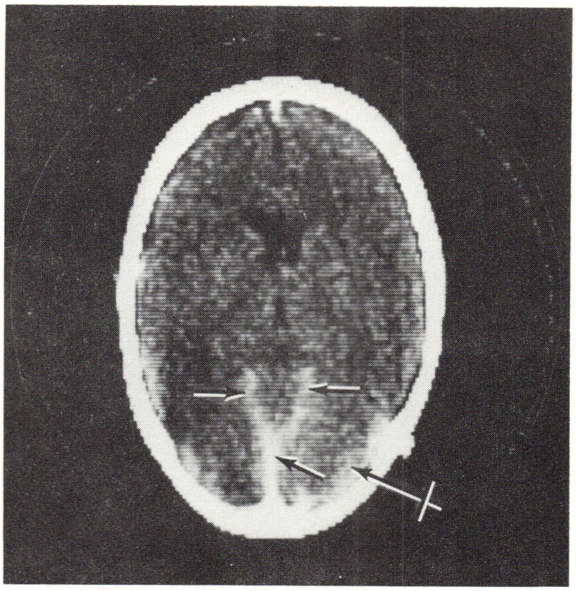

Figure 1–22

2A 2B

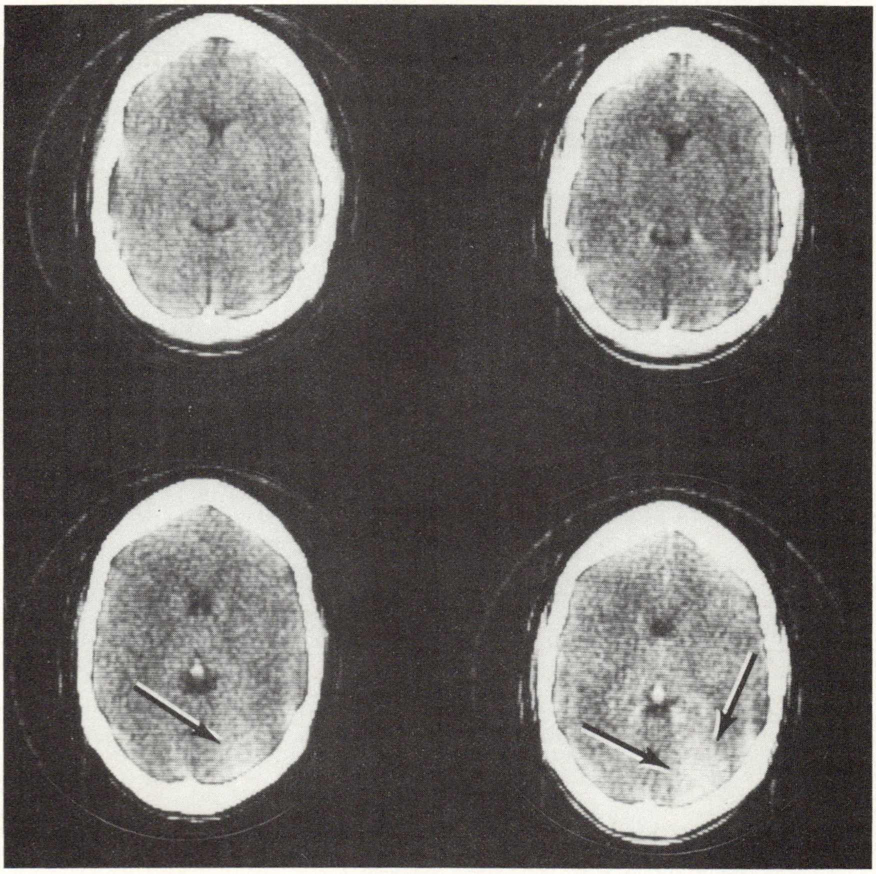

12A 12B

Figure 1–23

1B 11B

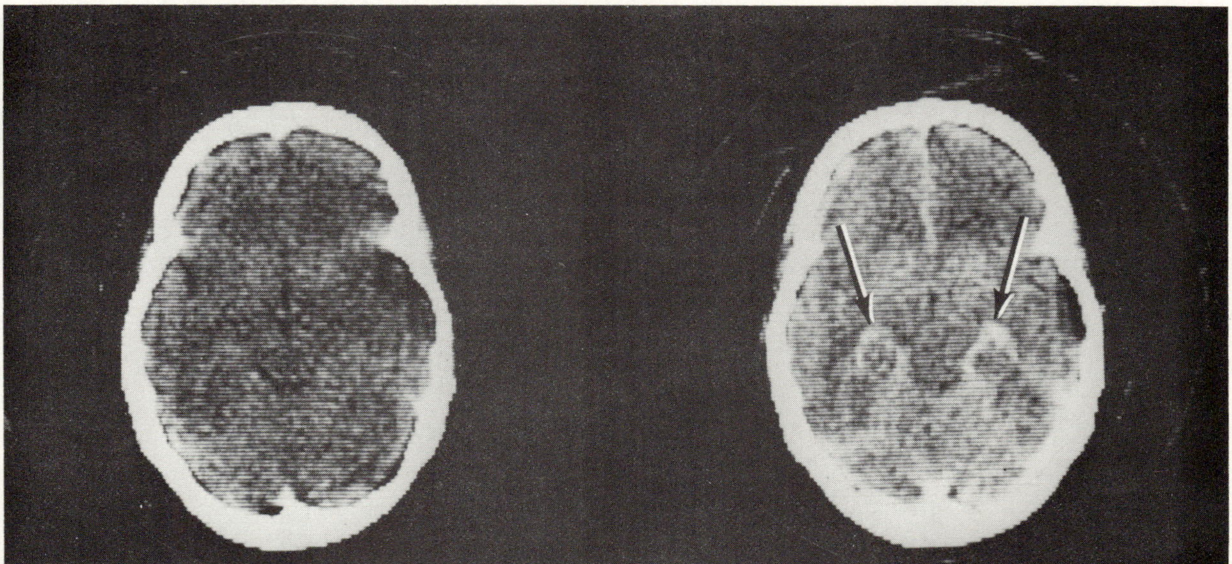

Figure 1–24

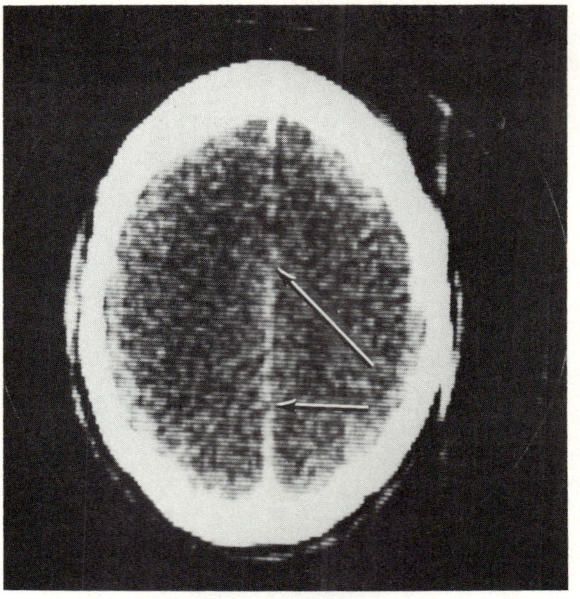

Figure 1–25

Postsurgical Changes

Surgery produces a variety of changes in the appearance of the CT scan. The changes are a reflection of the surgical procedure.

In Figure 1–26 are seen multiple round droplets of Pantopaque, which entered the cranial vault at the time of a previous myelogram. Notice the "computer artifact" produced by the high density of the foreign body (see arrow). In addition, on the higher cuts extensive calcification of the falx cerebri can be seen (crossed arrows).

In Figure 1–27, made after a shunt procedure, the metallic shunt tips can be seen (crossed arrows), and a good deal of air is present in the frontal horns and in the anterior tip of the left temporal horn (arrows). Notice that the low density of the air is surrounded by a thin white line. This also is a computer artifact.

PREFACE
to the Second Edition

Since the first edition of this book, there have been a number of advances in the field of computed tomography. However, it is worthwhile to reiterate the virtues of this technique before discussing these new developments. It is not an exaggeration to say that computed tomography has revolutionized our approach to the diagnosis of intracranial abnormalities. The technique is essentially noninvasive, provides more and better definition of the intracranial structures than any other method, and is particularly useful in defining midline lesions of the brain and abnormalities of the posterior fossa. Computed tomography outlines the exact pathologic condition better than any other method and makes anatomic abnormalities readily apparent. The examination is easily performed with essentially no discomfort to the patient, usually as an out-patient procedure. In addition to its importance in diagnosis, the method has proved of great value in treatment planning and in follow-up care.

Newer scanners provide even more precise anatomic definition and sensitivity than the earlier models. The new scanners are also much more rapid and versatile than the older models.

In addition to the chapters on computed tomography of the brain and orbit in this edition, new chapters have been added that provide an introduction to the newer techniques of ultrasonography of the neonatal brain, digital subtraction angiography, and nuclear magnetic resonance imaging.

This book is not meant to be a comprehensive textbook on any of these topics but rather a basic "handbook" or readily available information source about these techniques. In the case of computed tomography of the brain and orbits, the newer method of study is compared with the older, more established methods in the hope of correlating the CT scans with the type of studies with which many are already familiar. Medical students and residents in radiology, neurology, neurosurgery, internal medicine, and other medical specialties as well as technologists will find this book especially helpful. The practicing physician will also find this book useful as a day-to-day reference.

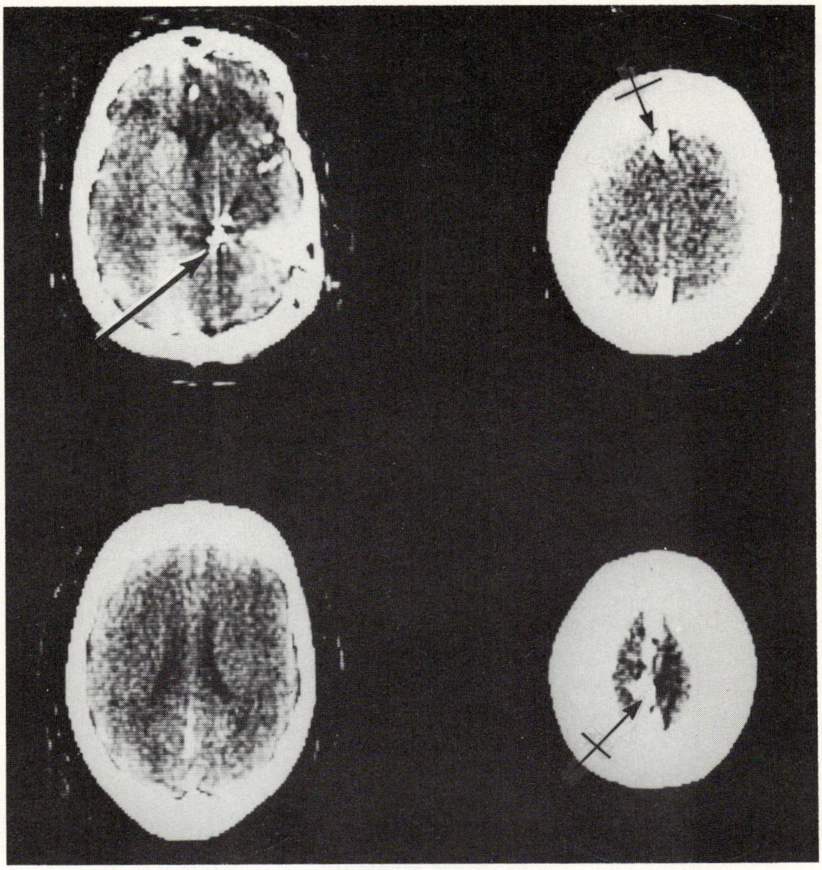

Figure 1–26

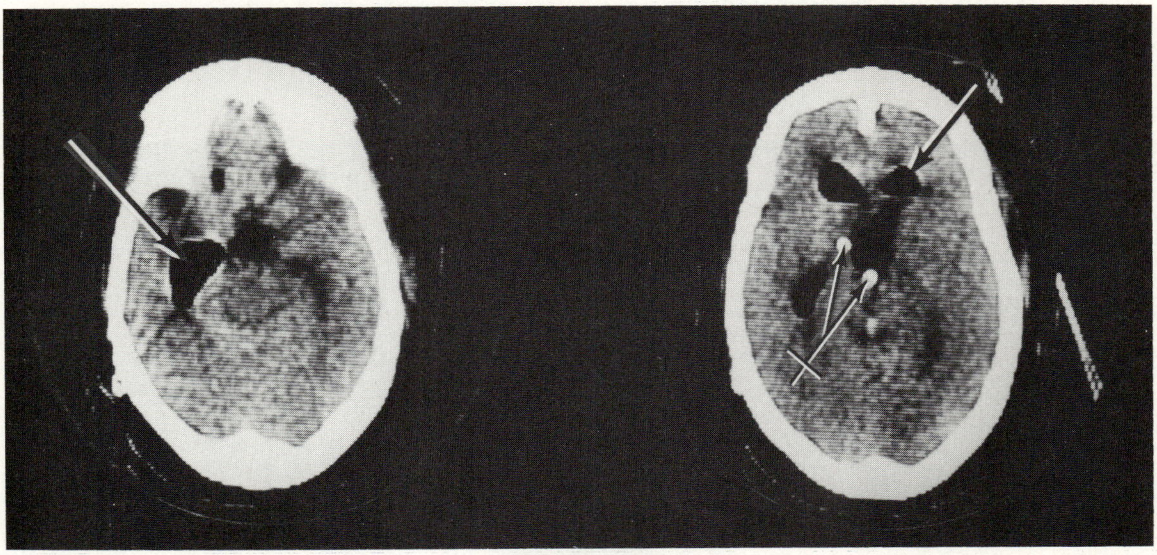

Figure 1–27

Figure 1–28 shows postsurgical changes with swelling in the soft tissues over the right side (arrows) and a small amount of air trapped in the skin flap (crossed arrow). There is slight compression of the right lateral ventricle. (The surgery was for repair of a carotid-cavernous fistula.)

Figure 1–29 shows a metallic foreign body—a bullet—which entered the left frontal region and came to rest adjacent to the right occipital bone. The "sunburst" pattern of computer artifact is quite apparent on an adjacent scan cut. Because of these computer artifacts, we have encouraged our surgeons to avoid using metallic vascular clips and intracranial Pantopaque when possible. In addition, it has proved impossible to scan patients who have metallic head plates.

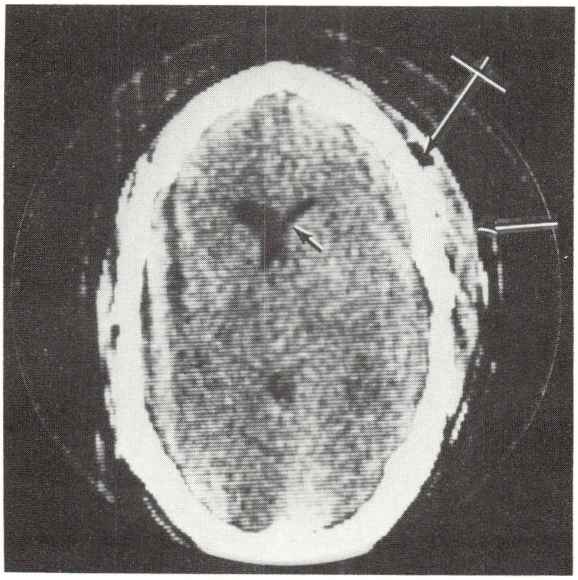

Figure 1–28

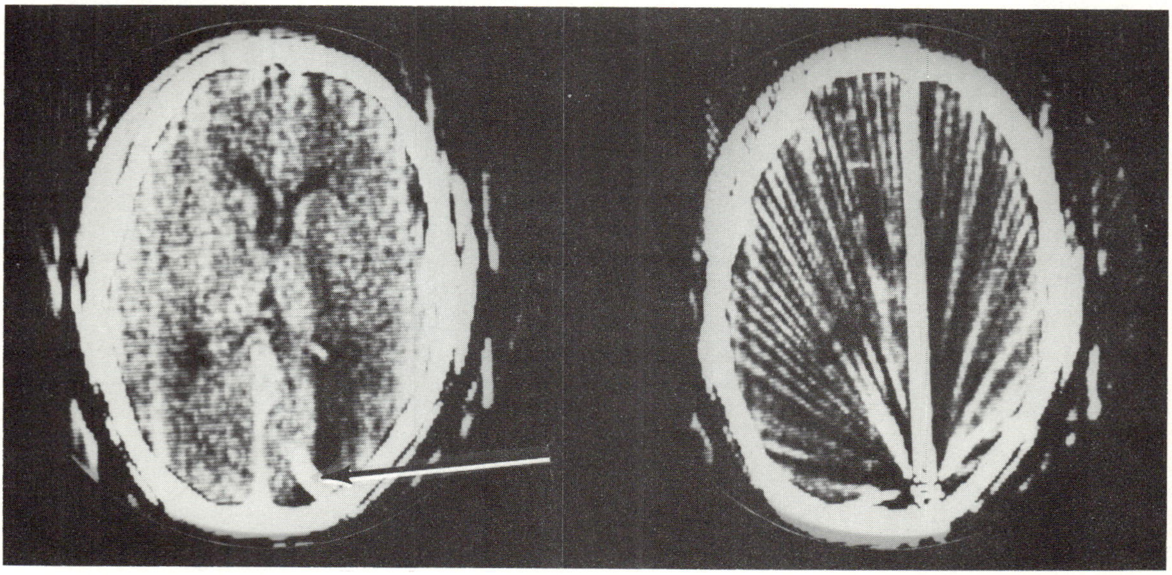

Figure 1–29

Figure 1–30 shows some typical findings seen after posterior fossa surgery. The bony defects are quite typical; the shunt tube artifacts are also quite typical. I do not believe that it is possible at all times to state the exact location of the end of the shunt tube device.

a. Craniectomy defect is noted in the posterior fossa, along with slight resultant deformity of the fourth ventricle (arrows) following removal of a medulloblastoma.

b. Sunburst computer artifact from a metallic portion of a shunt tube.

c. Shunt tube in place in the right lateral ventricle. Shunts can often be visualized on several adjacent cuts.

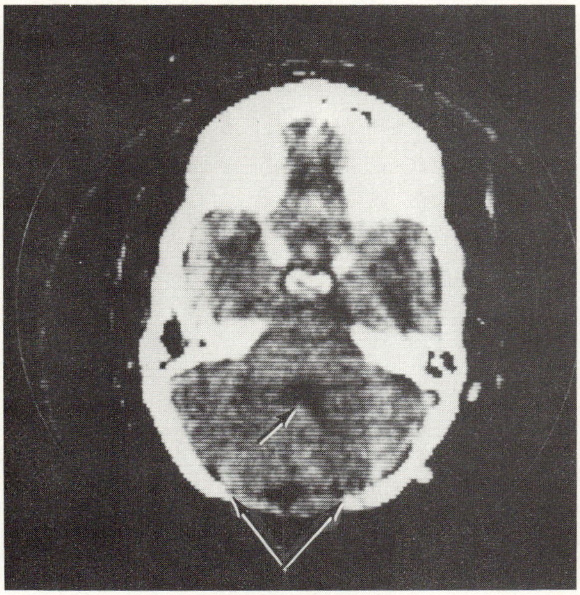

Figure 1–30a

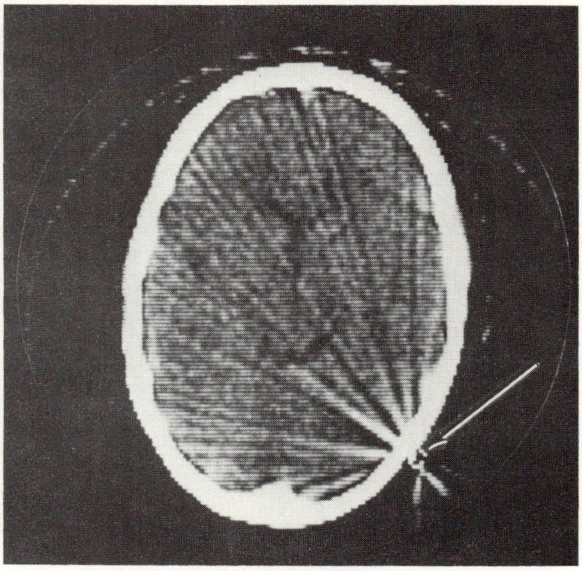

Figure 1–30b

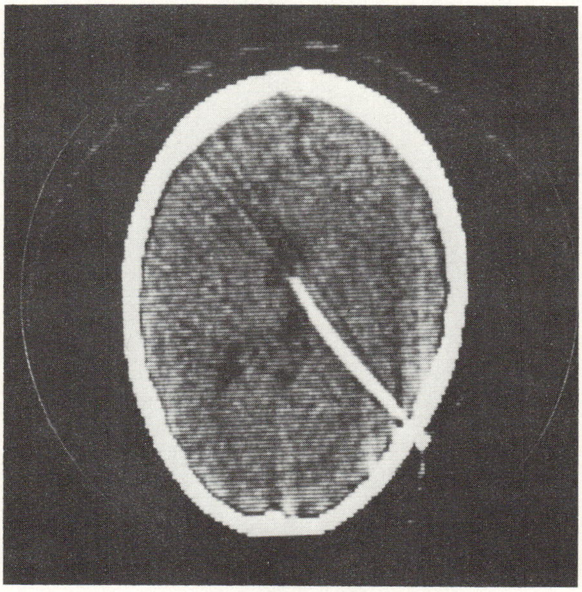

Figure 1–30c

CHAPTER 2
PRIMARY BRAIN TUMORS

Gliomas

Gliomas, in general, can present with a variety of appearances on computed tomograms. The most common appearance is that of a large lucent area with the tumor itself enhancing after the infusion of contrast material. The gliomas, at times, can appear as relatively dense areas; again they usually reveal definite enhancement after contrast enhancement. The glioblastomas most often appear as low density areas with a good deal of mass effect. The low density areas are often quite large, and the shift of the lateral ventricles and the third ventricle is secondary to the mass and the associated edema. The postinfusion scan outlines the actual area of tumor involvement, and the surrounding area of low density is the associated edema. It is interesting to note that a small tumor can be surrounded by a large area of edema. Correspondingly, it has been noted that the size of a mass at surgery is often much smaller than that outlined by arteriography or by radionuclide scan. The CT scan illustrates very graphically the actual tumor size as well as the surrounding edema and resultant mass effect; the CT scan also delineates to better advantage the actual position of the tumor relative to the mass effect, as the surrounding edema is not always symmetrical. If the tumor contains areas of hemorrhage, as occasionally happens, then areas of blood density will be apparent on the preinfusion scan. However, in addition to the area of blood density there are often other abnormal areas, which are clues to the presence of a tumor rather than a simple intracerebral hematoma. These clues are, first, a large area of surrounding edema, not closely associated with the area of hemorrhage, and, second, the enhancement of the remainder of the tumor after the infusion of contrast material.

Oligodendrogliomas calcify in a high percentage of cases, and this calcification is, of course, readily picked up on the initial CT scan. Astrocytomas also calcify in a certain percentage of cases, and again this calcification can be readily picked up on the initial scan. We have seen occasional, although rare, examples of gliomas in which a large lucent area with mass effect was present on the preinfusion scan but in which only minimal enhancement could be identified.

Although a histologic diagnosis cannot be made with certainty, the ring of enhancement of the tumor with an associated area of edema is quite typical of a glioblastoma. However, this ring of enhancement is not pathognomonic of glioblastoma and can also be seen with metastatic disease, with a brain abscess, or occasionally with a meningioma. We have noted that many of the grade I and II astrocytomas tend to have a very homogeneous blush similar to the meningiomas; their position deep within the brain, rather than closely associated with the dura, is the important differentiating point.

ASTROCYTOMA, GRADE II (Figure 2–1)

D. S. is a 13 year old male who had a history of a seizure disorder for approximately 7 years prior to admission. Over the preceding years he had had multiple arteriograms and two pneumoencephalograms. None of these studies were convincing of the presence of a tumor. The pneumoencephalogram done 4 years prior to the present admission revealed moderate hydrocephalus and what appeared to be a porencephalic cyst on the right side. Because of the hydrocephalus and the "porencephaly," the shunt tube was placed on the left side. This ultimately led to relative hemiatrophy on the left side. He was admitted at this time because of the remarkable findings on the CT scan—the symptomatology had not changed.

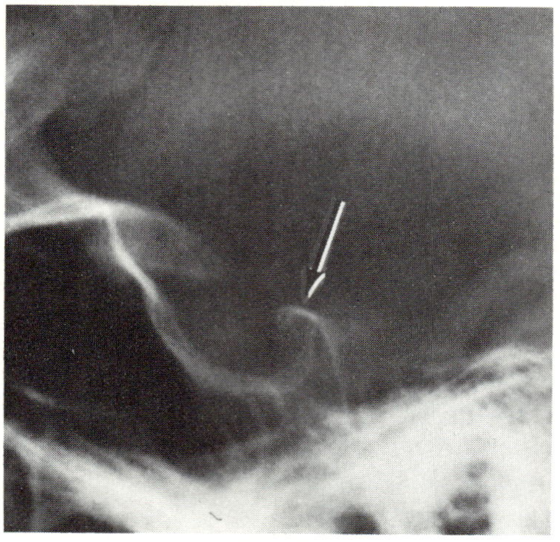

Figure 2–1a

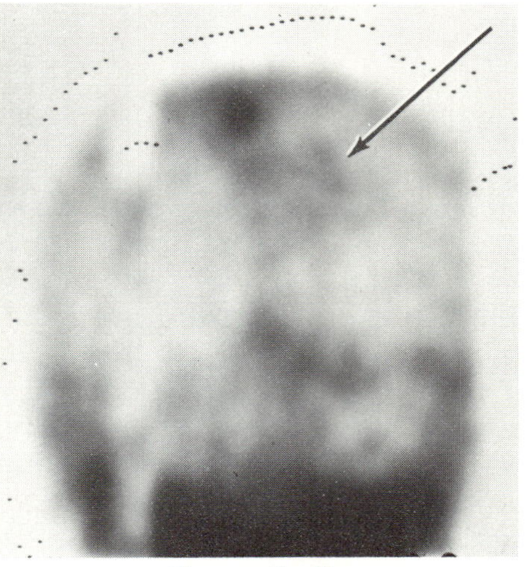

Figure 2–1b

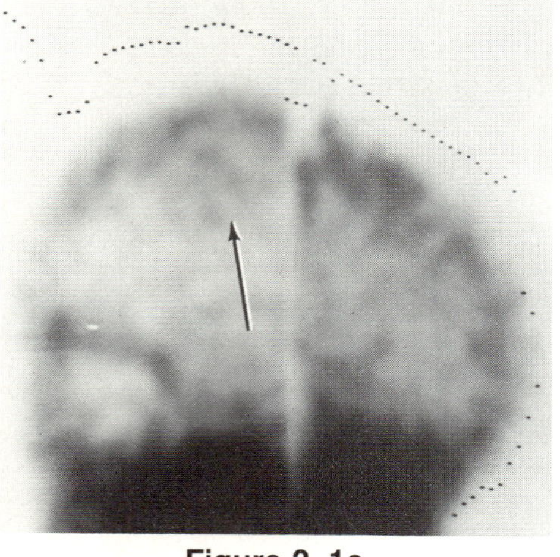

Figure 2–1c

a. The routine skull series reveals mild enlargement of the sella turcica and truncation of the dorsum sellae (see arrow); however, these changes had been present for several years.

b and c. Radionuclide scans available from 7 years prior to admission demonstrate an area of increased uptake in the right parietal area.

d and e. Right lateral (d) and vertex (e) views obtained at this time again show the abnormal area of increased uptake deep in the right parietal lobe. The size appears essentially unchanged since the initial study.

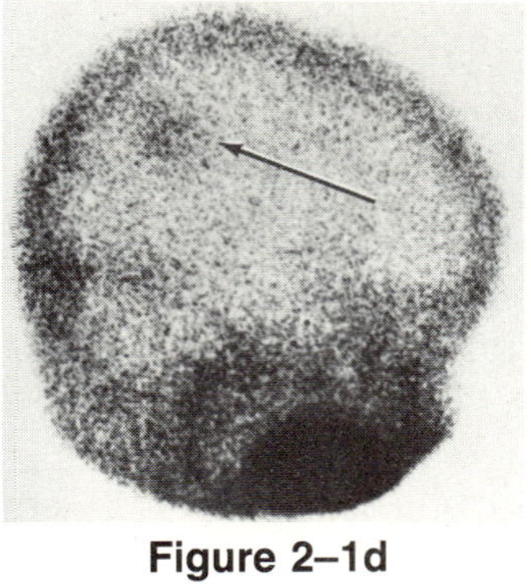

Figure 2–1d

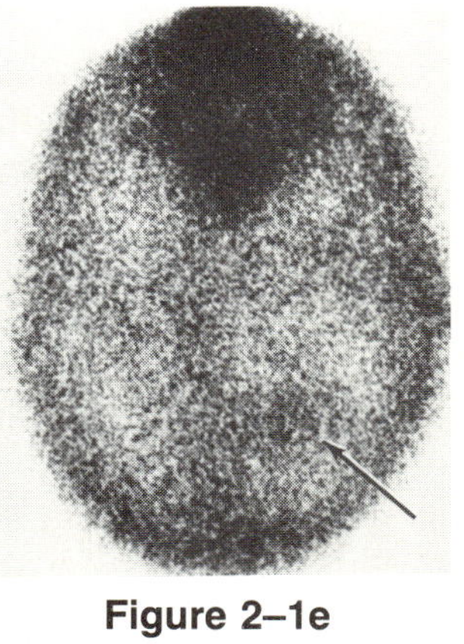

Figure 2–1e

f. The initial CT scan is spectacularly abnormal. A very large calcified mass appears deep in the right parietal lobe. The density of the calcifications ranges from 40 to 120 u. The mass is surrounded by a large low density area with a well-defined margin and appears to be a cystic component of the tumor rather than surrounding edema. This cystic area may well have been the "porencephaly" noted on the earlier pneumoencephalogram.

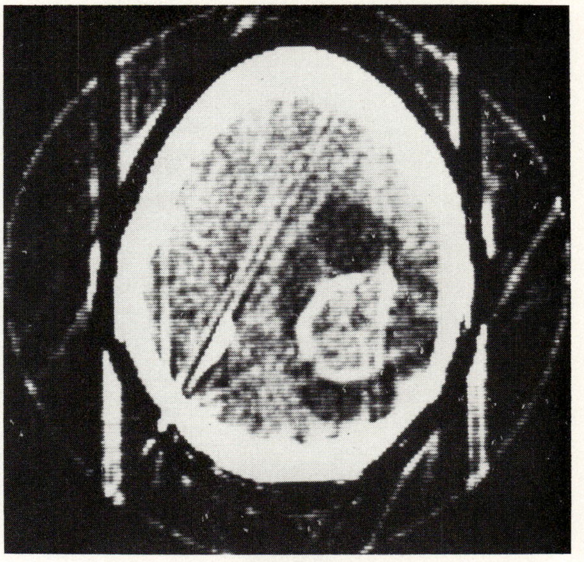

Figure 2–1f

g. The right carotid arteriogram at this time is grossly abnormal. There is shift to the left; however, the amount of shift is deceptive because of the hemiatrophy on the left. A large mass lesion can be identified in the parietal area with spreading of the vessels in this area (arrows).

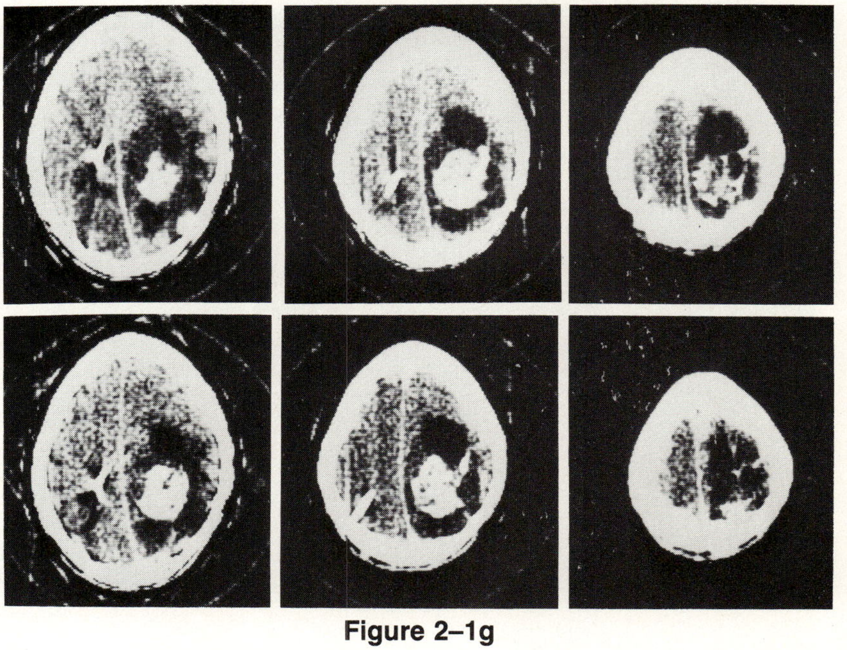

Figure 2–1g

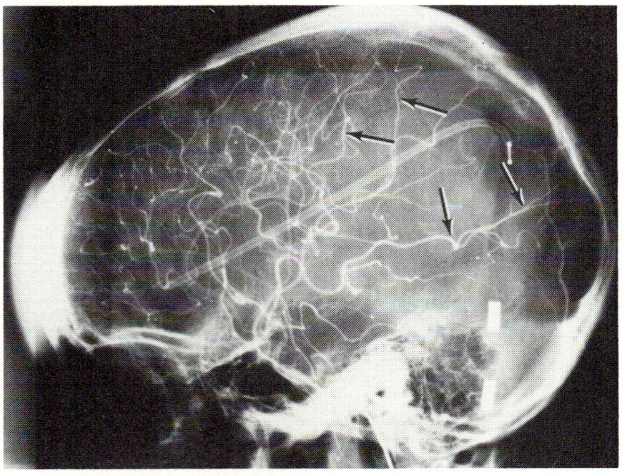

Figure 2–1h

h. A speckled irregular area of tumor blush is noted on the late arterial and venous phases (arrows).

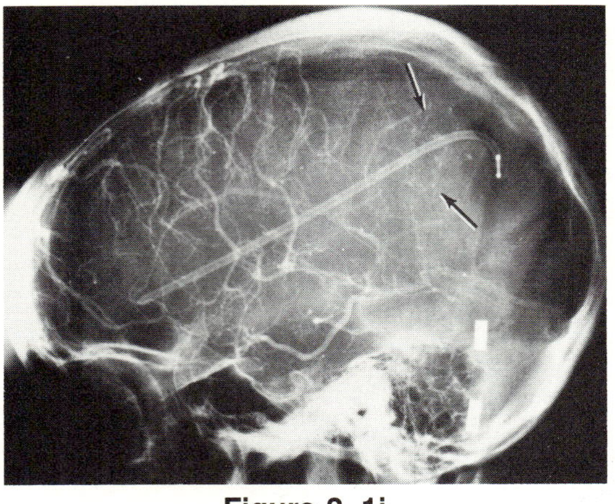

Figure 2–1i

i. The subtraction view shows the blush to better advantage. Shunt tubing device is noted in place on the left side.

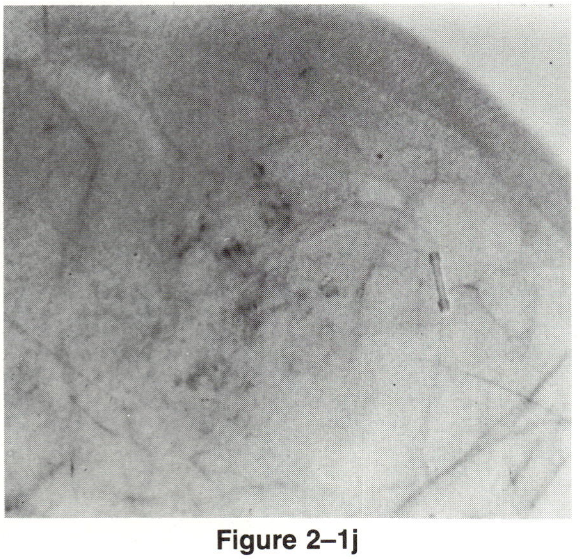

Figure 2–1j

j. There is puddling of contrast in the region of the tumor.

Surgery with gross total removal revealed a calcified astrocytoma, Grade II.

GLIOBLASTOMA MULTIFORME (Figure 2–2)

W. B. is a 51 year old man with a recent onset of somnolence and a right-sided headache for 8 days prior to admission.

a and b. The anterior (a) and right lateral views reveal a focal discrete intracerebral mass situated in the right temporal-parietal region.

c. The initial CT scan discloses a large lucent area involving the right frontal, temporal, and parietal lobes. There is shift toward the left. No evidence of calcification is apparent. On cut 2A one can see some curvilinear areas of increased density (arrow) within the area of lucency. This is the actual tumor mass within an area of surrounding edema.

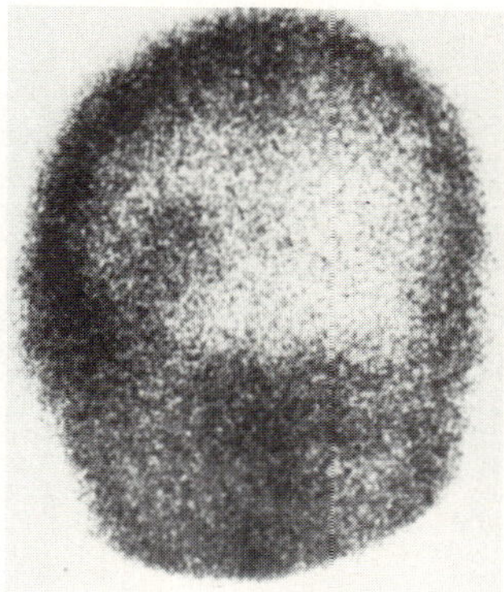

Figure 2–2a

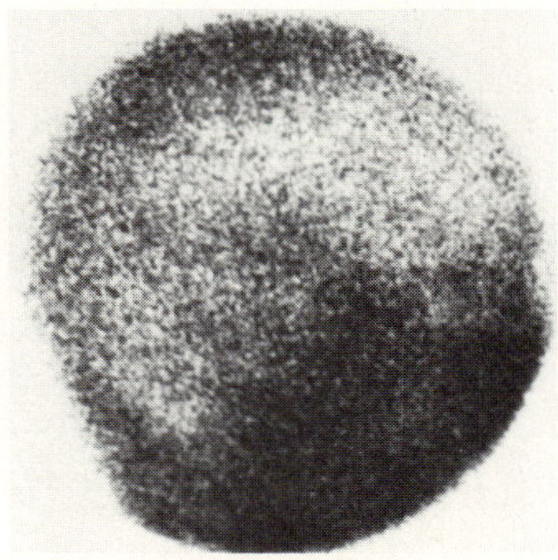

Figure 2–b

1A 2A

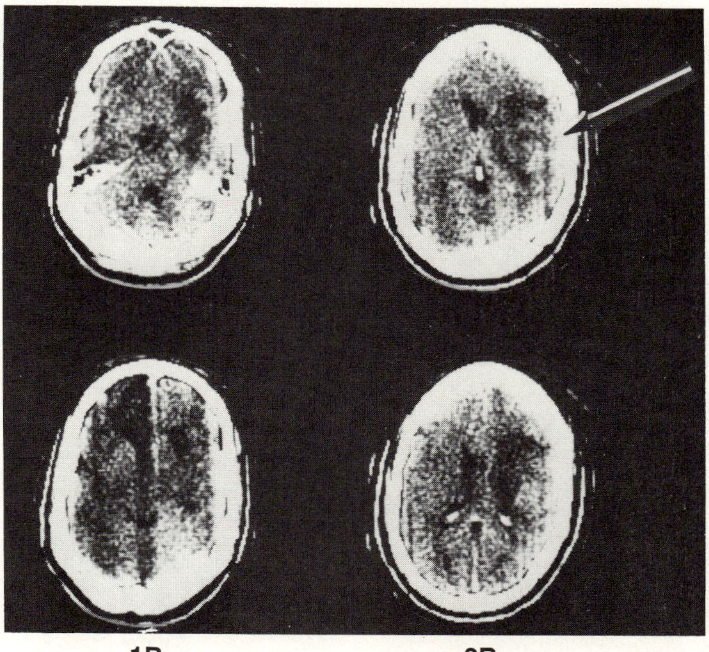

1B 2B

Figure 2–2c

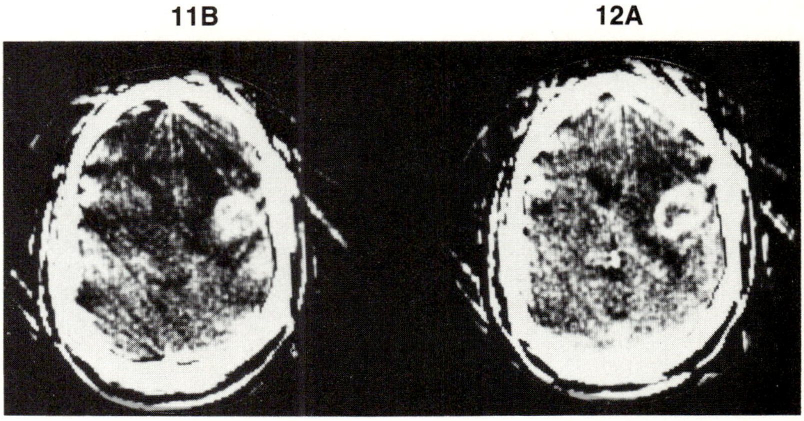

Figure 2–2d

d. Cuts 11B and 12A show marked contrast enhancement of the tumor, which appears to have a "ring" of enhancement. This ring, although quite typical with gliomas, is not, unfortunately, pathognomonic. We have seen this with abscesses and metastatic tumors as well. The surrounding lucent area represents edema associated with the tumor. The mass effect is secondary to the edema as well as the mass itself.

e. The AP arterial phase of the right carotid arteriogram reveals multiple small tumor vessels just inferior and lateral to the sylvian point (arrows). Medial displacement of the sylvian point has occurred, along with a slight shift of the anterior cerebral artery (crossed arrow).

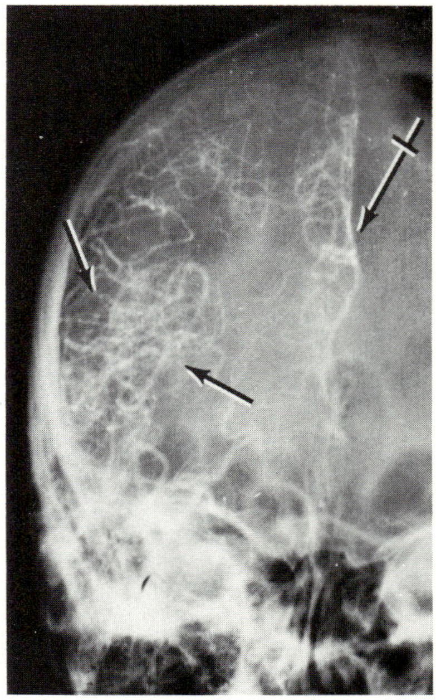

Figure 2–2e

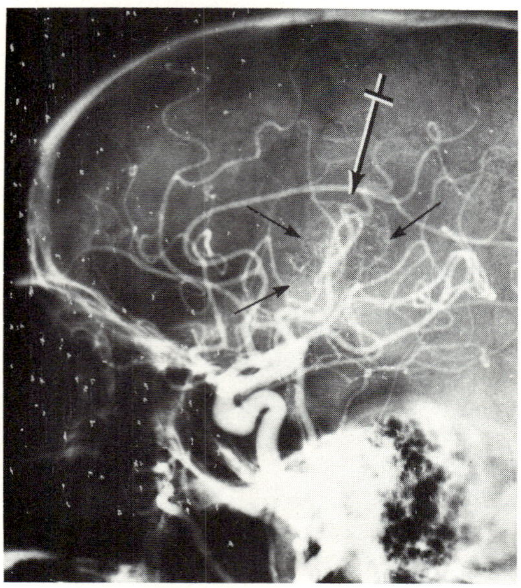

Figure 2–2f

f. The arterial phase on the lateral view again reveals the multiple small neoplastic vessels (arrows) associated with upward displacement of one of the vessels of the sylvian triangle (crossed arrow).

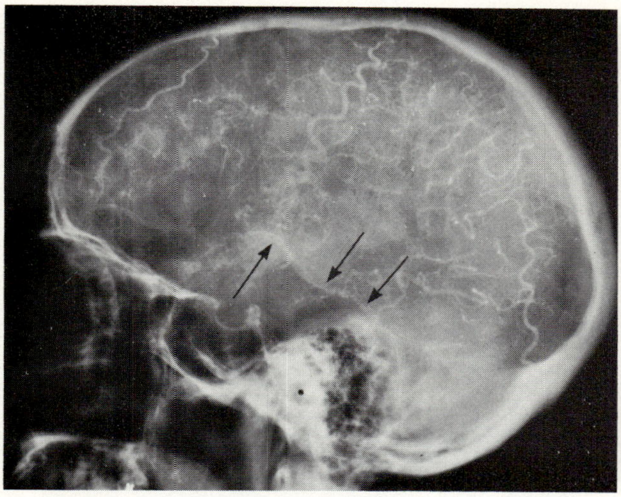

Figure 2–2g

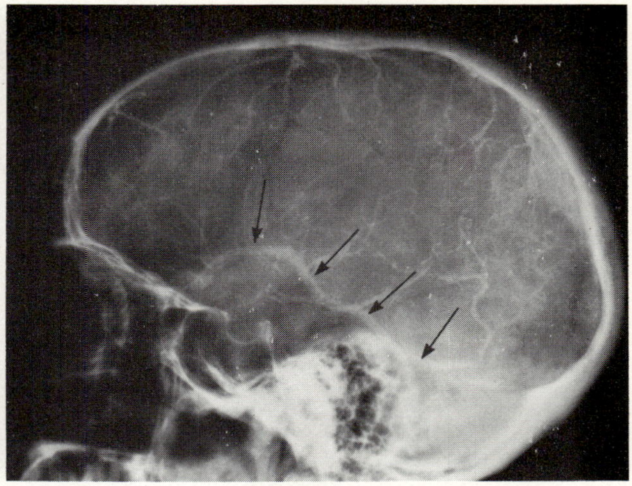

Figure 2–2h

g. The late arterial phase shows an early draining vein originating from the bed of the tumor.

h. The venous phase reveals the early vein better. These are classic findings in a glioblastoma.

i. Surgical exploration was unsuccessful in localizing the tumor. The arteriogram was repeated several weeks later, revealing an increase in the size of the mass (arrows) and a more marked shift of the anterior cerebral artery under the falx cerebri (crossed arrow).

j. The lateral view reveals increased disruption of the sylvian triangle (arrows) and even earlier filling of the early draining vein than was noted on the earlier study.

This was presumed to be a glioblastoma multiforme. Radiation and chemotherapy were given.

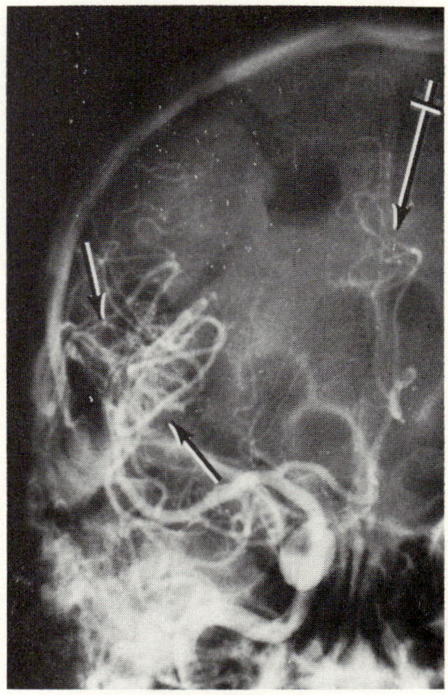

Figure 2–2i

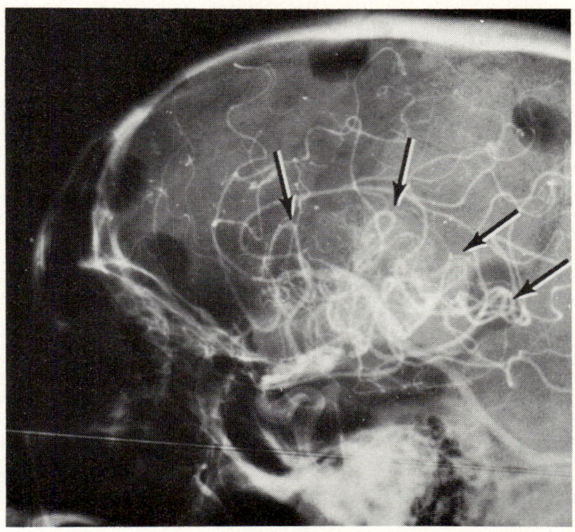

Figure 2–2j

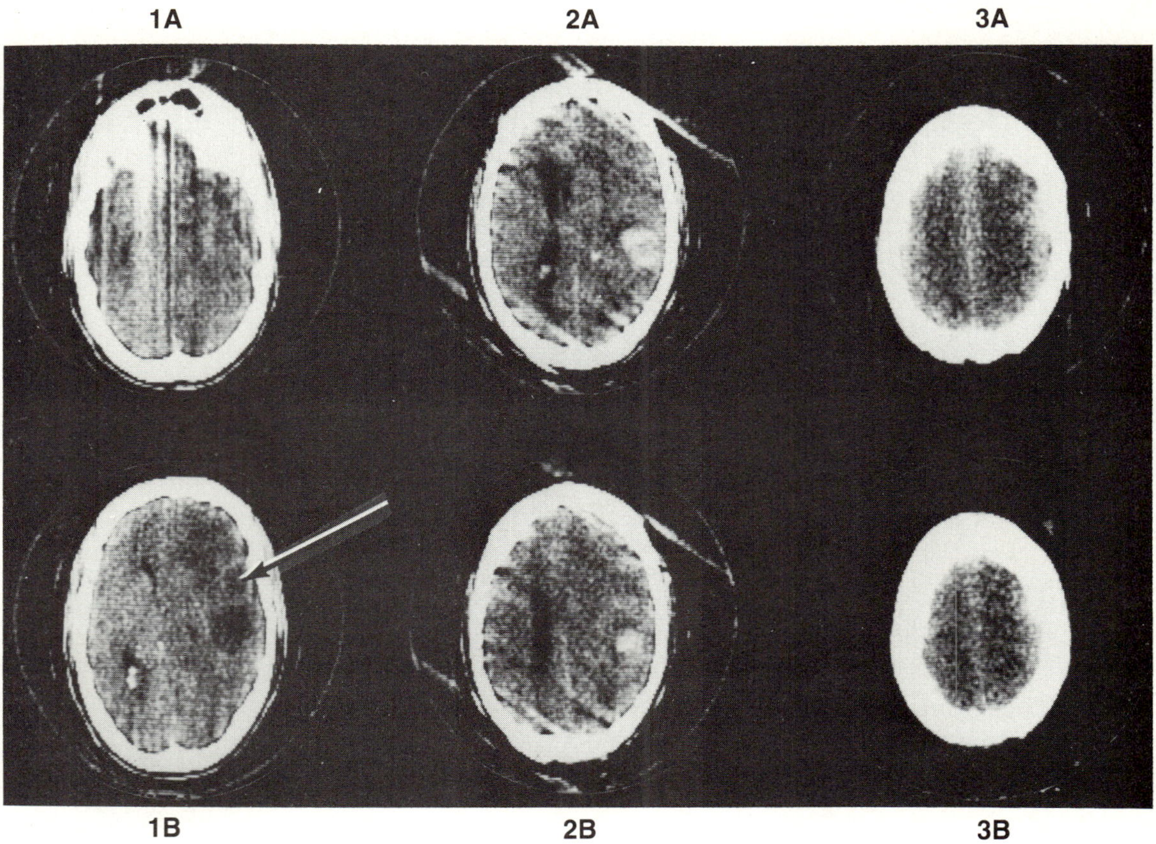

Figure 2–3a

HEMORRHAGIC GLIOBLASTOMA MULTIFORME (Figure 2–3)

R. G. is a 22 year old man with left arm and leg weakness, associated with confusion. The onset had been rather insidious.

a. The initial CT scan reveals a large area of lucency in the right temporal, frontal, and parietal lobes. This lucency is best seen on cut 1B (arrow). There is a marked shift from right to left. In addition a rounded area of increased density is seen in the parietal lobe on cut 2A measuring from 42 to 74 u. The smaller, higher extension of this area can be seen on cut 2B. This is an area of hemorrhage within the tumor mass.

b. The postinfusion scan reveals a ring of enhancement best seen on cut 11B (arrow). A curvilinear area of enhancement can be seen around the area of hemorrhage as well. These findings are consistent with an area of hemorrhage within a glioblastoma. The clinical history, the area of edema, and the ring of enhancement differentiate this from a simple spontaneous intracerebral hematoma.

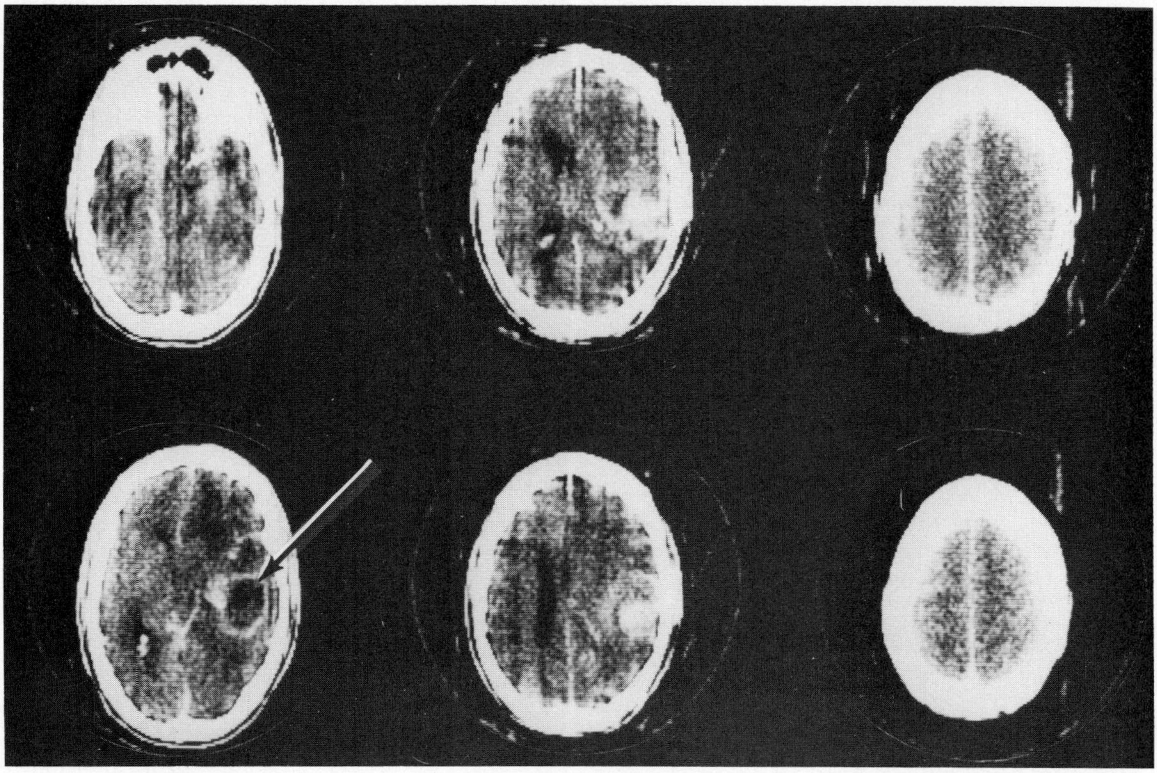

Figure 2–3b

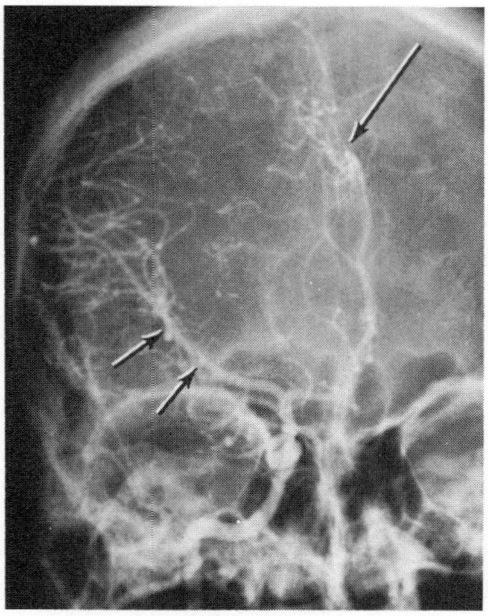

Figure 2–3c

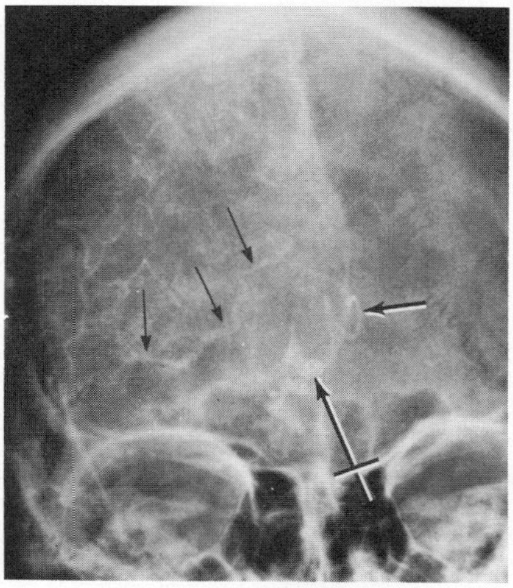

Figure 2–3d

c. The AP arterial phase demonstrates a distal shift of the anterior cerebral artery under the falx cerebri (upper arrow) and medial displacement of the trifurcation of the middle cerebral artery (lower arrows).

d. The late arterial phase reveals an early draining vein (arrows) that drained into the shifted internal cerebral vein (short arrow) and the vein of Galen (crossed arrow).

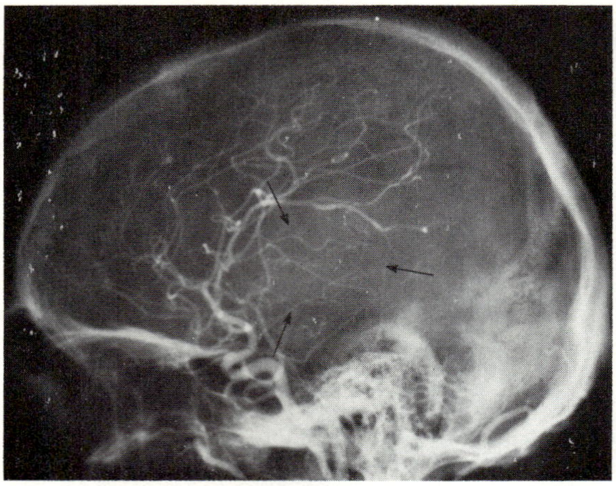

Figure 2–3e

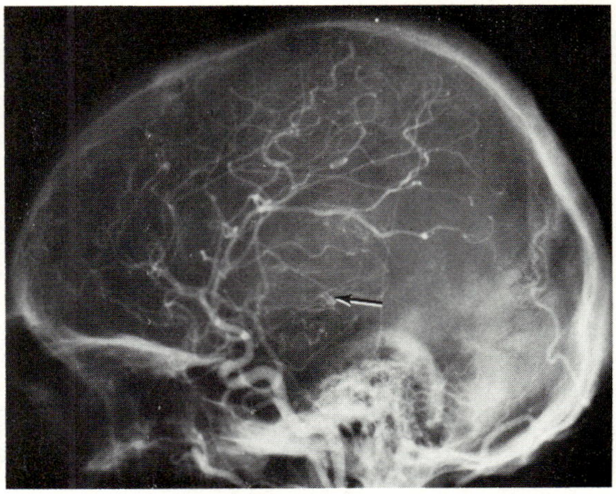

Figure 2–3f

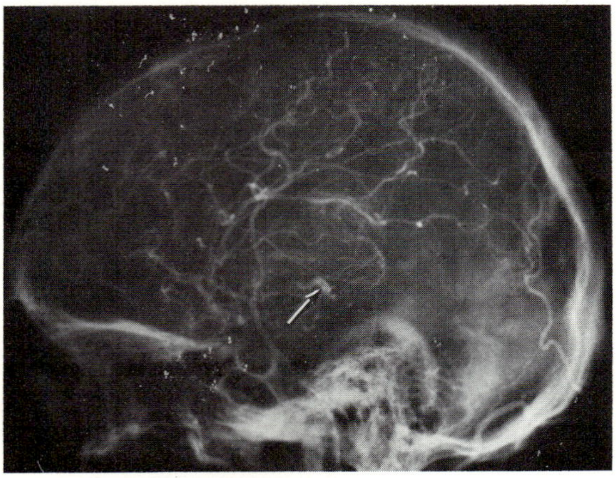

Figure 2–3g

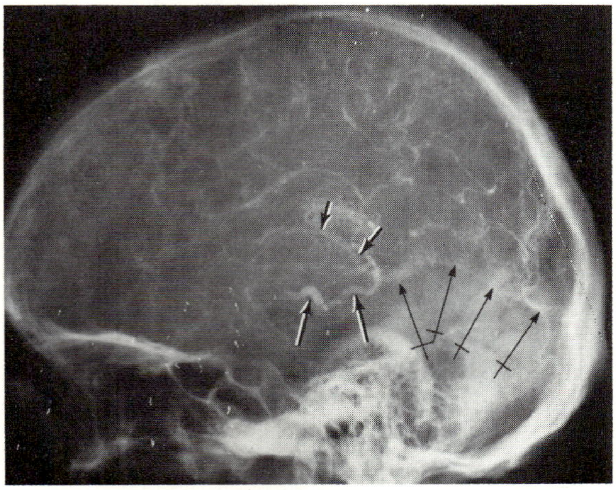

Figure 2–3h

e. The early arterial phase shows elevation and disruption of the sylvian triangle. Neovascularity can be seen in the infrasylvian region (arrows).

f. The later arterial phase reveals the initial filling of what is to be an early draining vein (arrow).

g. More neovascularity and the early draining vein (arrow).

h. The late arterial phase reveals the early draining vein (arrows) that drained into the internal cerebral vein (short arrows) and vein of Galen and the straight sinus (crossed arrows).

Surgery, with gross total removal, revealed a large glioblastoma multiforme with areas of hemorrhage.

GLIOBLASTOMA MULTIFORME (Figure 2–4)

G. J. is a 19 year old female who presented with right arm paresis and mild dysphasia. She dated her present problem from an incident of minor head trauma sustained in an automobile accident 4 months previously. In addition to the right arm weakness, physical examination revealed a mild right facial paresis and a slight increase in the knee jerk on the right side.

a to c. Vertex (a), anteroposterior (b), and left lateral (c) views of the radionuclide scan reveal an area of increased uptake deep in the left parietal lobe (arrows).

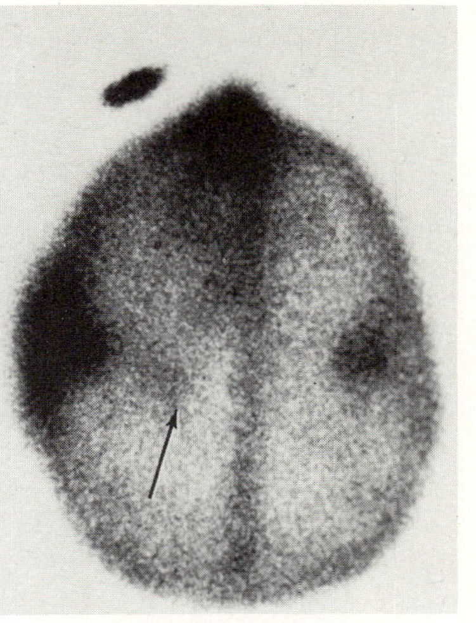

Figure 2–4a

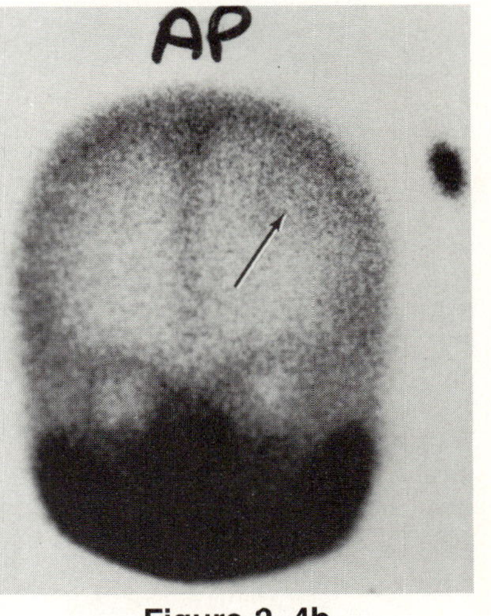

Figure 2–4b

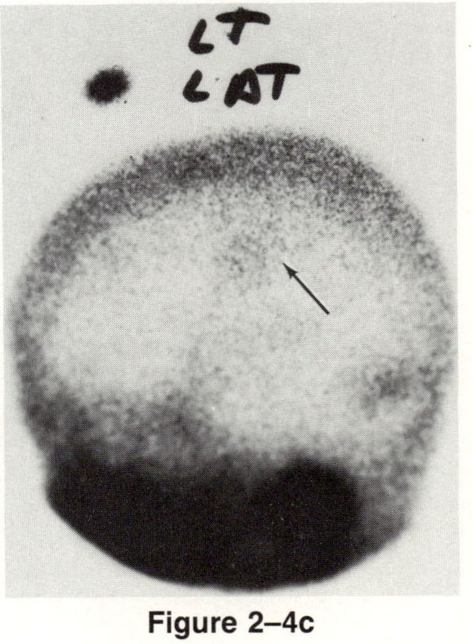

Figure 2–4c

d. The routine CT scan reveals a mass in the left parietal lobe that measures 34 to 48 u. The density is not markedly different from that of the normal brain; however, there is an area of surrounding edema (arrows on 3A and 3B). The frontal horns of the lateral ventricles are shifted from left to right (arrow on 2A).

2A 3A 2B 3b

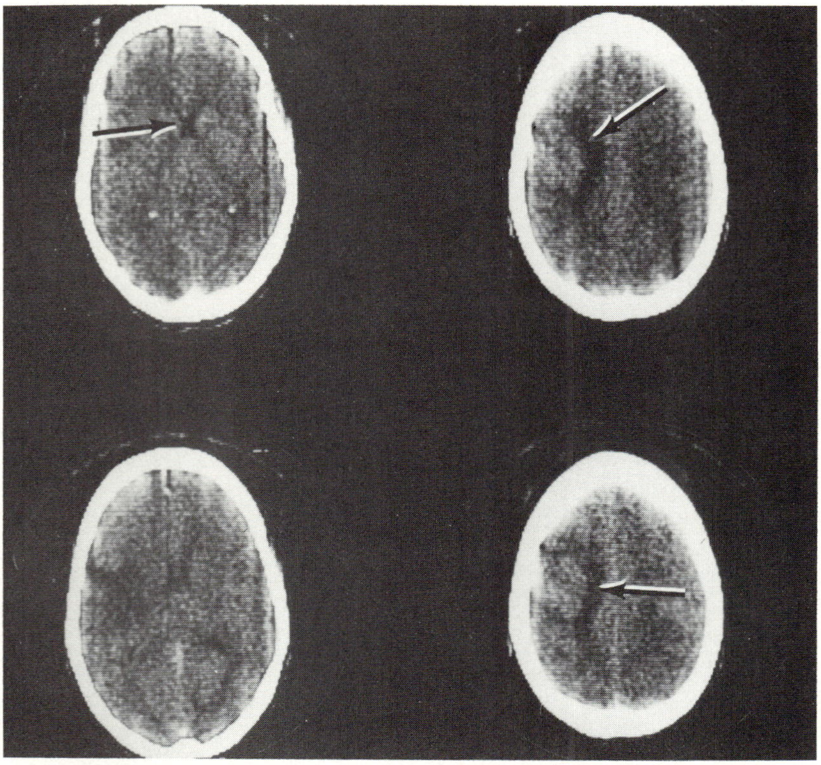

Figure 2–4d

12A 13A x2B 13B

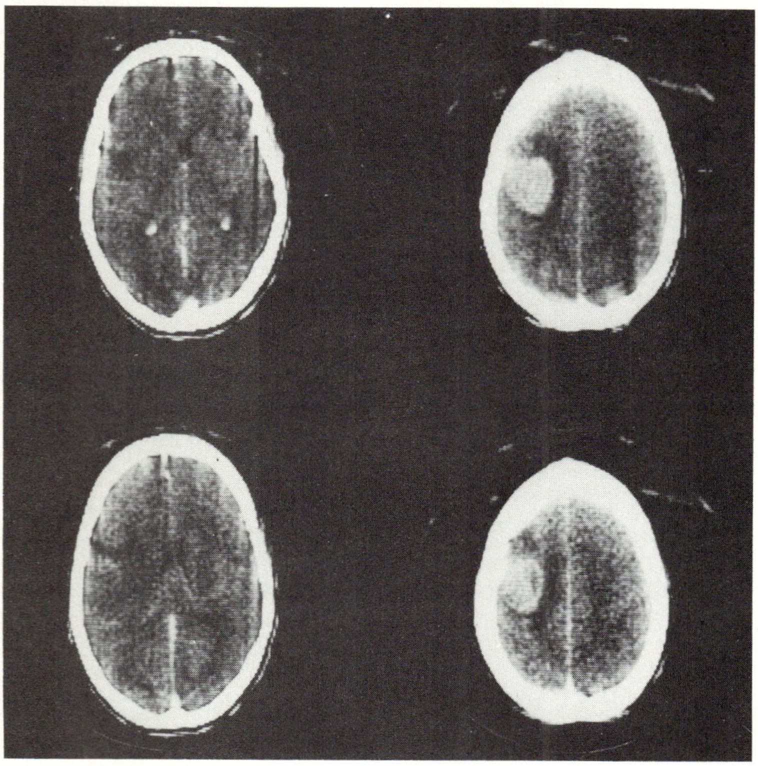

Figure 2–4e

e. Following the infusion of contrast material, the tumor enhanced in a homogeneous fashion. The density increased to 70 u. We have seen this pattern of homogeneous enhancement most often in the low grade gliomas and in meningiomas. This mass appeared to be seated within the cerebral tissue, and so meningioma appeared unlikely. Surgery with gross total removal revealed a glioblastoma multiforme.

f. The anteroposterior arterial phase shows a mild shift of the anterior cerebral artery under the falx cerebri (arrow). The sylvian point is depressed (short arrow).

g. Surprisingly there is almost no venous shift.

h. The lateral arterial phase reveals downward displacement of the entire sylvian triangle and mild splaying of the opercular branches of the middle cerebral artery.

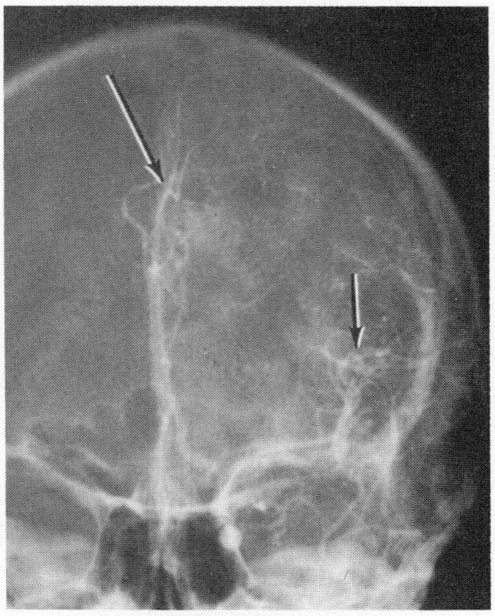

Figure 2–4f

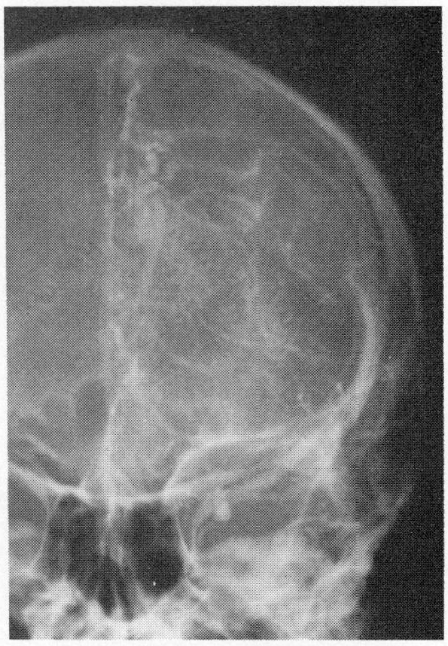

Figure 2–4g

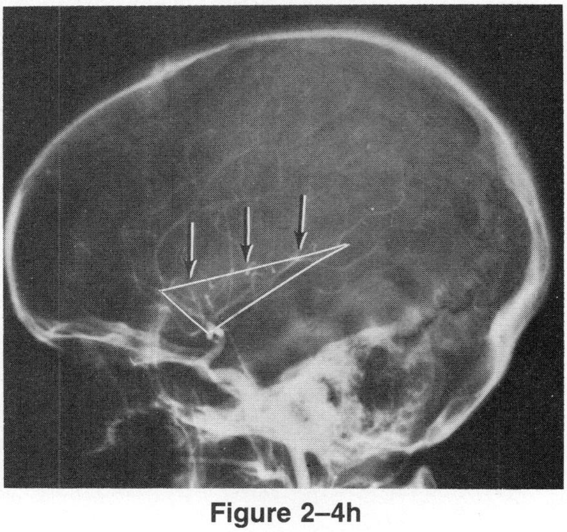

Figure 2–4h

ASTROCYTOMA, GRADE II (Figure 2–5)

S. B. is a 3 year old female with failure to reach the normal developmental milestones and an enlarging head.

1A 2A 3A

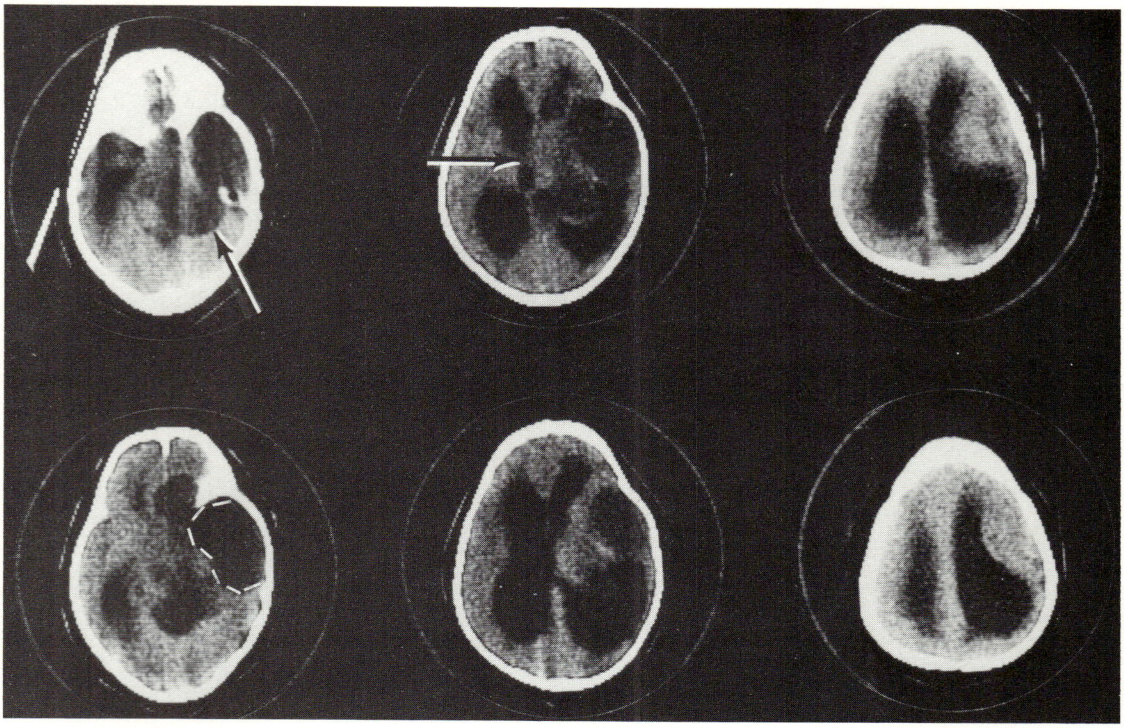

1B 2B 3B

Figure 2–5a

11A 12A 13A

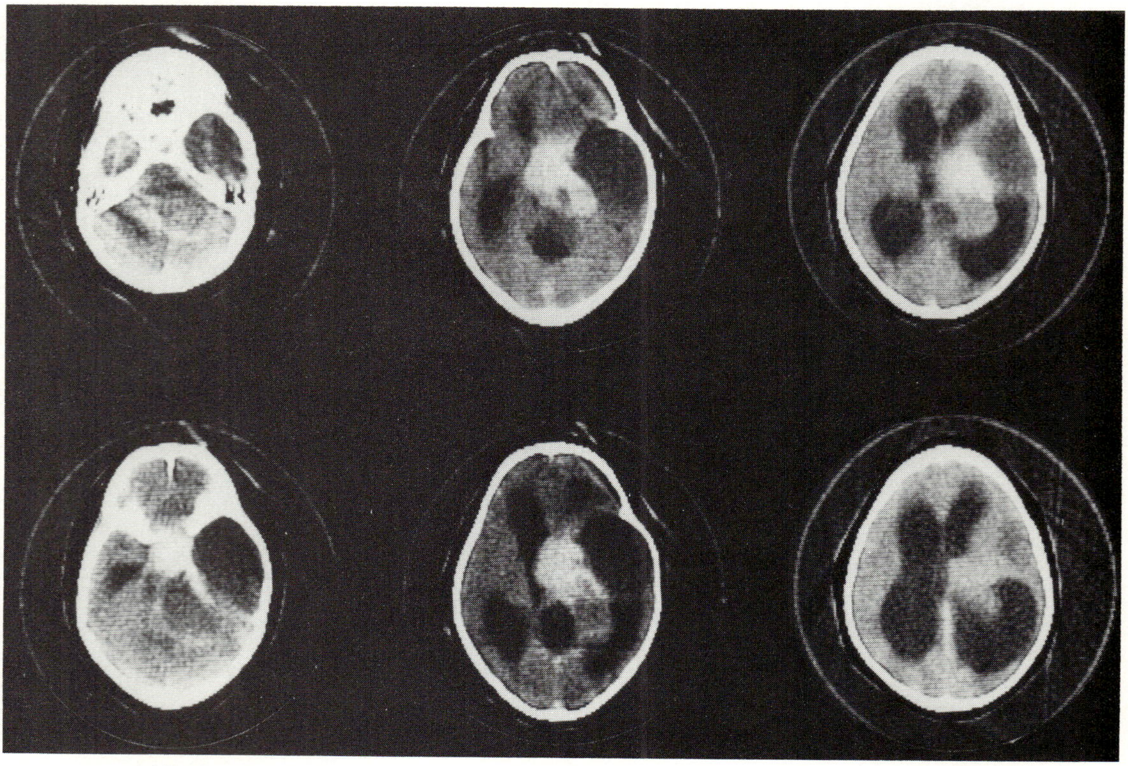

11B 12B 13B

Figure 2–5b

a. The routine CT scan shows a markedly distorted intracranial architecture. Both ventricles were dilated and the right ventricle was distorted. There was mild shift of the third ventricle from right to left (horizontal arrow on 2A). A large cyst in the right temporal fossa could be seen on cuts 1A through 2A. The cyst is outlined with a dashed line in 1B. The cyst fluid measured 5 to 15 u, which is higher than cerebrospinal fluid. The abnormality appeared to extend into the posterior fossa (arrow on 1A).

b. After contrast infusion there was homogeneous enhancement of the tumor mass, which was midline in position, extending off to the right, with the large cystic component described above. The tumor increased from a preinfusion density of 16 to 32 u to a postinfusion density of 44 to 70 u.

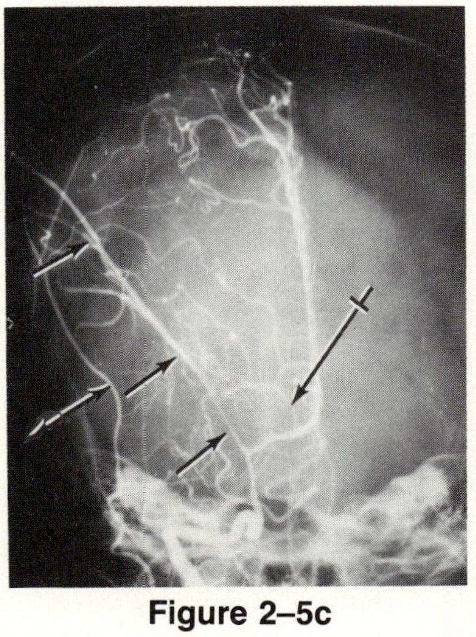

Figure 2–5c

c. The AP arterial phase reveals a mild shift of the anterior cerebral artery. There was marked elevation of the entire middle cerebral artery group (arrows). The vessels were noted to be displaced from the inner table of the skull (double-headed arrow). In addition there was marked enlargement of the recurrent artery of Heubner (crossed arrow).

d. The lateral view, arterial phase, demonstrates elevation of the middle cerebral artery and thinning of the origins of the anterior and middle cerebral arteries and the supraclinoid internal carotid artery (arrows). The hypertrophied recurrent artery of Heubner (crossed arrow) is again seen.

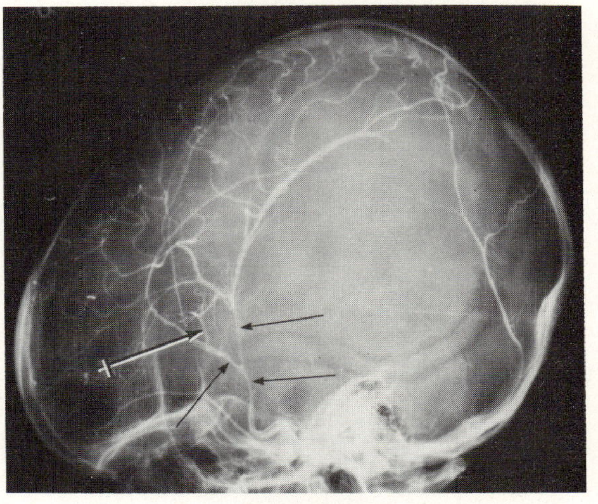

Figure 2–5d

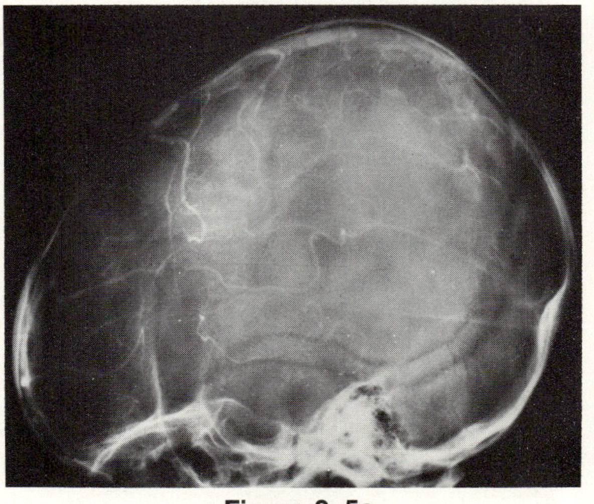

Figure 2–5e

e. The later arterial phase reveals a distorted architecture, but no neovascularity or early draining veins.

The arteriographic picture is distinctly unusual. Surgical biopsy following drainage of the large cyst revealed an astrocytoma, Grade II.

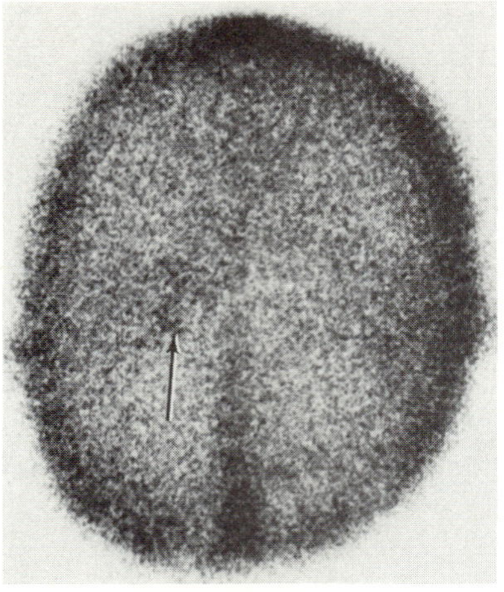

Figure 2–6a

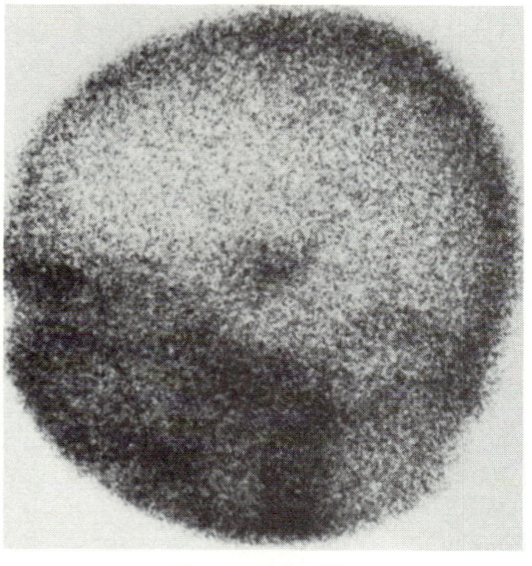

Figure 2–6b

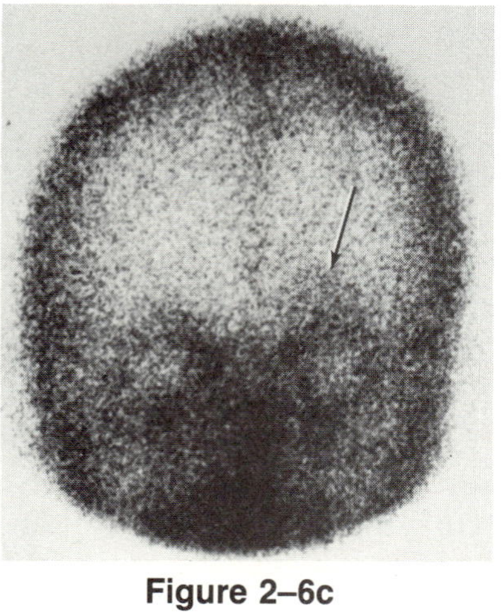

Figure 2–6c

ASTROCYTOMA, GRADE II (Figure 2–6)

P. M. is a 34 year old male with suspected neurofibromatosis and memory loss of 8 years' duration. His physical examination was entirely within normal limits.

a to c. Radionuclide scan: The vertex (a), left lateral (b), and anterior (c) views reveal an area of increased uptake deep in the left temporal-basal ganglia region (arrows).

d. The routine CT scan shows a mottled area of lucency deep in the hemisphere on the left side (arrow on 1A). The density measured from 18 to 30 u. There appears to be a smaller lucent area with a well-defined anterior border just above and anterior to this area. This may represent a small cystic component of the tumor or perhaps the dilated anterior tip of the temporal horn.

e. After contrast enhancement, the tumor enhanced in a homogeneous fashion. A small tongue of tumor tissue extended to the midline adjacent to the third ventricle (arrows on 11B and 12A). The density increased to 48 to 84 u. The cause of the ventricular enlargement is uncertain.

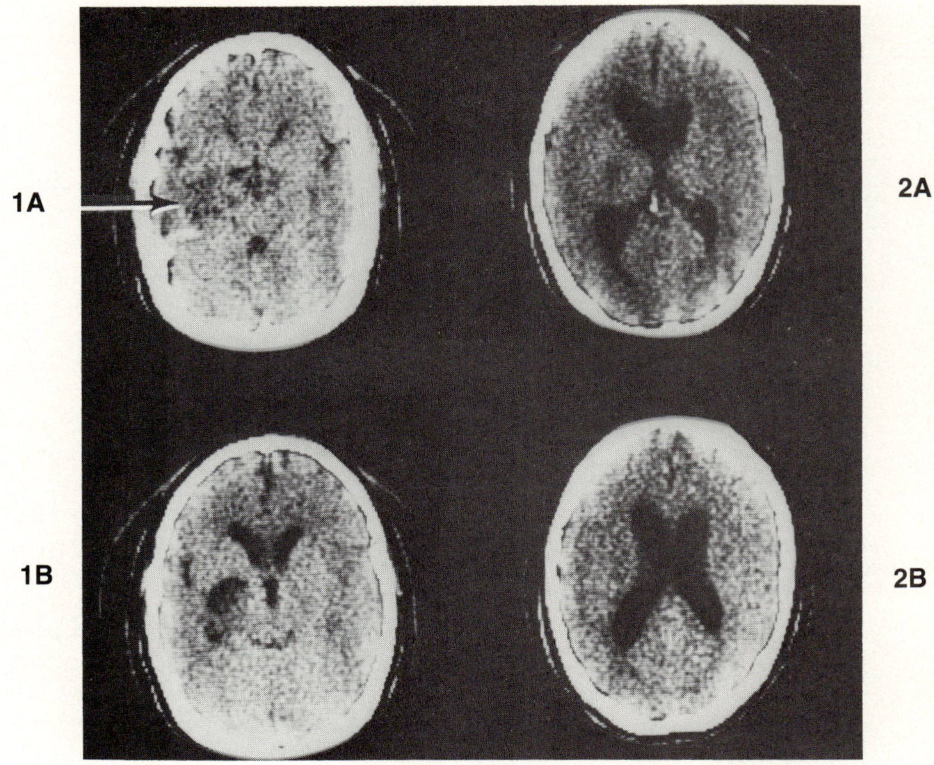

Figure 2–6d

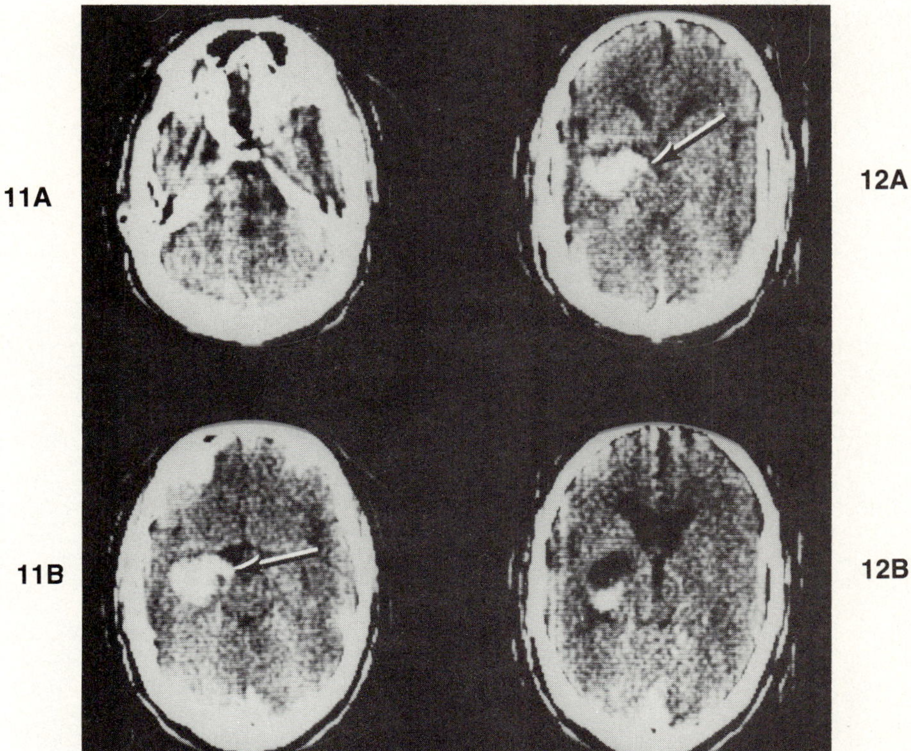

Figure 2–6e

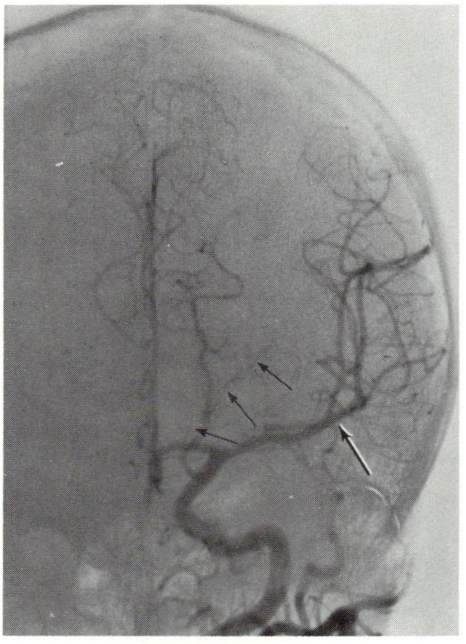

Figure 2–6f

f. The anteroposterior arterial phase demonstrates mild elevation of the distal horizontal portion of the middle cerebral artery (large arrow). Note the medial displacement of the anterior choroidal artery (small arrows).

g. The AP venous phase reveals mild hydrocephalus with outward bowing of the thalamostriate vein (long arrows). The basal vein of Rosenthal appears in normal position (lower arrows).

h. The lateral arterial phase reveals upward bowing of one of the middle cerebral artery vessels (arrow), but is otherwise unremarkable.

i. In the lateral venous phase, mild upward displacement of the anterior end of the basal vein of Rosenthal is seen (arrow).

At surgery, gross total removal with histologic sections disclosed an astrocytoma, Grade II.

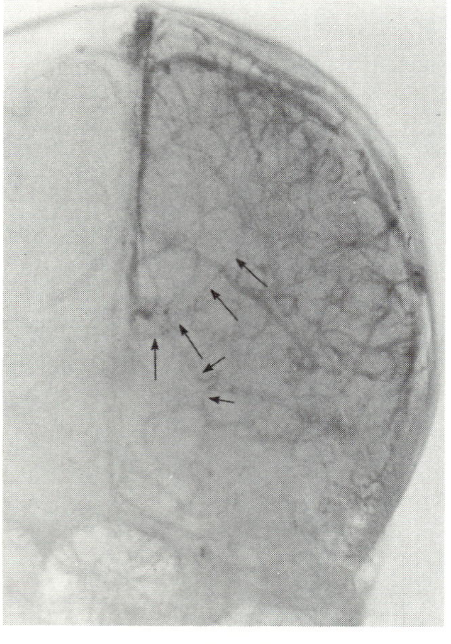

Figure 2–6g

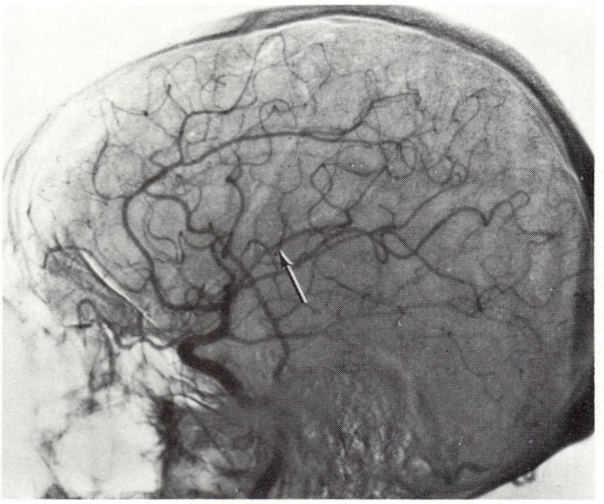

Figure 2–6h

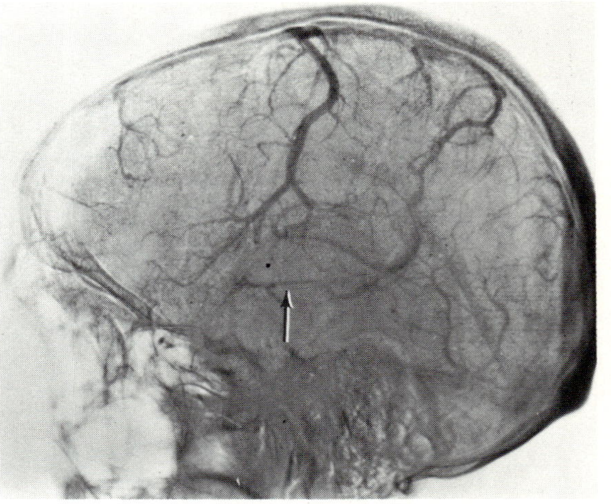

Figure 2–6i

ASTROCYTOMA, GRADE II (Figure 2–7)

A. D. is a 16 year old female who had a long history of left arm focal motor seizures. She was known to have neurofibromatosis.

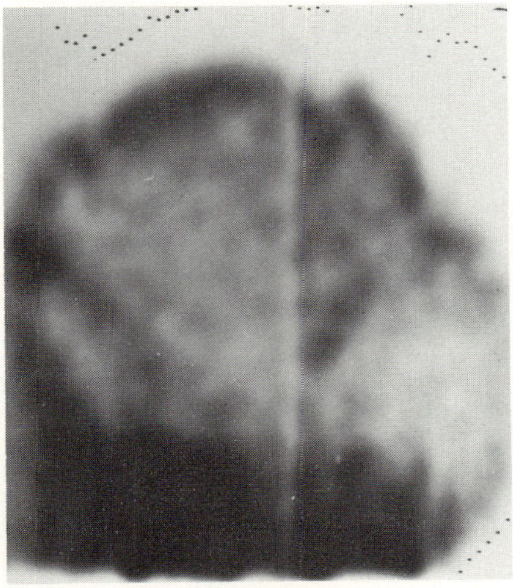

Figure 2–7a

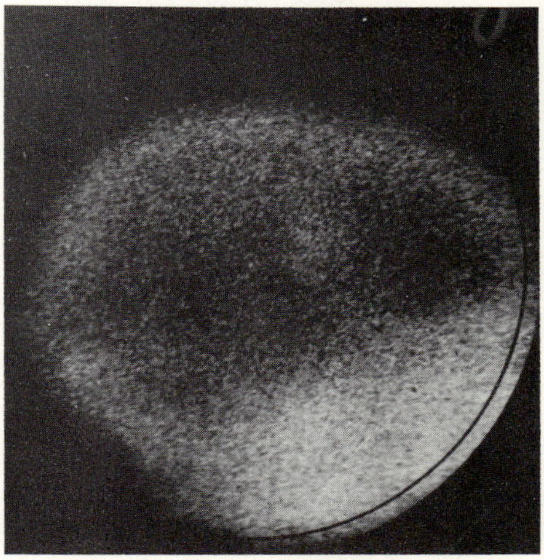

Figure 2–7b

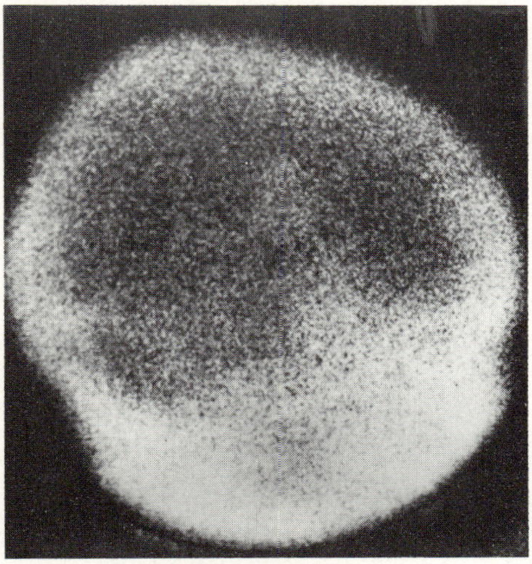

Figure 2–7c

a. A radionuclide scan, obtained 10 years prior to this admission, shows an abnormal area of uptake in the right posterior frontal region.

b. A radionuclide study taken 7 years previously is essentially unchanged from the initial study.

c. A radionuclide study at the time of this admission again discloses the abnormal area of uptake, and again this appears little changed from the initial studies obtained 7 and 10 years ago.

1A 2A 3A

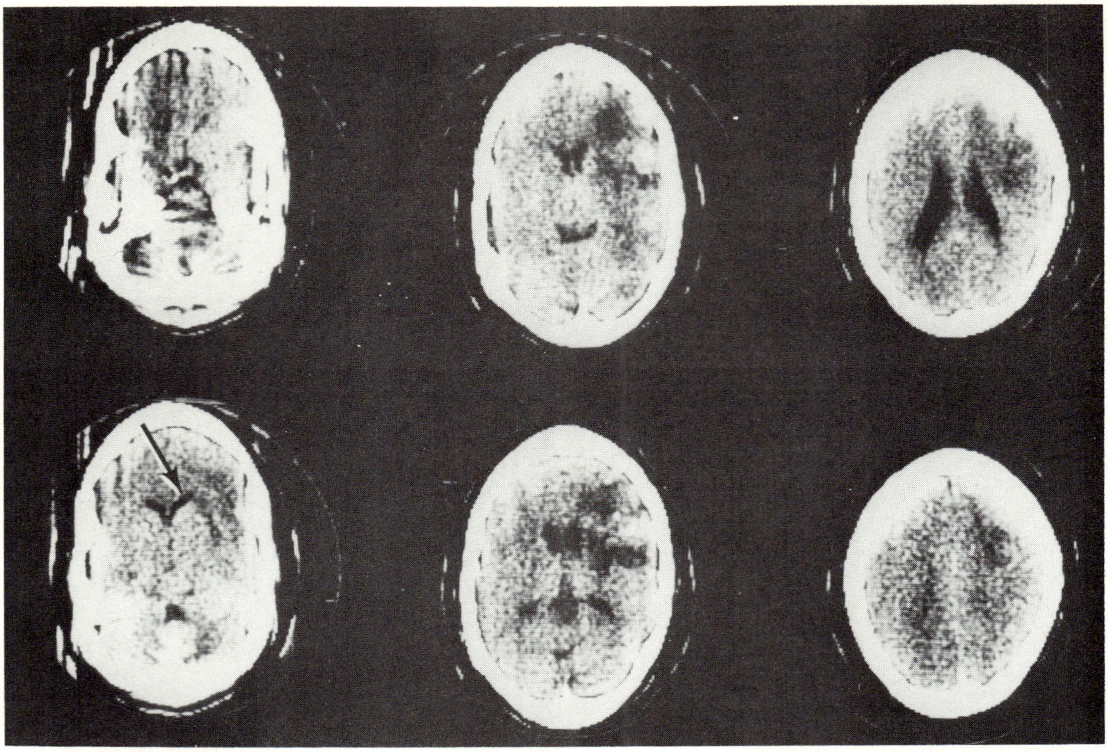

1B 2B 3B

Figure 2–7d

d. The routine CT scan reveals a large calcified tumor mass adjacent to the right sphenoid wing and surrounded by a large area of edema. Interestingly, there is mild anterior displacement of the anterior tip of the right frontal horn (arrow on 1B) but no other evidence of shift. The calcification measured from 30 to 130 u.

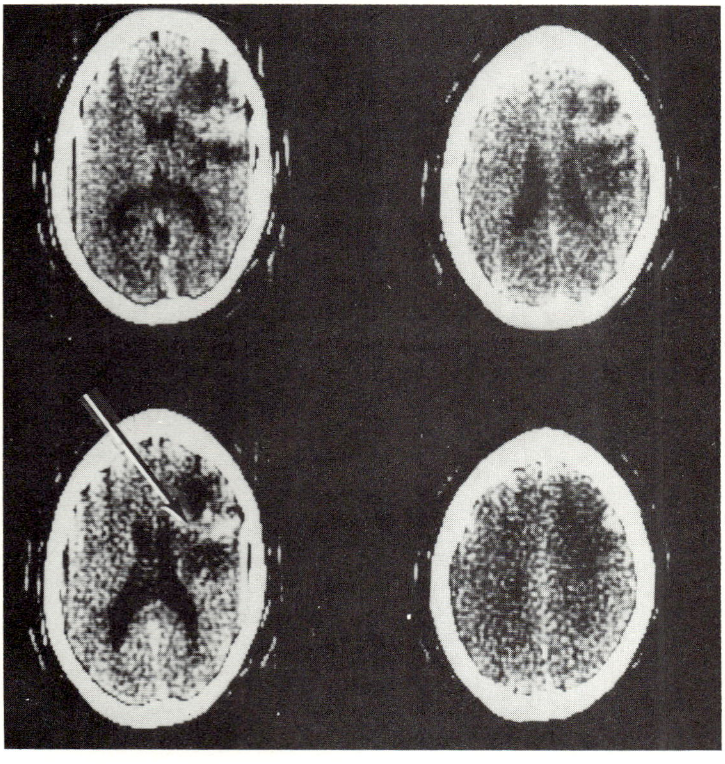

e. Following contrast enhancement, a small area just medial to the area of calcification was noted to enhance to a density of 38 to 64 u. It appears as if this small "active" area of contrast enhancement is the area that was seen on the radionuclide scan (arrow).

Figure 2–7e

f. The lateral arterial phase discloses downward displacement of the midportion of the sylvian triangle (dashed line) and splaying of the opercular branches of the middle cerebral artery group (arrows).

g. The AP arterial phase reveals that the anterior cerebral artery was bowed mildly across the midline.

Surgery was performed, but only partial removal was possible because of the infiltrative nature of the tumor. This was an astrocytoma, Grade II.

h. Follow-up scan after radiation therapy shows a large low density area, 16 to 26 u. Again, there is no gross mass effect. However, after contrast enhancement a definite rim of enhancement is noted. Density, 36 to 50 u. This area appears to represent remaining and/or recurrent tumor in the original tumor site.

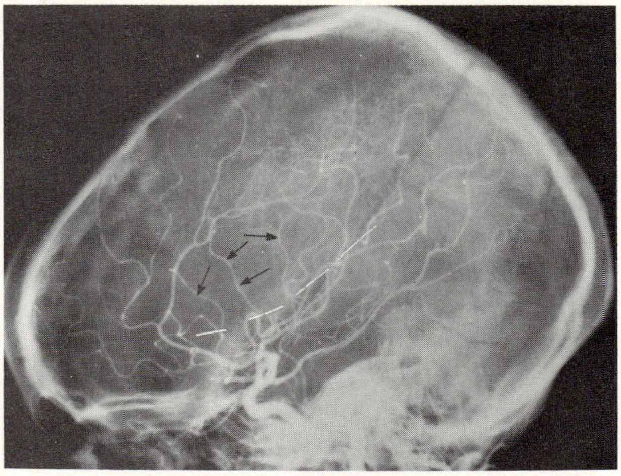

Figure 2–7f

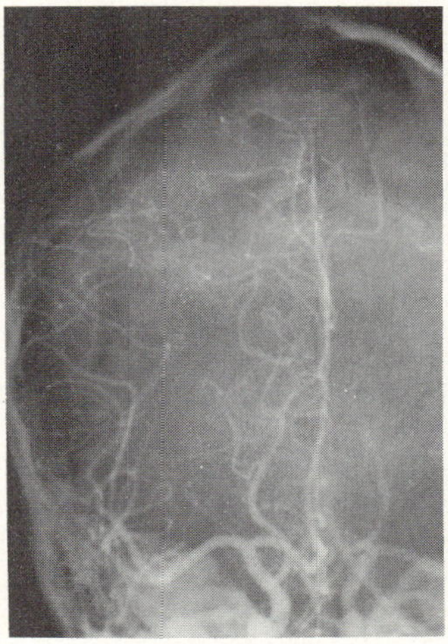

Figure 2–7g

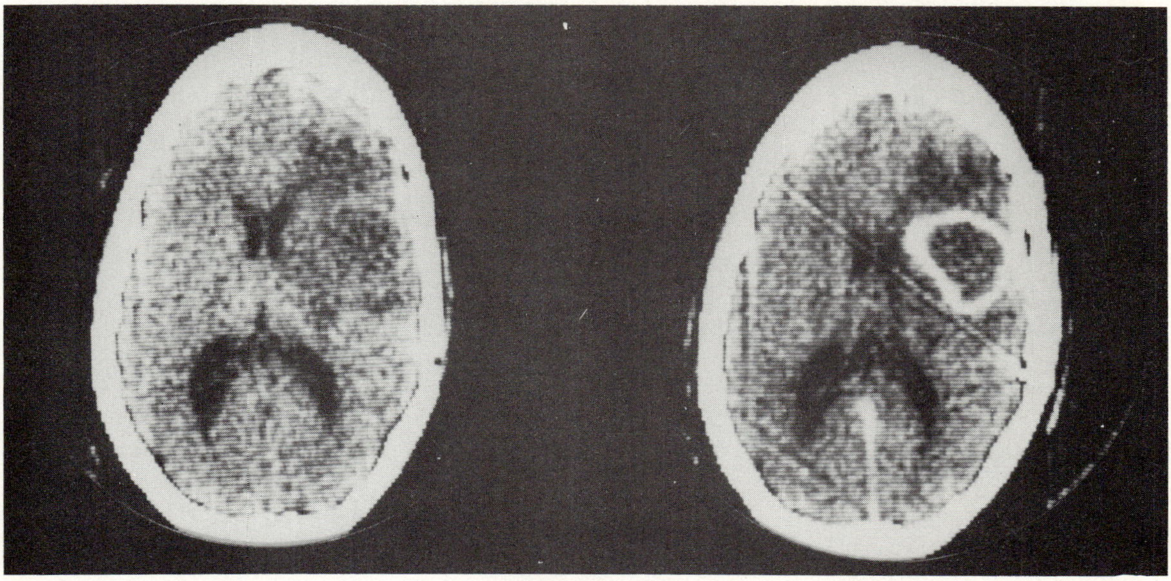

Figure 2–7h

GLIOBLASTOMA MULTIFORME (Figure 2–8)

L. B. is a 70 year old man with a history of 8 days of increasing fatigue, confusion, and ataxia. His past history is significant because of his having had a gastric resection for adenocarcinoma 3 years prior to this admission. The physical examination revealed ataxia but no papilledema.

a and b. The right lateral (a) and posterior (b) views disclose a large area of increased uptake deep within the brain in the right posterior parietal region. The mass has a doughnut appearance. This doughnut appearance is associated with metastatic lesions or occasionally a glioblastoma, as well as the typical brain abscess. Because of the patient's past history this was felt to be an area of metastases.

c. In the routine CT scan a large area of lucency in the right parietal area is seen, with shift toward the left and obliteration of the right lateral ventricle by the mass effect.

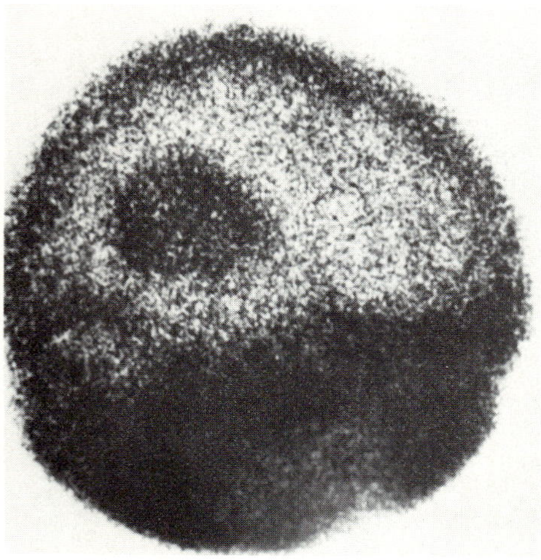

Figure 2–8a

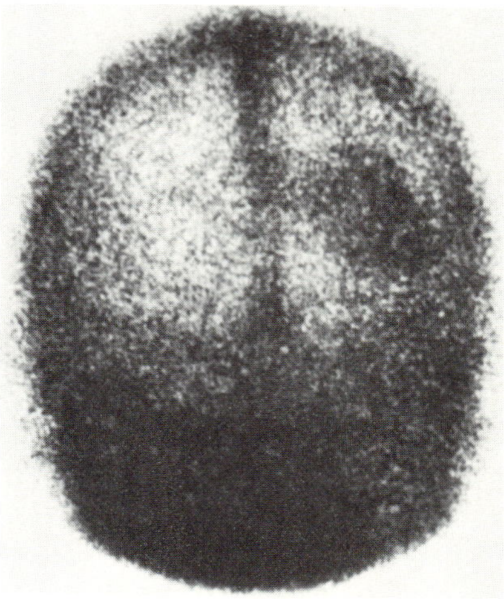

Figure 2–8b

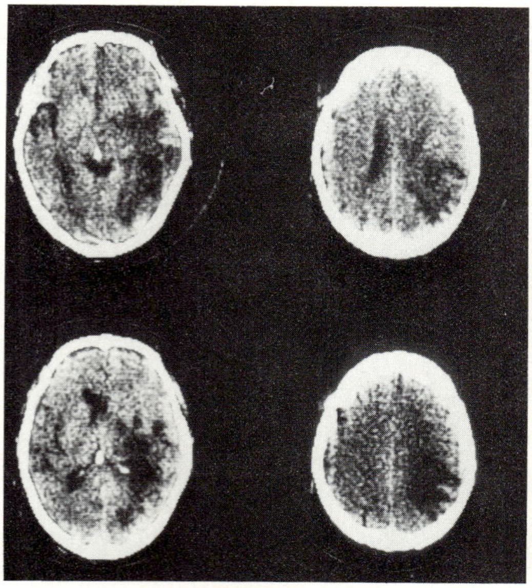

Figure 2–8c

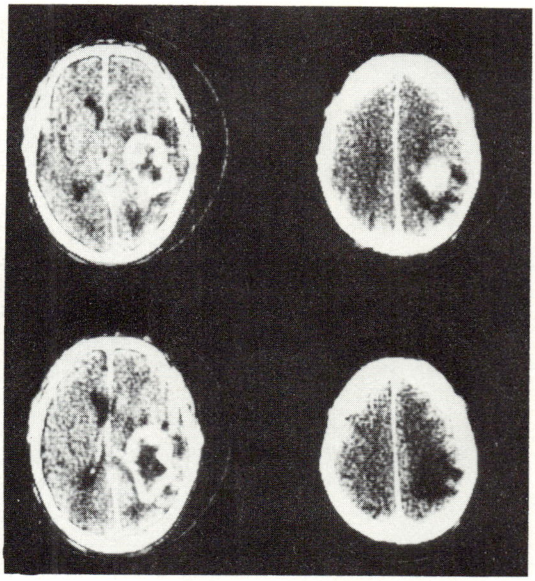

Figure 2–8d

d. The contrast enhancement views reveal a large irregular ring of enhancement. This was originally felt to be secondary to central necrosis, but the tumors do not have to have this central necrosis to have a "ring" sign.

Surgery revealed a glioblastoma multiforme.

THALAMIC GLIOMA (Figure 2–9)

T. B. is a 9 year old female with a 1-year history of right arm monoparesis.

a. The left lateral view of the radionuclide scan shows a small area of increased uptake in the left temporal region. This was not seen on the other views.

b. On the routine CT scan, areas of edema are seen anterior to and lateral to a mass in the left thalamic region (the cross on 2A is on the thalamic mass).

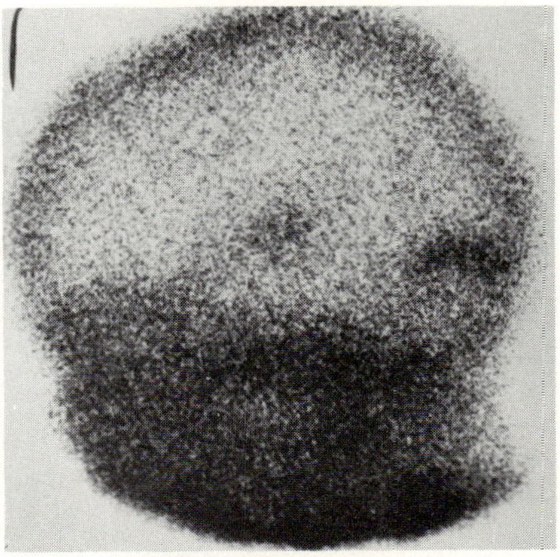

Figure 2–9a

1A 2A

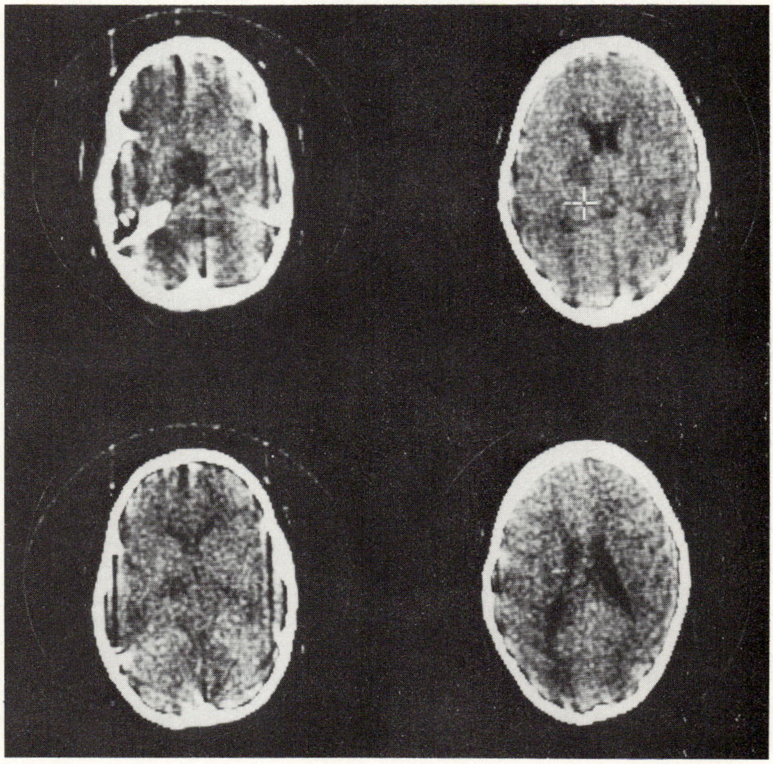

1B 2B

Figure 2–9b

c. The postinfusion views reveal enhancement of a small mass lesion in the thalamus on the left side. This is best seen on cut 12A (arrow).

d. The lateral arterial phase appears within normal limits.

e. The late venous phase reveals poor venous filling, but there does appear to be separation between the internal cerebral vein and the basal vein of Rosenthal (arrows). A mild shift of the internal cerebral vein is noted on the anteroposterior view. A vertebral arteriogram was not done.

This was presumed to be a left thalamic glioma, and radiation treatment was administered.

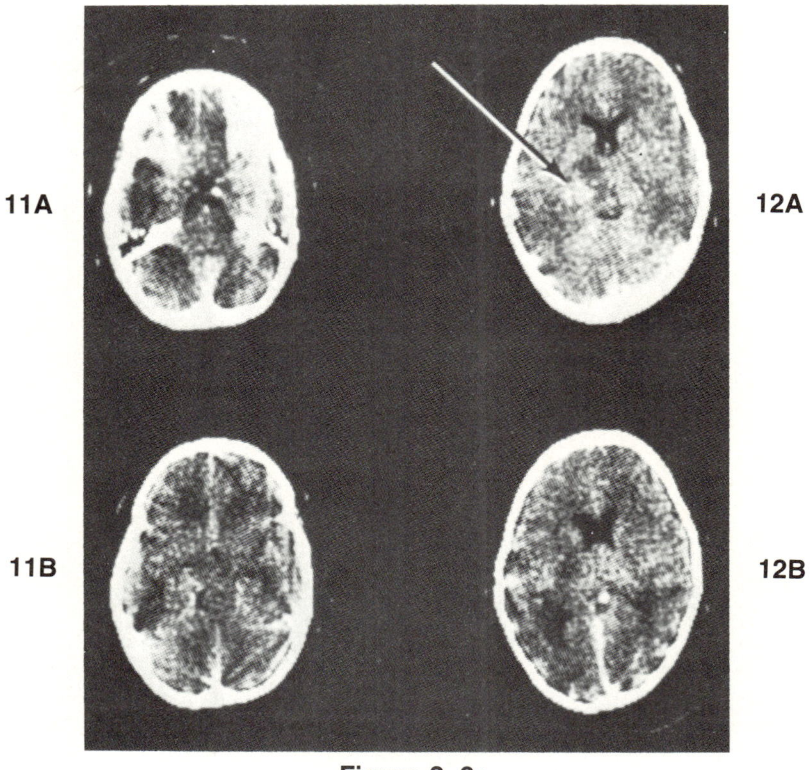

Figure 2–9c

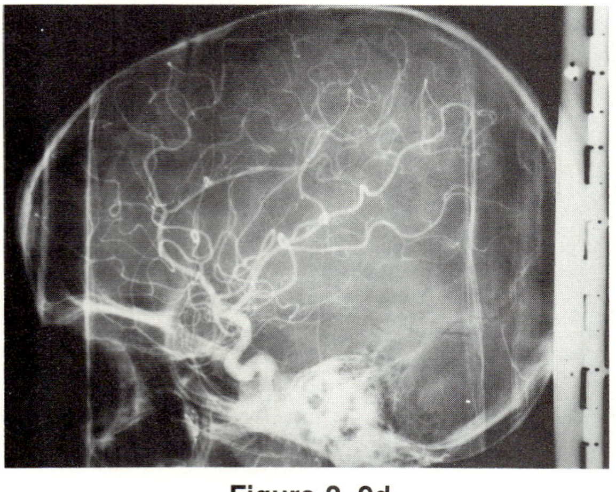

Figure 2–9d

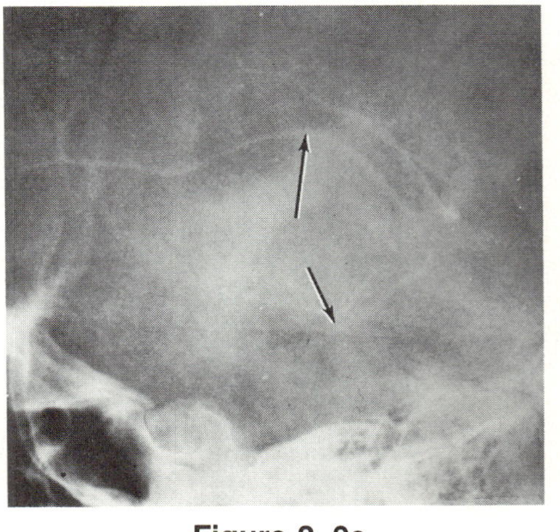

Figure 2–9e

GLIOBLASTOMA MULTIFORME (Figure 2–10)

A. B. is an elderly man with confusion and a left hemiparesis.

a. The routine scan reveals much motion artifact because the patient was unable to cooperate. However, a large area of lucency can be identified in the right posterior parietal and occipital regions (arrow).

b. After contrast enhancement a large double-ringed (arrow) area of enhancement can be identified in spite of the marked motion artifact.

c. The anteroposterior late arterial phase demonstrates spectacular neovascularity, which is more apparent on the lateral views. There is a shift of the internal cerebral

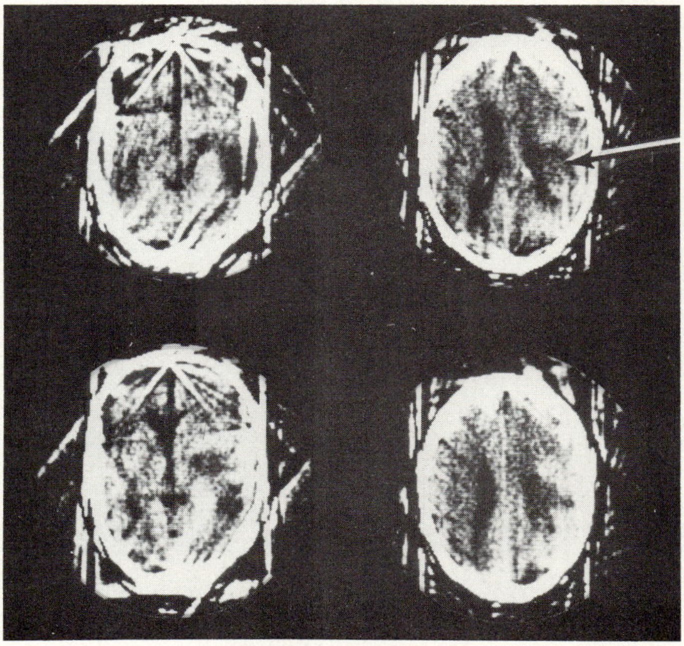

Figure 2–10a

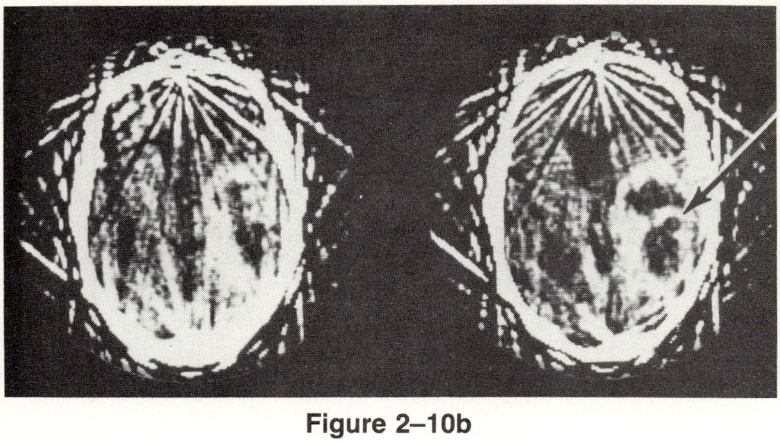

Figure 2–10b

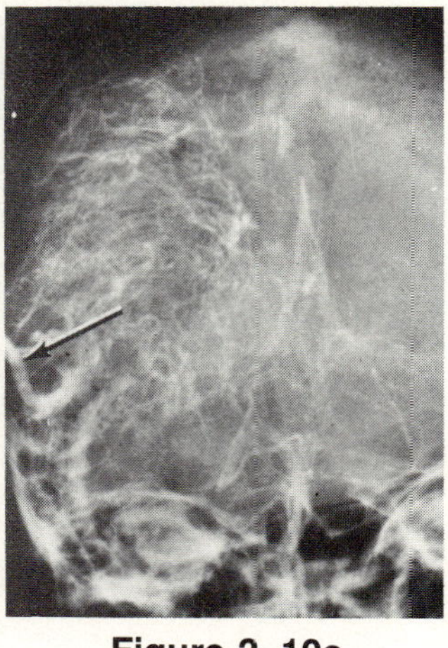

Figure 2–10c

vein and a large early draining view noted superficially (arrow).

d. The early arterial view reveals enlargement of the feeding branches of the middle cerebral vessels as well as hypertrophy of the posterior cerebral vessel (arrows). The neovascular stain is already present.

e. In the later arterial phase, a spectacular neovascular blush is seen, occupying almost the entire right parietal and occipital lobes. An early draining vein of Labbé is also noted (arrows).

f. The early draining vein is again seen (arrows).

Note that there is no filling of the anterior cerebral artery, possibly because of stealing of the blood by the large vascular tumor. The enlarged feeding arteries seen here are much more commonly associated with arterial malformations, but can occasionally be found with glioblastoma multiforme.

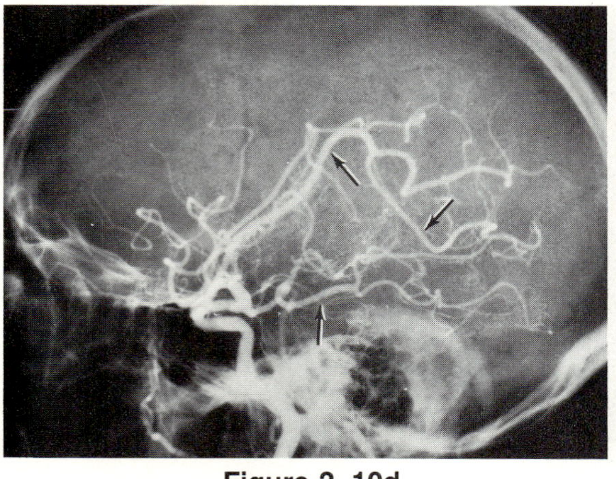

Figure 2–10d

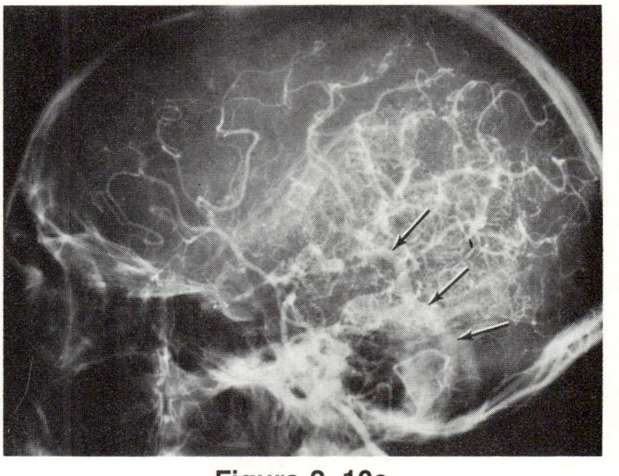

Figure 2–10e

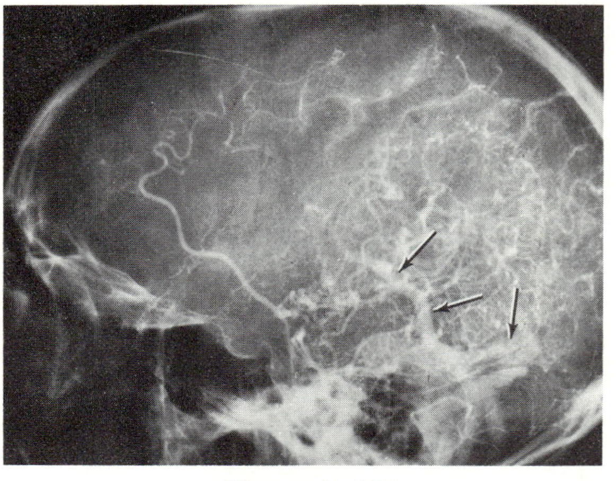

Figure 2–10f

GLIOBLASTOMA MULTIFORME (Figure 2–11)

B. S. is a 29 year old man with headaches and papilledema.

a. The routine CT scan reveals a large area of lucency in the left posterior parietal and occipital region, with obliteration of the left lateral ventricle. Cuts 12A and 12B demonstrate marked enhancement of a large cauliflower-like mass in the left parieto-occipital region. After surgical removal of this glioblastoma multiforme, a large area of postsurgical porencephaly could be seen on cuts 112A and 112B (arrows). The density of the fluid in this cystic area was similar to that of cerebrospinal fluid. There was no evidence of remaining tumor.

b. This shows the somewhat unusual cauliflower appearance to better advantage.

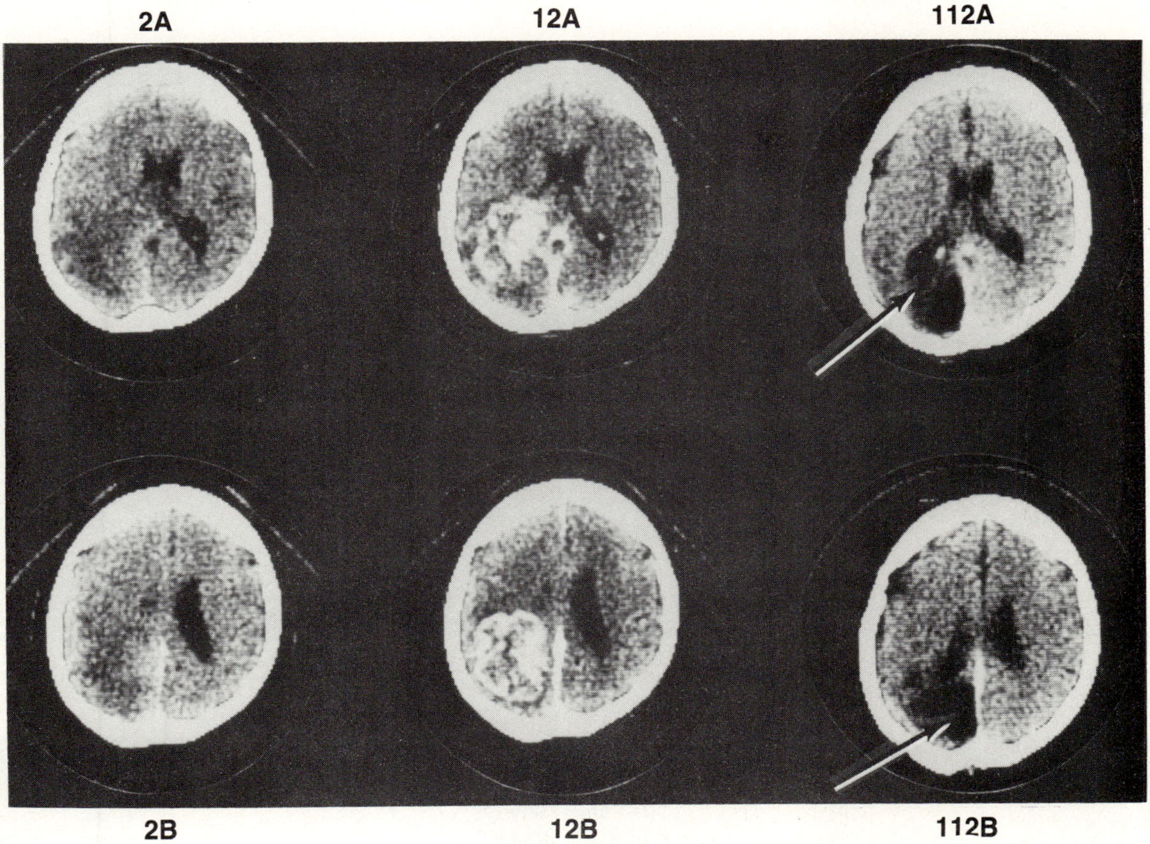

Figure 2–11a

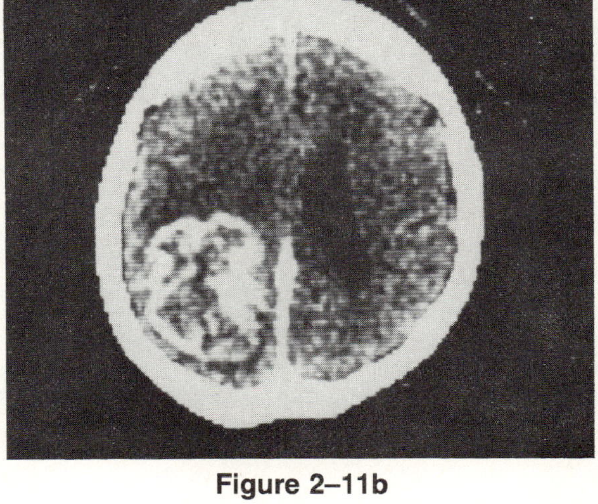

Figure 2–11b

ATYPICAL GLIOBLASTOMA MULTIFORME (Figure 2–12)

C. V. S. is a 37 year old man who had had a convulsive disorder for many years. Post radionuclide scans had all been negative. The recent onset of depression, crying, and other personality changes, along with the physical finding of right leg weakness, prompted the CT scan.

a. The routine CT scan reveals a large irregular area of lucency in the left hemisphere. There is shift from left to right.

b. The contrast enhancement shows shift of the falx cerebri (arrow) but otherwise no real change.

Although the lack of enhancement is unusual, this was assumed to be a glioma and radiation therapy was given without a biopsy.

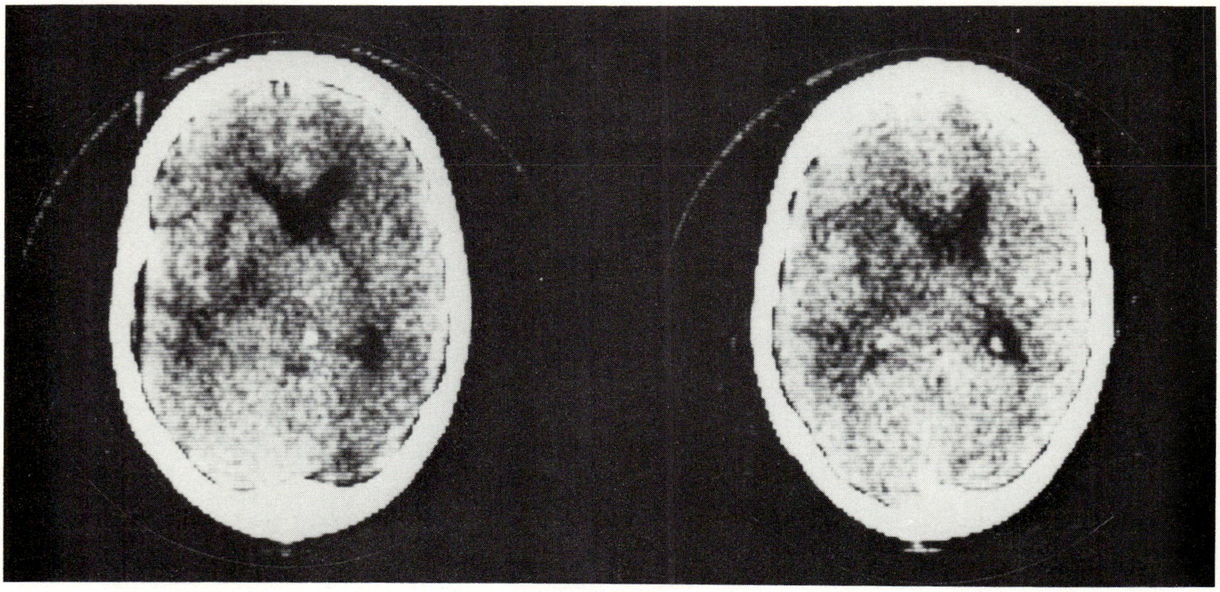

Figure 2–12a

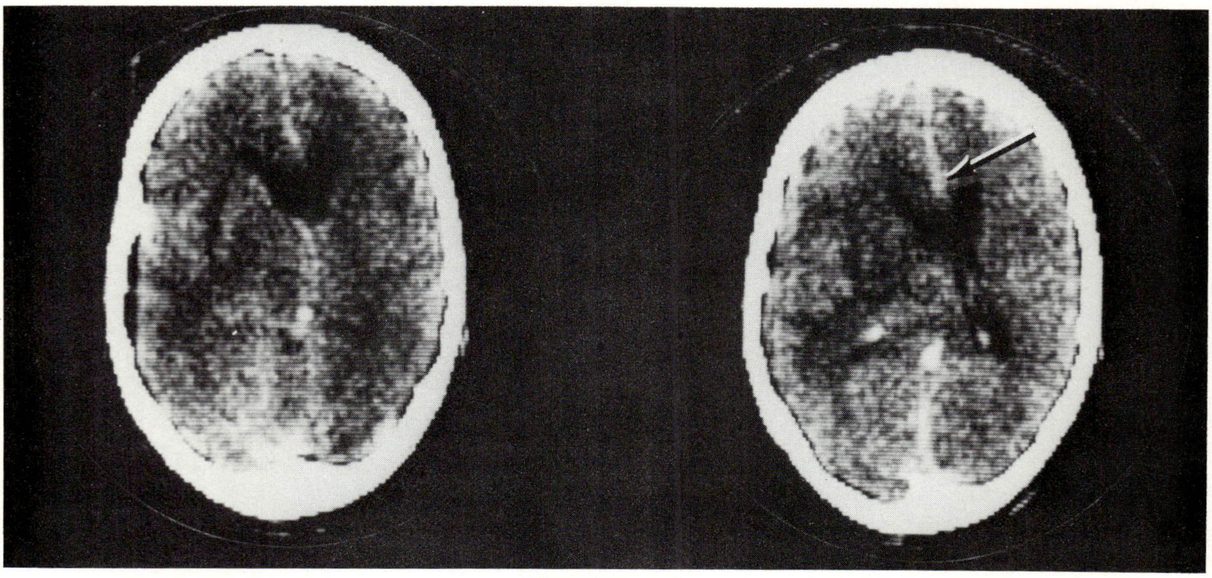

Figure 2–12b

GLIOBLASTOMA MULTIFORME (Figure 2–13)

J. M. is a 29 year old man who entered with a history of uncinate fits for 6 months prior to admission. At the onset of this disorder a radionuclide scan, arteriogram, and computed tomogram had all been normal.

a. The initial CT scan reveals an area of lucency with an onion peel pattern in the right temporal lobe region (arrows on 1A and 1B). Shift of the lateral ventricles to the left is demonstrated, as well as obliteration of the right lateral ventricle.

b. Following contrast enhancement an area of enhancement is seen surrounded by edema in the right temporal lobe region. The enhancement was homogeneous, with a small ring best seen in cut 11A (arrow). This is a glioblastoma multiforme.

It is interesting to note that when the patient first presented 6 months prior to this admission all the diagnostic tests were normal, whereas on this admission the radionuclide scan, computed tomogram, and angiogram all were abnormal.

1A 2A

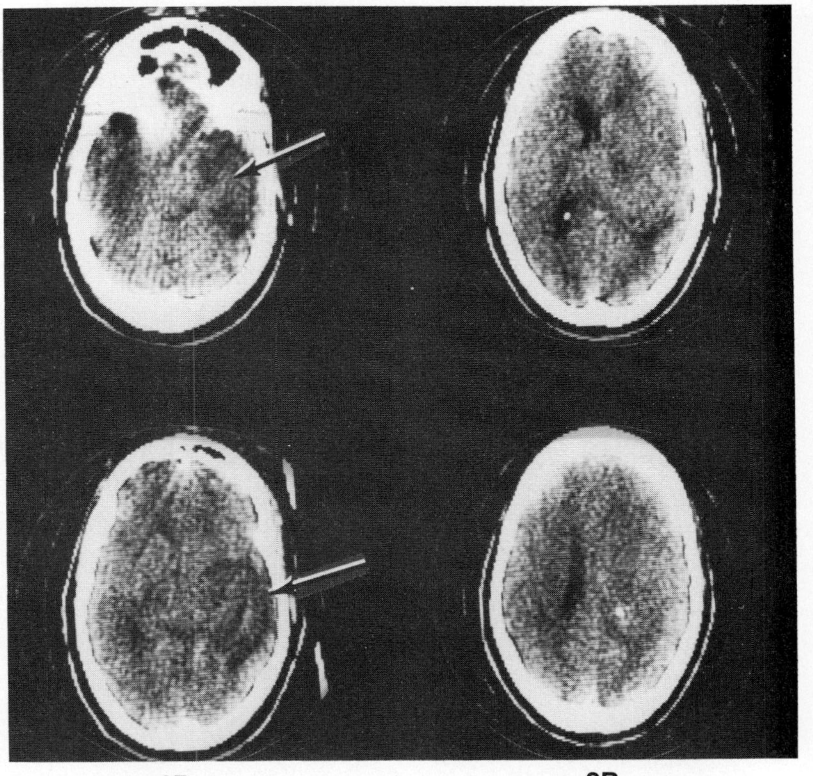

1B 2B

Figure 2–13a

12A 11A

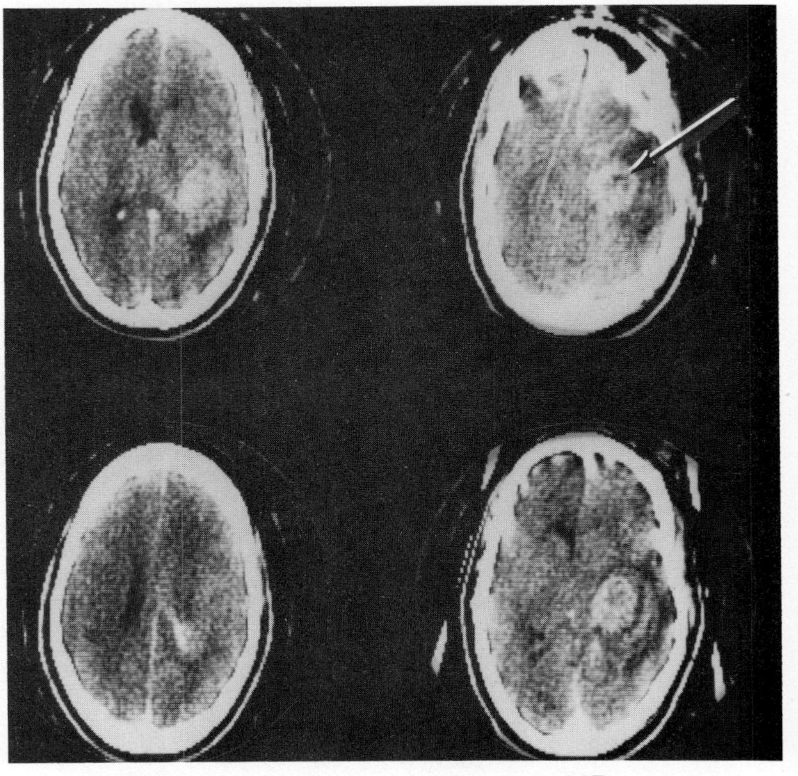

12B 11B

Figure 2–13b

PINEALOMA (Figure 2–14)

R. K. is a 30 year old man who was involved in an automobile accident 2 months prior to admission. Following the accident, in which he sustained severe head injuries, the patient developed bilateral hearing loss, left-sided hypalgesia, left hyper-reflexia, and Parinaud's syndrome. Over a period of several weeks the symptoms gradually resolved, only to recur 1 week prior to admission.

a. The routine CT scan reveals an area of increased density in the region of the quadrigeminal plate. The density measured from 40 to 62 u. Several small areas of cal-

2A

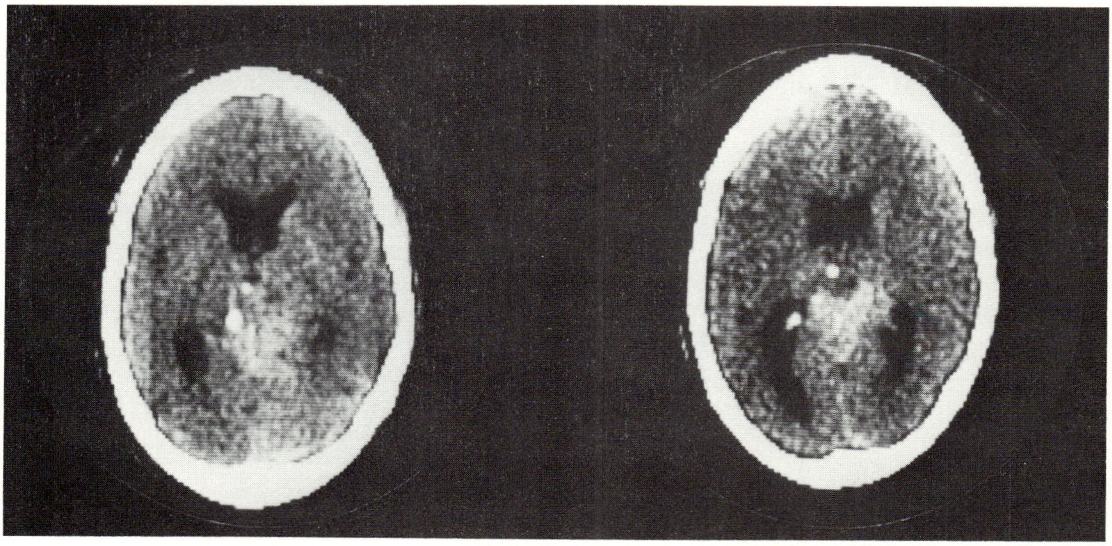

2B

Figure 2–14a

11A

12A

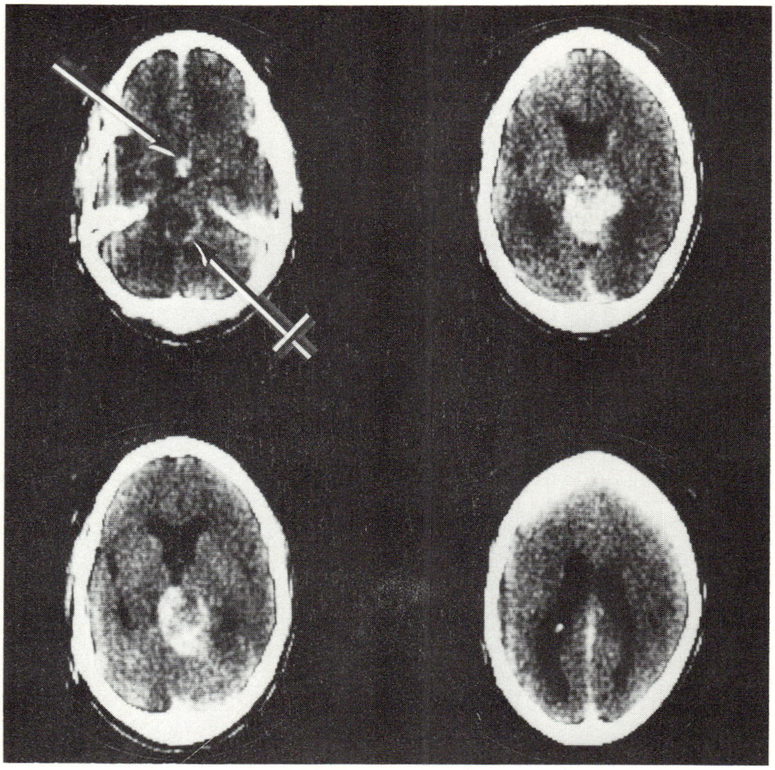

11B

12B

Figure 2–14b

cification are associated with the lesion. There is moderate obstructive hydrocephalus.

b. After infusion the density increased to 44 to 78 u. The lesion has an irregular outline, and appears to be "hollowed out" on cut 11B. There is a "drop metastasis" in the suprasellar cistern (arrow) on cut 11A. In addition, there appears to be a small infratentorial component (crossed arrow). The findings were felt to be consistent with a pinealoma.

c. The anteroposterior arterial phase of a right brachial arteriogram reveals slight spreading of the posterior cerebral arteries (arrows), although the right posterior cerebral never visualized well, possibly secondary to local pressure by the tumor or early transtentorial herniation. This seemed unlikely, however, because the patient had no visual disturbance other than Parinaud's syndrome. There is no neovascularity.

d. The AP venous phase demonstrates hydrocephalus but is otherwise unremarkable. The arrows are on the thalamostriate vein, which is bowed outward.

e. The lateral arterial phase shows no neovascularity and slight downward displacement of the posterior cerebral arteries (arrow), but no other abnormalities.

f. The lateral venous phase reveals hydrocephalus, but there is elevation of the internal cerebral

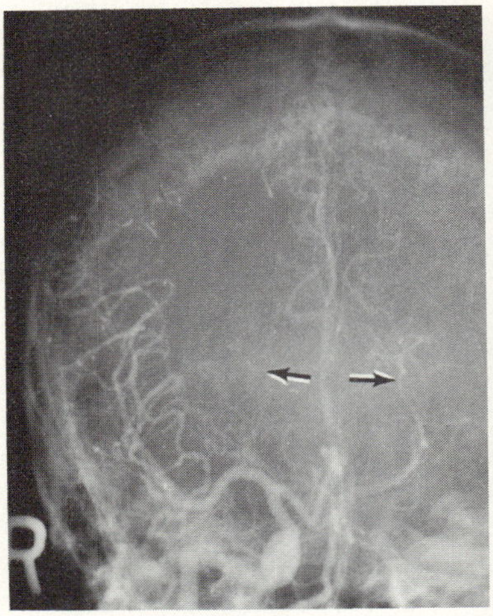

Figure 2–14c

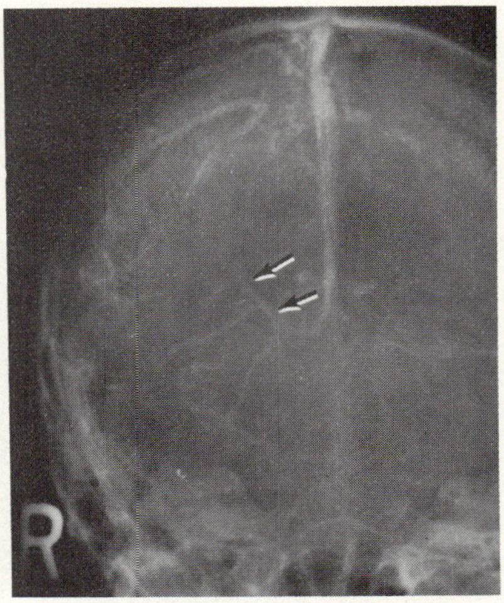

Figure 2–14d

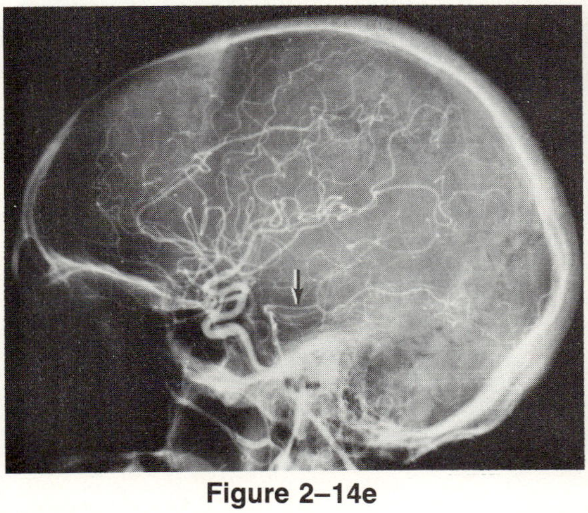

Figure 2–14e

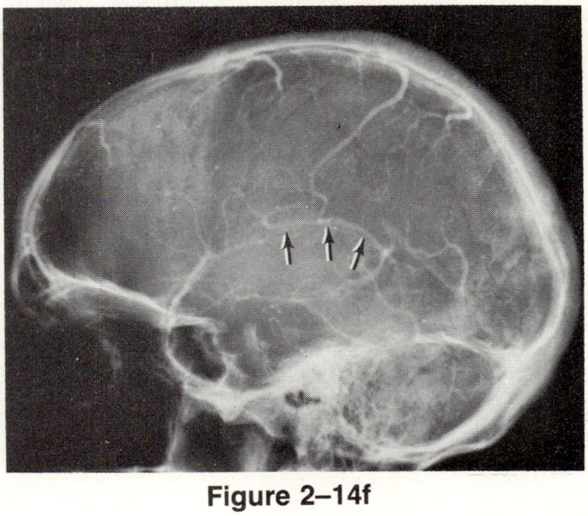

Figure 2–14f

vein (arrows), rather than the depression that one usually anticipates with hydrocephalus. The elevation is presumably secondary to extension of the tumor into the third ventricle.

Surgery with partial removal of the tumor revealed a pineal tumor, germinoma type. Radiation therapy was planned. The bilateral deafness was felt to be secondary to involvement of the inferior colliculi by the tumor.

HYPOTHALAMIC GLIOMA (Figure 2–15)

P. C., a 23 year old woman, had a 1-year history of amenorrhea and a 1-week history of severe headaches and vomiting. There was a bitemporal visual field deficit. Routine skull films revealed truncation of the dorsum sellae.

The routine CT scan (top row) reveals a mass in the suprasellar region that was slightly more dense than in normal brain (arrow on 1A). In addition, symmetrical hydrocephalus is seen secondary to obstruction of the ventricles at the level of the foramen of Monro. After contrast infusion, marked enhancement of the oval-shaped midline tumor is noted, best seen on cuts 11A and 11B. The third ventricle is seen to be flattened just anterior to the mass on cuts 1B and 11A (arrow).

Bilateral carotid and vertebral arteriography revealed hydrocephalus but was otherwise unremarkable. A pneumoencephalogram was not done. The mass was thought to be a hypothalamic glioma. Following a shunt procedure radiotherapy was planned.

1A 1B 2B

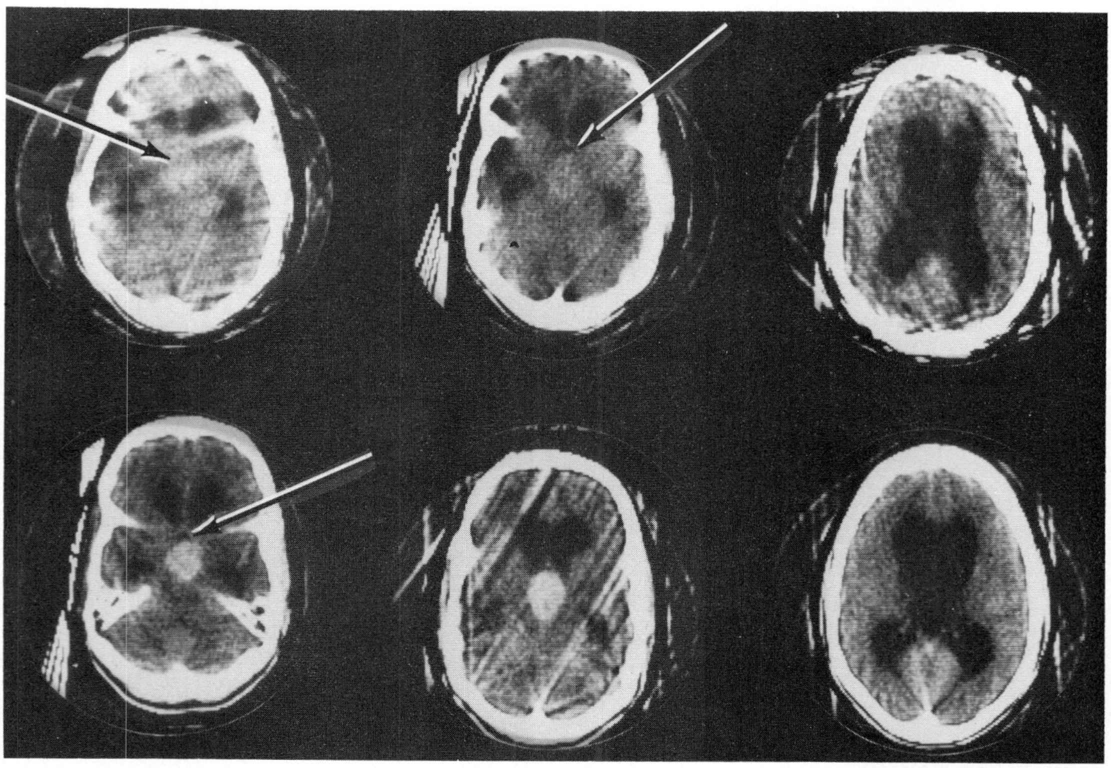

11A 11B 12B

Figure 2–15

HYPOTHALAMIC GLIOMA (Figure 2–16)

J. B. is a 29 year old woman with a 2½-week history of headaches and ataxia. Physical examination disclosed bilateral papilledema. Routine skull films were normal. A right brachial arteriogram revealed hydrocephalus but was otherwise unremarkable.

Cut 2A reveals that the patient has been shunted, and the tip of the shunt tube device can be seen in the anterior tip of the right lateral ventricle. Note that the right lateral ventricle is smaller than the left. Great care must be exercised in such cases, because serious consequences with herniation toward the shunted side may ensue if there is compromise of the communication between the lateral ventricles at the level of the foramen of Monro. Both lateral ventricles may have to be shunted at the same time. The preinfusion density was 24 to 40 u, and increased to 48 to 76 u.

Surgery revealed a glioblastoma multiforme; radiation therapy was given.

GLIOBLASTOMA MULTIFORME (Figure 2–17)

J. S. is a 54 year old man who initially presented with the following chief complaint: "I was sitting and eating dinner when I lost my vision between 12 o'clock and 3 o'clock." With the exception of the visual field defect, his physical examination was entirely within normal limits.

a and b. A radionuclide scan obtained acutely revealed a small rounded area of increased radio-

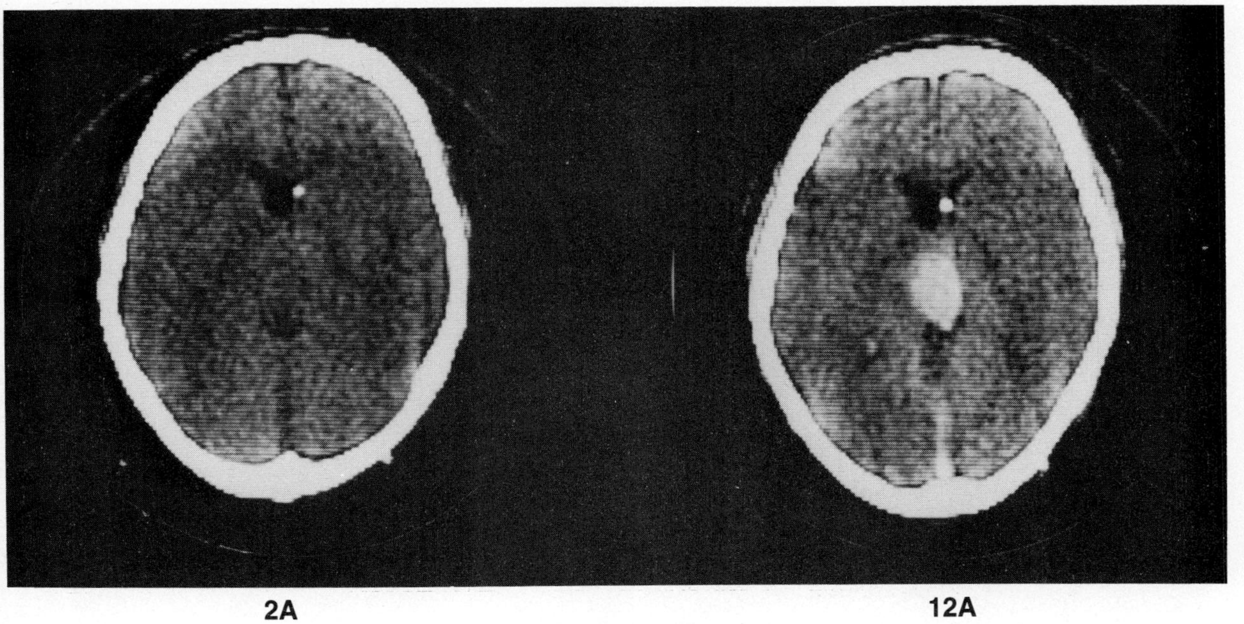

2A 12A

Figure 2–16

activity in the temporal lobe on the left side. This could not be seen on the posterior view, probably because of the overlying transverse sinus (b).

c. The CT scan obtained at the same time showed a small area of lucency, density 20 to 28 u (arrow on 2A), which increased to 40 to 66 u postinfusion. There was no mass effect. The diagnostic possibilities were thought to be a small infarct with luxury perfusion or an early glioma.

d to j. Left carotid and vertebral arteriography as well as pneumoencephalography were within normal limits.

d. Left carotid arteriogram, lateral view, arterial phase.

e. Left carotid arteriogram, lateral view, venous phase.

f. Left carotid arteriogram, anteroposterior view, arterial phase.

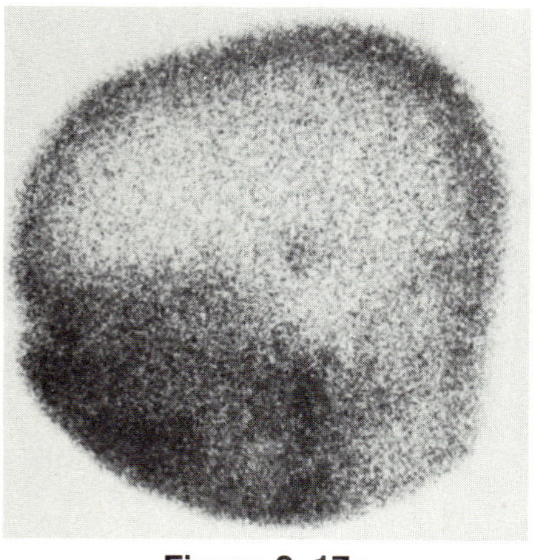

Figure 2–17a

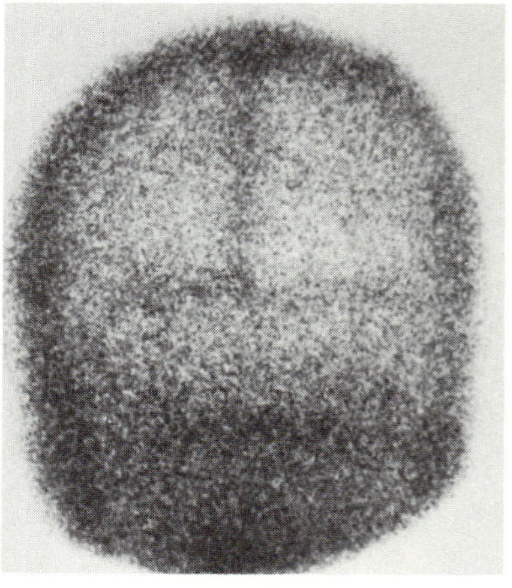

Figure 2–17b

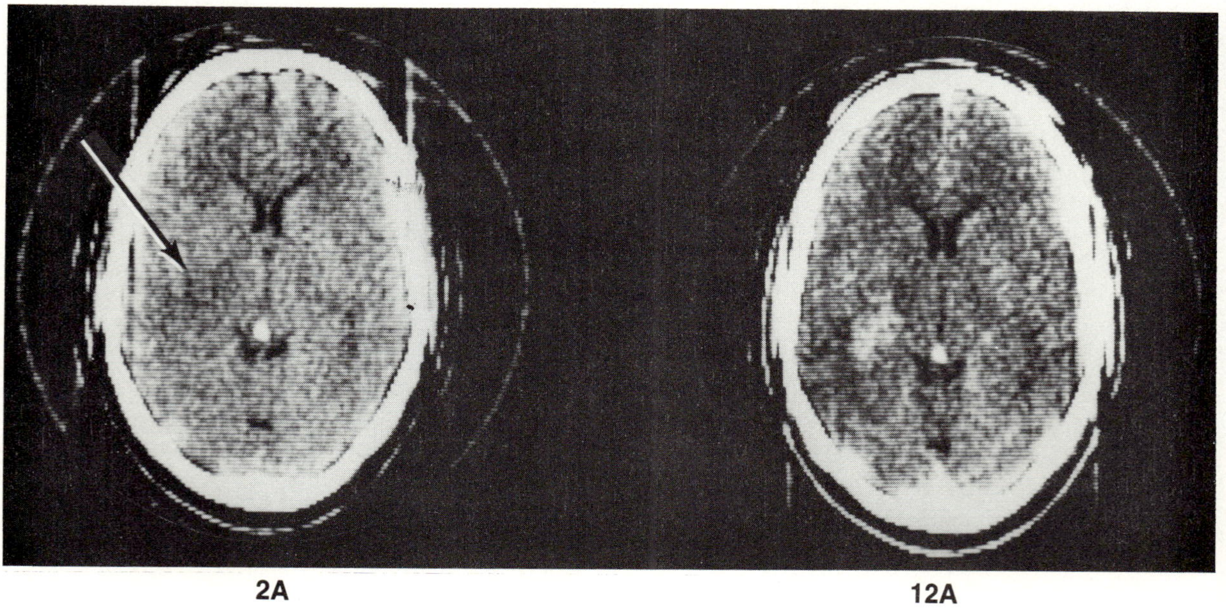

2A

12A

Figure 2–17c

g. Left vertebral arteriogram, arterial phase.

h. Pneumoencephalogram, midline tomogram, brow down.

i. Pneumoencephalogram, antero-posterior view, brow up; note symmetry of temporal horns (arrows).

j. Pneumoencephalogram, Towne's view, brow down.

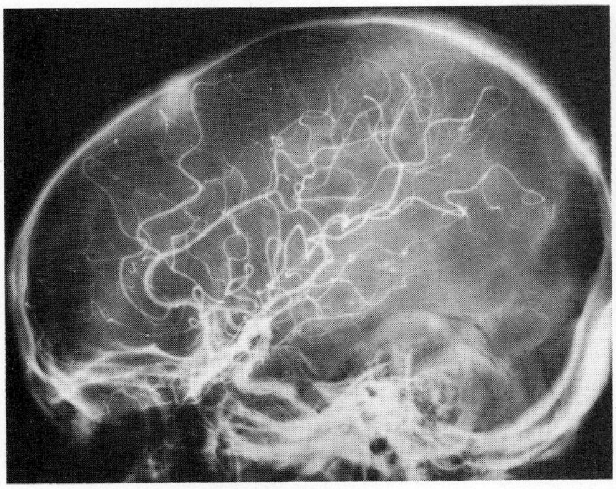

Figure 2–17d

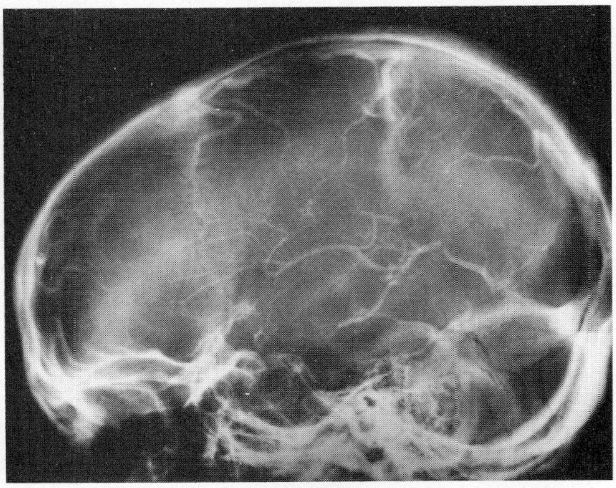

Figure 2–17e

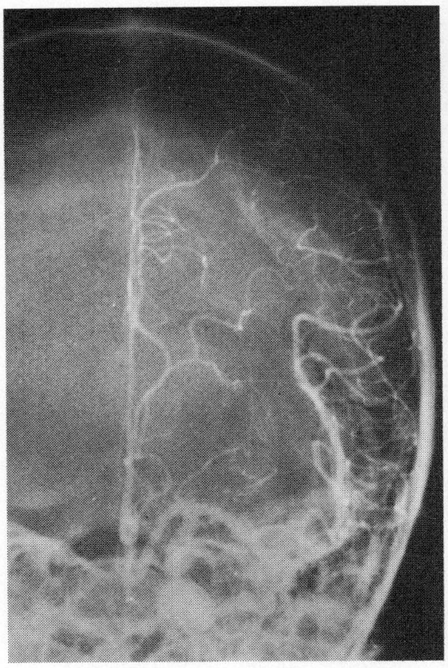

Figure 2–17f

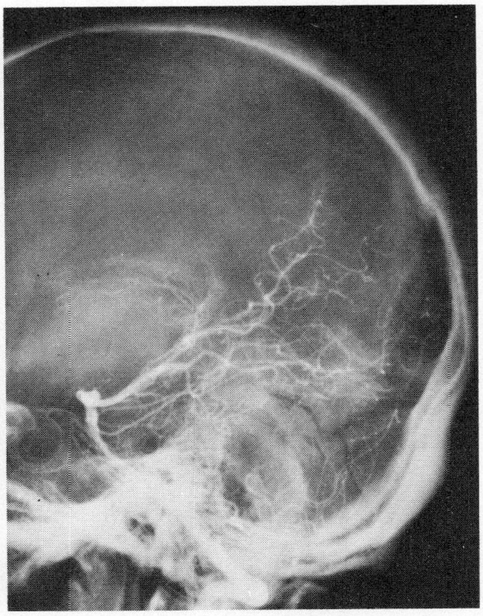

Figure 2–17g

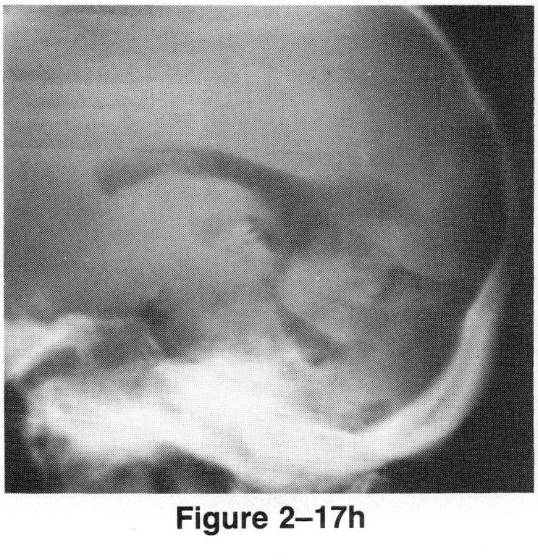

Figure 2–17h

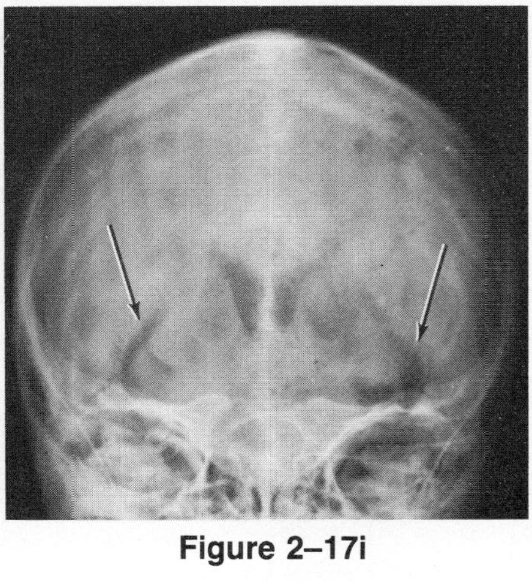

Figure 2–17i

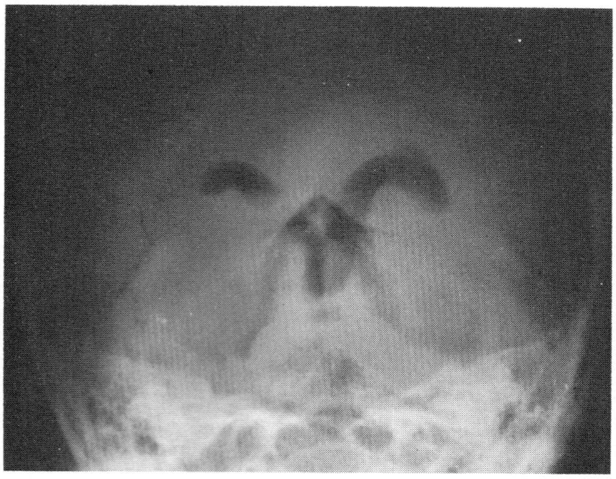

Figure 2–17j

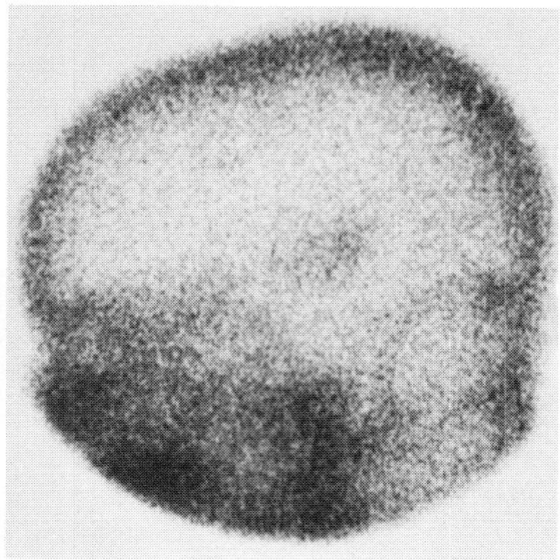

Figure 2–17k

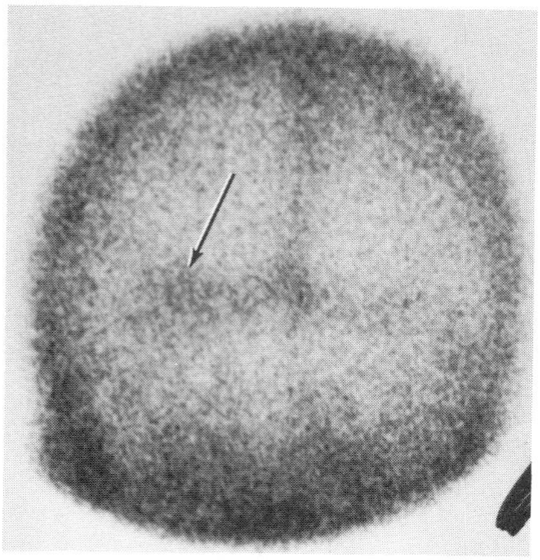

Figure 2–17l

k and l. Two months later, the radionuclide scan again revealed the area of increased uptake in the left temporal region, which appeared more prominent than previously. In addition, the area was now visible on the posterior view (arrow).

m. The CT scan at this time again revealed a small area of lucency on the preinfusion scan, measuring from 12 to 30 u. This increased to 40 to 86 u after the infusion of contrast material. It was noted, however, that the configuration had changed somewhat—the area of enhance-

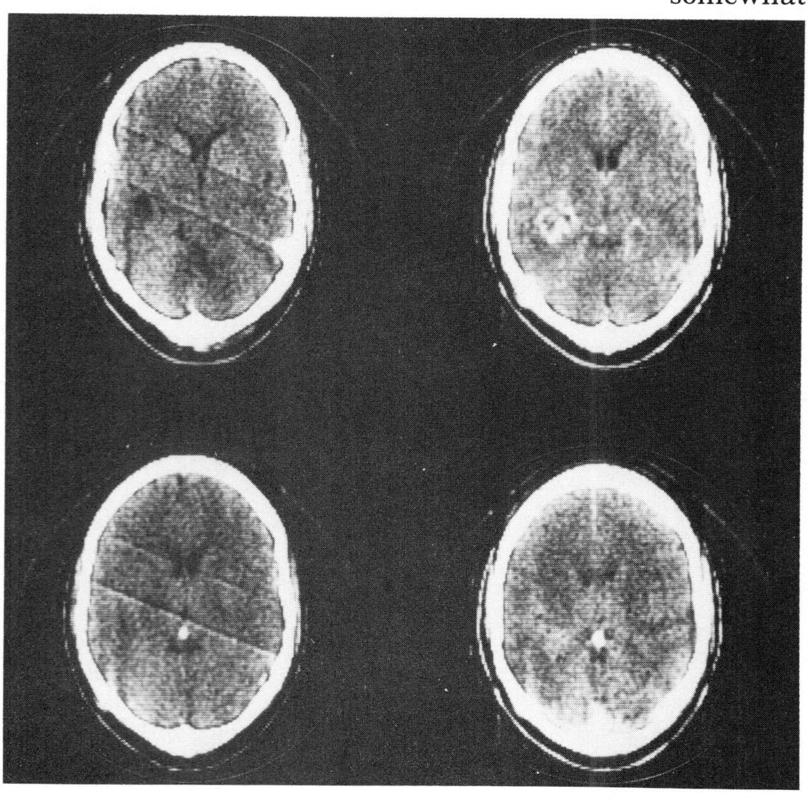

2A

12A

2B

12B

Figure 2–17m

ment now had a circular configuration. The patient's symptom complex was unchanged, and the differential diagnosis was still between an area of infarction with luxury perfusion and an early glioma.

The patient returned 2½ months later with classic aphasia and right-sided weakness.

n and o. The left lateral (n) and anterior (o) views of the radionuclide scan now reveal a large area of uptake deep in the left hemisphere.

p. The routine CT scan shows marked dilatation of the left temporal horn in the anterior temporal region (arrow), as well as a large irregular area of lucency in the left parietal lobe. There is now a marked shift from left to right.

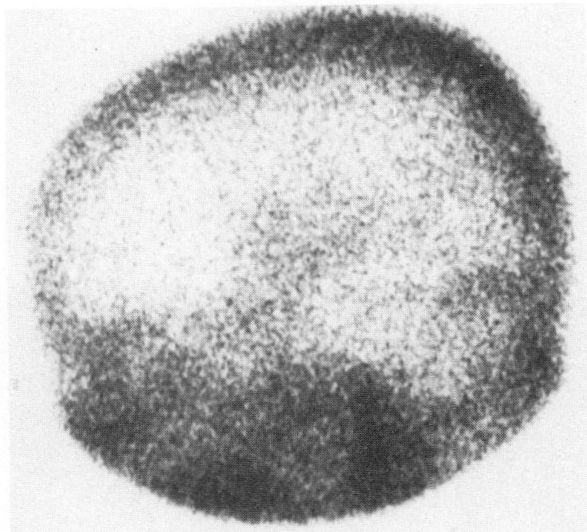

Figure 2–17n

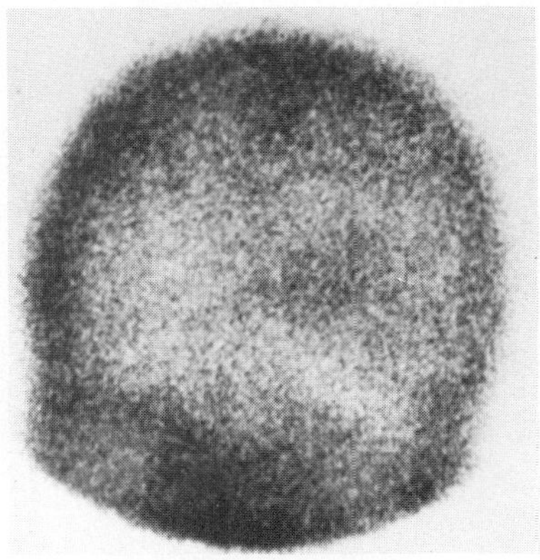

Figure 2–17o

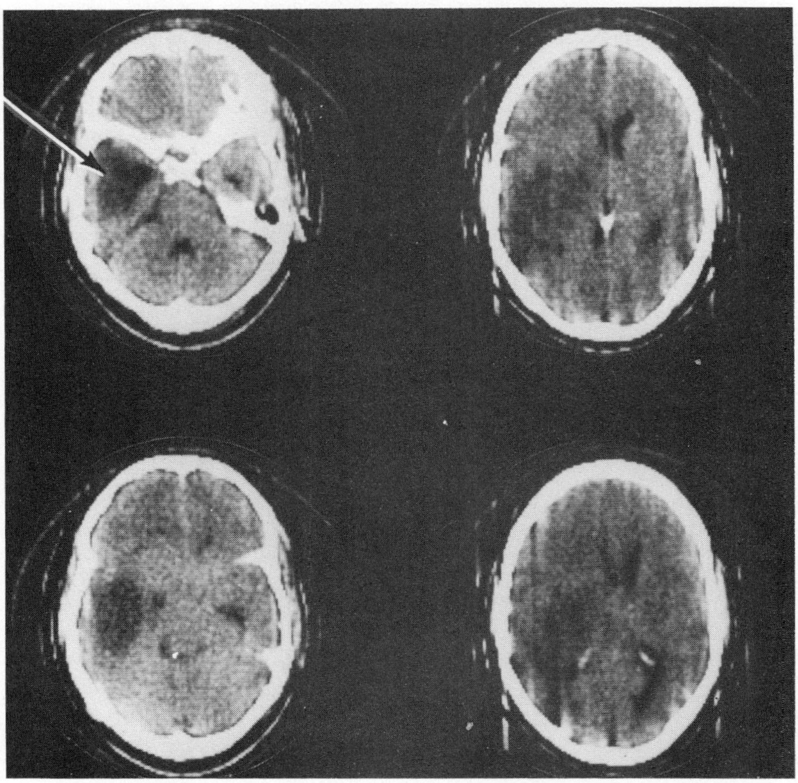

Figure 2–17p

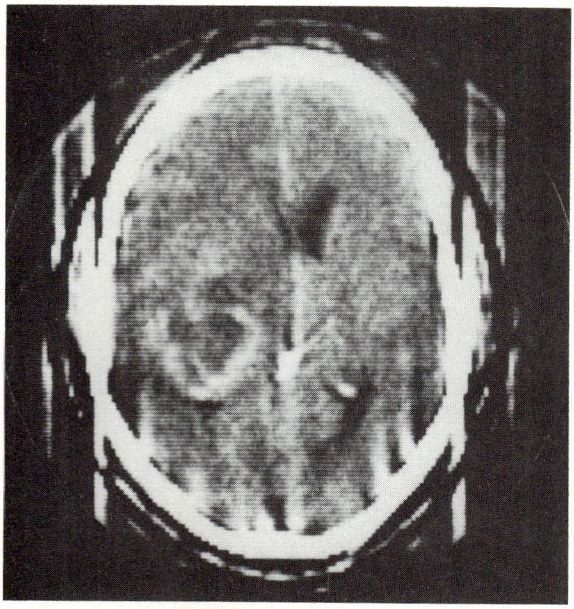

Figure 2–17q

q. Following the infusion of contrast material, there is marked enhancement of a "ring" of tumor deep in the left parietal lobe. The tumor is surrounded by an area of edema.

Surgical decompression was performed in an attempt to drain the obstructed temporal horn and improve the patient's symptoms. The tumor was histologically a Grade II to III astrocytoma.

This case illustrates the rather rapid clinical course that can be seen with glioblastoma multiforme. From the initial symptoms—which appeared to be quite typical for a cerebrovascular accident—to the typical findings of a glioblastoma, only 2½ months had elapsed. Had the tumor been in a more accessible area, surgical removal could conceivably have provided cure. It is hoped that computed tomography will assist in early diagnosis of brain tumor and ultimately lead to better survival.

Pituitary Tumors

Computed tomography is an excellent modality for evaluating pituitary tumors. Not only can a mass be demonstrated, but the bony changes around the sella turcica are also readily evaluated. These bony changes can be noted by viewing the various scan cuts at appropriate window widths and levels. Direct coronal cuts are also helpful for precise evaluation of tumor size. Most pituitary tumors enhance densely and homogeneously on the postinfusion portion of the examination and are therefore readily identified. On the other hand, these tumors may be cystic and thus very difficult to detect. Such cysts occur because of hemorrhage into the adenoma, which then subsequently undergoes cystic change. Suprasellar and parasellar meningiomas may mimic pituitary adenomas; meningiomas, however, usually contain a small amount of calcification.

Giant aneurysms, larger than 2½ cm, may also mimic a pituitary adenoma. Aneurysms usually have a peripheral rim of calcification, however, and enhance homogeneously on the postinfusion scan. If partially thrombosed, aneurysms will enhance homogeneously on the postinfusion portion of the examination.

The introduction of metrizamide cisternography has also greatly facilitated the visualization of pituitary adenomas. With this technique, a lumbar puncture is performed and 5 ml of 190 mgm of iodine per ml solution of metrizamide (Amipaque—Winthrop Labs) is instilled in the subarachnoid space. The contrast material is then allowed to flow immediately cephalad and to accumulate in the basilar cisterns. The patient is kept in the head-down position at an angle of 45 to 60° with the head straight for 5 minutes and is then scanned using the CT scanner through the region of the sellar and suprasellar cistern. In this way the suprasellar extent of the tumor can be evaluated.

The newer CT scanners, which can perform direct coronal cuts or reconstruction views in the coronal and sagittal planes, are very helpful for diagnosis, and in many cases can eliminate the need for cisternography. In any patient with undiagnosed visual symptoms, a metrizamide cisternogram is justified to rule out a mass lesion.

Lesions that may be differentiated from pituitary tumors include pituitary abscesses (by cisternogram), adenoma (by axial and reconstructed views), empty sella, and microadenoma.

PITUITARY ADENOMA (Figure 2–18)

J. B. is a 30 year old male who presented with an 8-year history of "visual difficulties" and a recent history of rapidly decreasing vision. Physical examination revealed that his "visual difficulties" consisted of a bitemporal hemianopsia. In addition, he had almost no development of secondary sex characteristics.

a. The routine skull series reveals a markedly enlarged sella turcica. The floor of the sella is depressed, and the posterior clinoids and dorsum sellae are thinned and displaced posteriorly (arrows). There is undercutting of one of the anterior clinoids (short arrows). The findings are typical of an expanding intrasellar mass lesion.

b to e. The radionuclide scan discloses a large area of increased uptake of the radionuclide in the region of the sella. Incidentally, the abnormal area appears to extend slightly more to the right side on the anterior view (arrow on b).

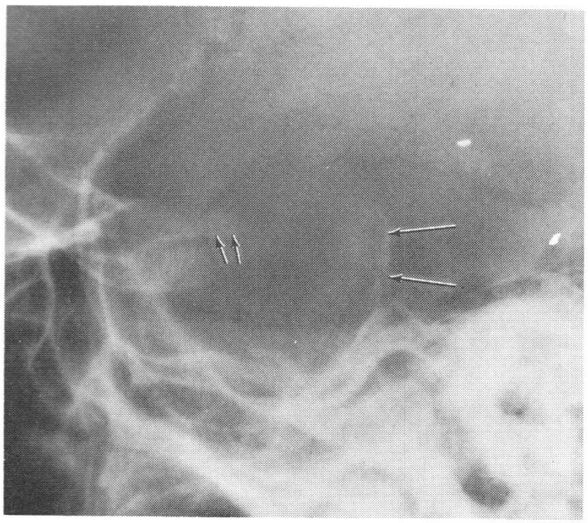

Figure 2–18a

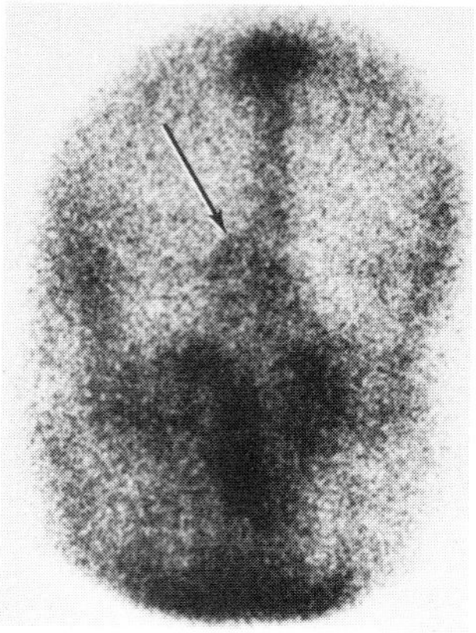

Figure 2–18b

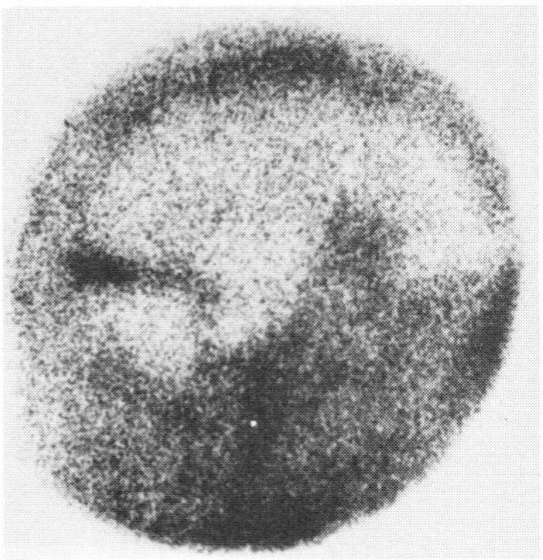

Figure 2–18c

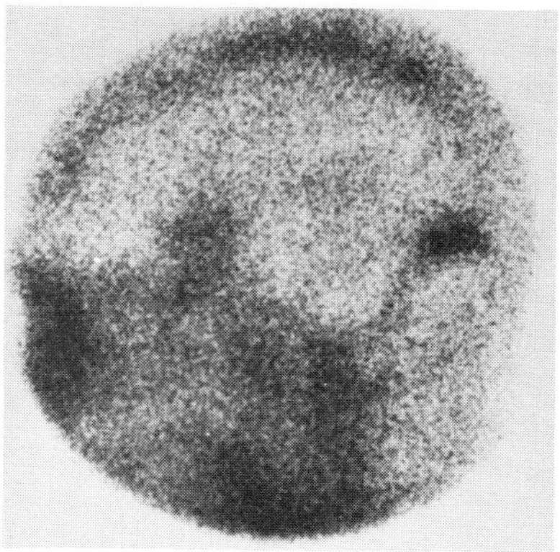

Figure 2–18d

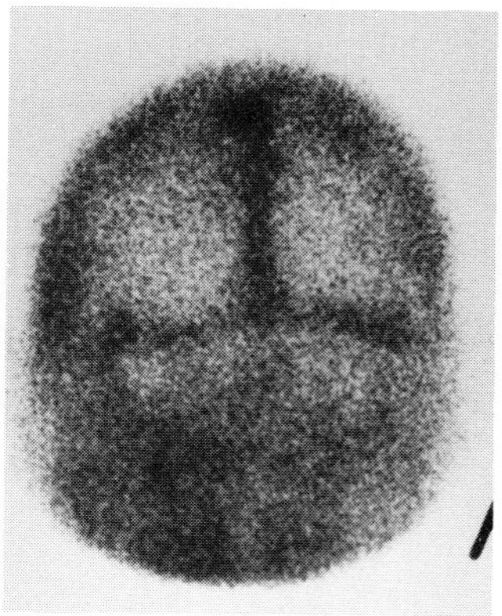

Figure 2–18e

f and g. The routine scan reveals a dense tumor mass in the region of the sella that measured from 40 to 66 u. This can best be seen on cuts 1A and 1B (arrows). There is no evidence of hydrocephalus. Following contrast enhancement, the mass increased greatly in density to 62 to 92 u. On the postinfusion scan, the slightly irregular outline of the tumor becomes more apparent. On cut 12A it can be seen that the tumor mass extends slightly more superiorly on the right side than it does on the left (arrow). The findings are typical of a large pituitary adenoma.

1A 2A

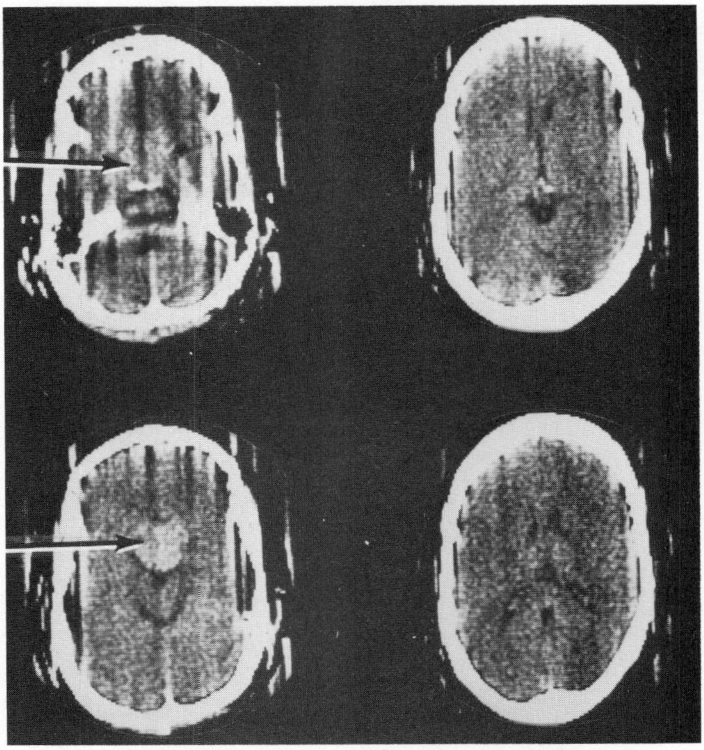

1B 2B

Figure 2–18f

11A 12A

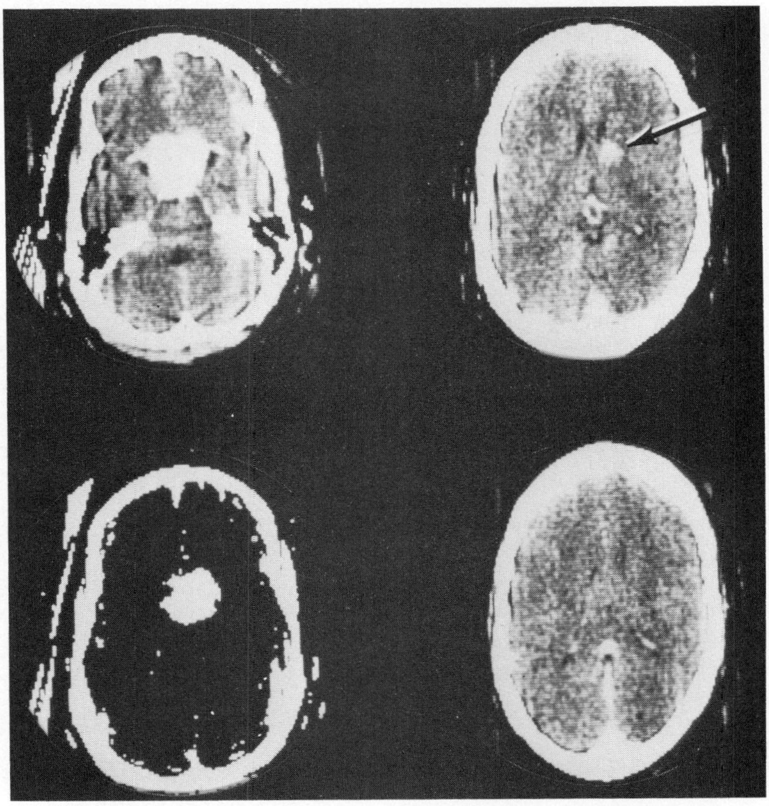

11B 12B

Figure 2–18g

h to k. Bilateral carotid arteriography reveals elevation of the horizontal portions of the anterior cerebral arteries bilaterally (upper arrows on h and i). There is lateral displacement of the cavernous portions of the internal carotid arteries as well (lower arrows on h and i). The lateral view (j) discloses opening of the carotid siphon (see arrow). Vertebral arteriography (k) reveals backward displacement of the basilar artery; however, the basilar artery remains closely applied to the dorsum sellae, implying that the tumor does not extend posterior to the dorsum.

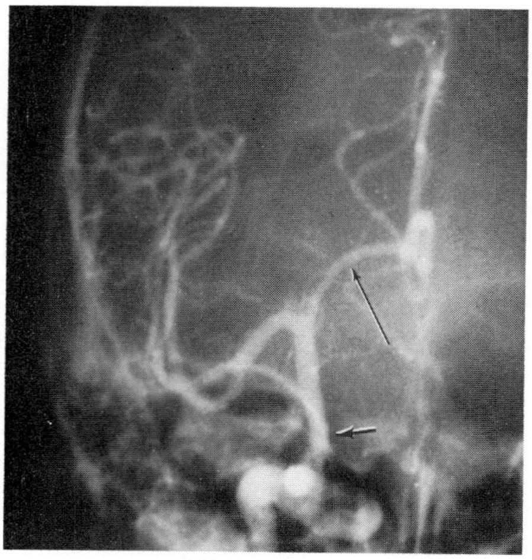

Figure 2–18h

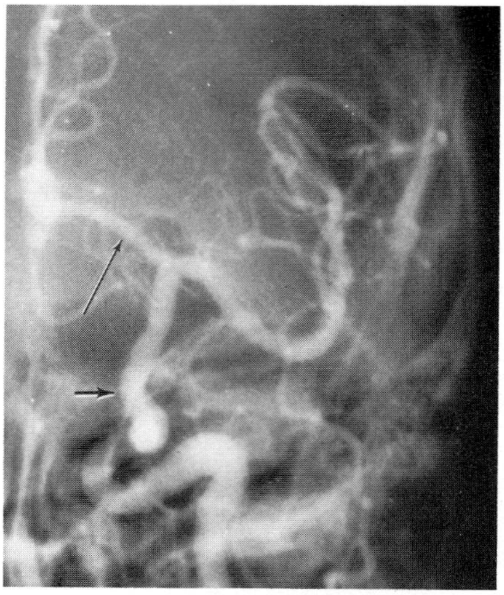

Figure 2–18i

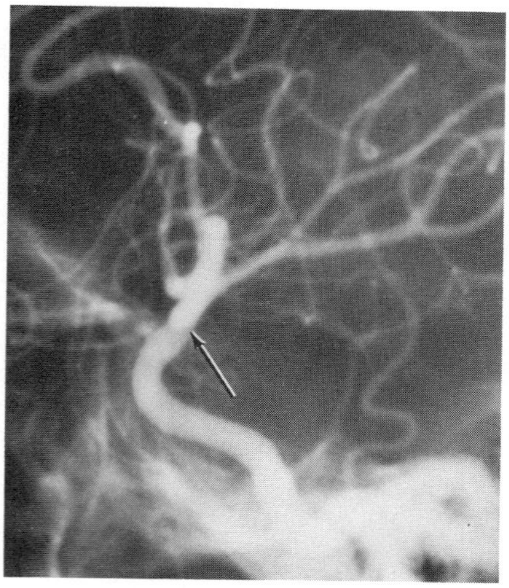

Figure 2–18j

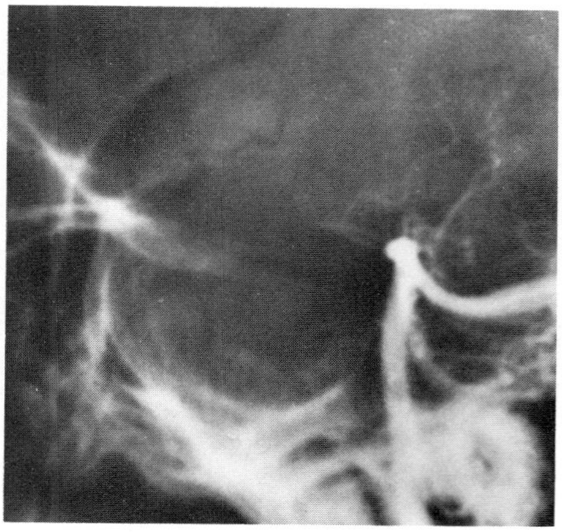

Figure 2–18k

The tumor was removed through a craniotomy and was histologically a chromophobe adenoma.

PITUITARY ADENOMA (Figure 2–19)

This 45 year old female presented with a history of headaches and decreasing vision. Physical examination revealed that the patient had a bitemporal hemianopsia.

a. Direct coronal cuts through the region of the sella turcica reveal a homogeneously enhancing intrasellar mass (X) that extends into the suprasellar cistern. The mass is convex superiorly (arrow). The carotid arteries are visualized bilaterally (C). The bifurcation into the anterior and middle cerebral arteries can also be easily seen (A and M).

b. Further posteriorly, the basilar artery is visualized as it is surrounded by the cerebrospinal fluid in the prepontine cistern (open arrow).

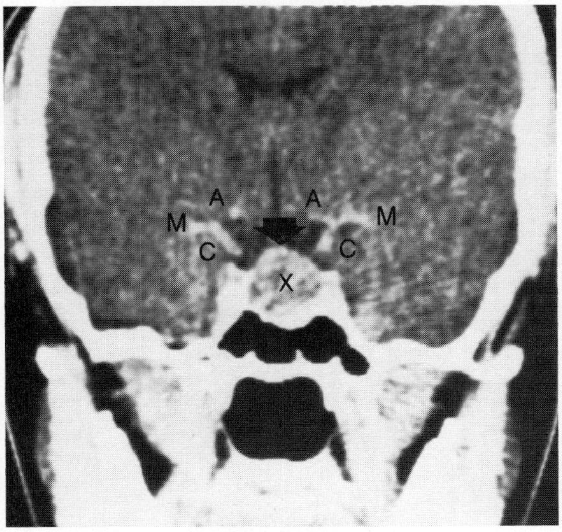

Figure 2–19a

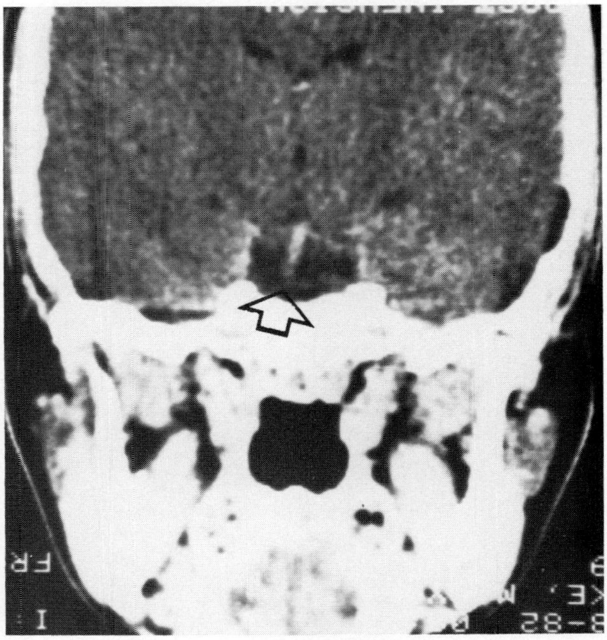

Figure 2–19b

c. The pituitary tumor measures 20 mm in height. The normal gland in a female should not measure greater than 8 mm; it should be <7 mm in a male.

d. The width of the tumor is also demonstrated, as it extends from one cavernous sinus to the other (CS).

Surgery proved this to be a pituitary adenoma.

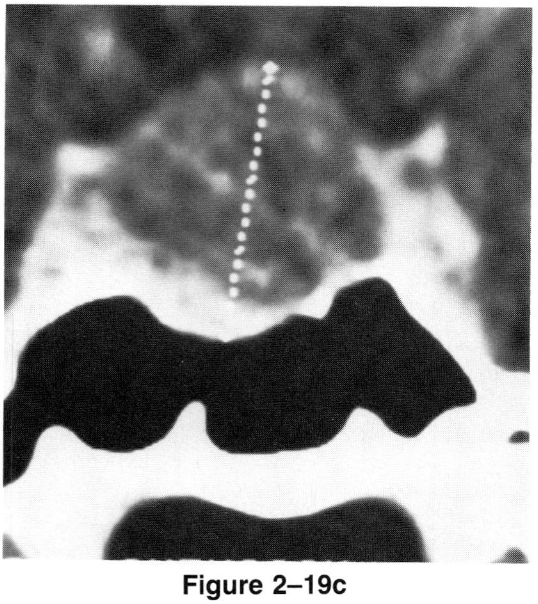

Figure 2–19c

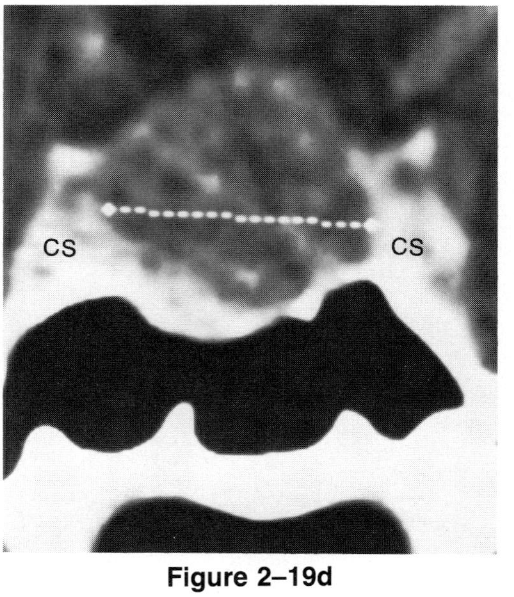

Figure 2–19d

PITUITARY ADENOMA (Figure 2–20)

This 36 year old female presented with a history of gradually decreasing vision in the left eye.

a. The preinfusion scan reveals a bilobed mass in the region of the pituitary that extends into the left medial temporal region. There is obliteration of the normal suprasellar cistern.

b. The postinfusion portion of the examination reveals homogeneous enhancement of the tumor.

c. The internal carotid angiogram reveals a prominent meningohypophyseal trunk (arrowhead) that drapes over the tumor mass (curved arrows).

Surgery proved this to be a pituitary adenoma. Note that the bilobed configuration is somewhat unusual but not inconsistent with a pituitary adenoma.

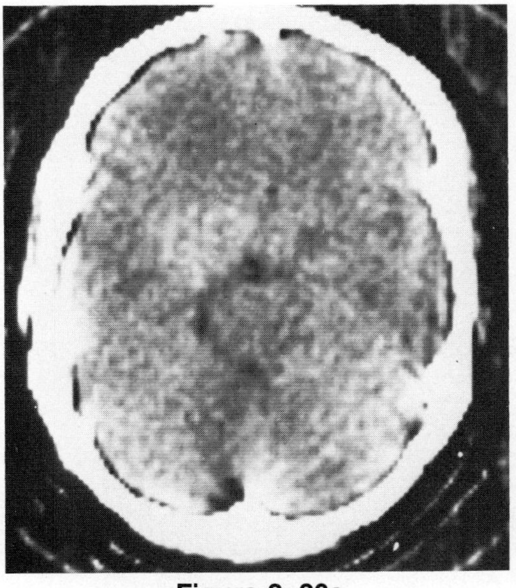

Figure 2–20a

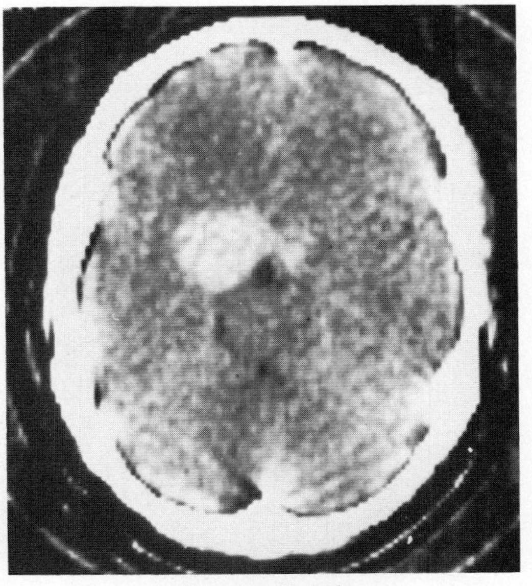

Figure 2–20b

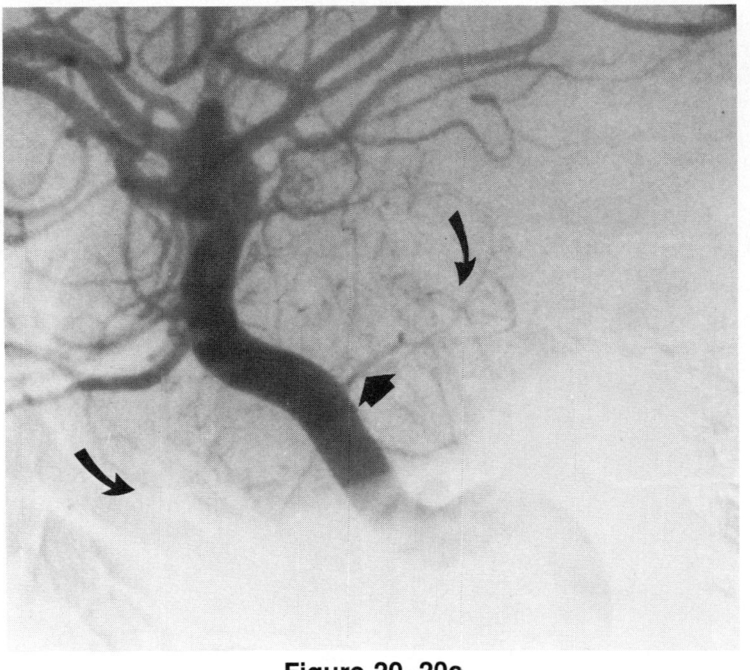

Figure 20–20c

CYSTIC PITUITARY ADENOMA (Figure 2–21)

a and b. This 65 year old female was experiencing gradually decreasing visual acuity. The initial scan appears normal through the region of the suprasellar cistern. The lowest cut (a) does demonstrate some rounding of the anterior portion of the suprasellar cistern (arrows). The second scan (b) was originally thought to be normal, but note the slight but definite fullness of the anterior portion of the third ventricle (arrows).

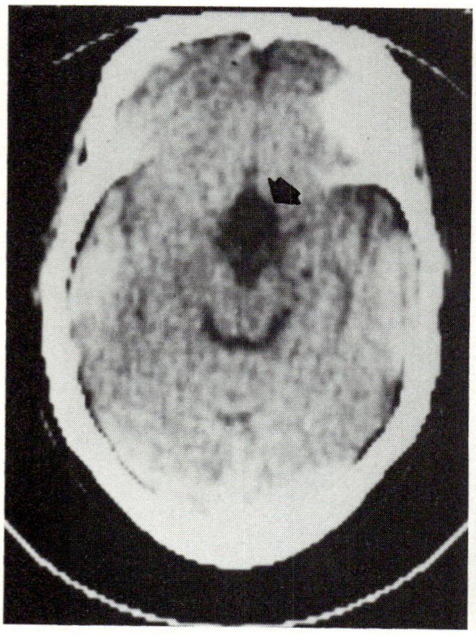

Figure 2–21a

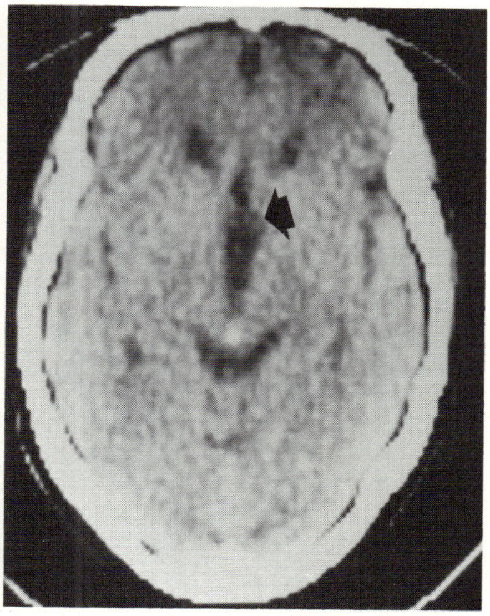

Figure 2–21b

c to e. A follow-up examination (c and d) was obtained 2 years after the initial study and appears basically unchanged (arrows). Metrizamide cisternography (e) was also performed. After the lumbar injection of 5 ml of a 190 mg of iodine per ml solution of metrizamide and allowing the patient to remain in the 45° head-down position for 5 minutes, the last CT scan was obtained. This demonstrated a well-defined cystic lesion that extends into the suprasellar cistern (arrow).

Surgery revealed a cystic pituitary tumor. Cystic tumors develop because pituitary adenomas can undergo hemorrhage (or apoplexy), which causes degenerative change and ultimately the formation of a thin-walled cyst of the pituitary gland. The postinfusion scan often does not demonstrate enhancement of the wall of the cyst. While the newer, more versatile scanners can perform coronal cuts that probably show the abnormality, if the available scanner does not have these features, metrizamide cisternography should be performed in any patient with decreasing vision. We have also seen pituitary abscesses with a similar appearance.

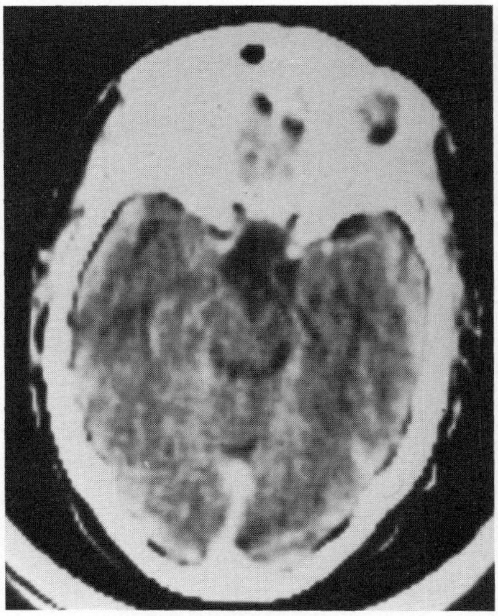

Figure 2–21c

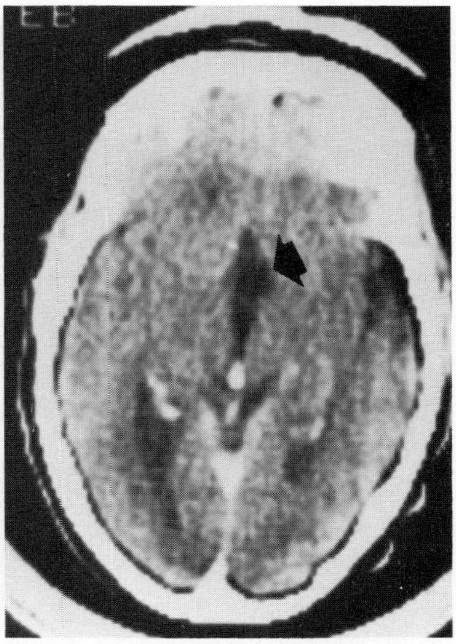

Figure 2–21d

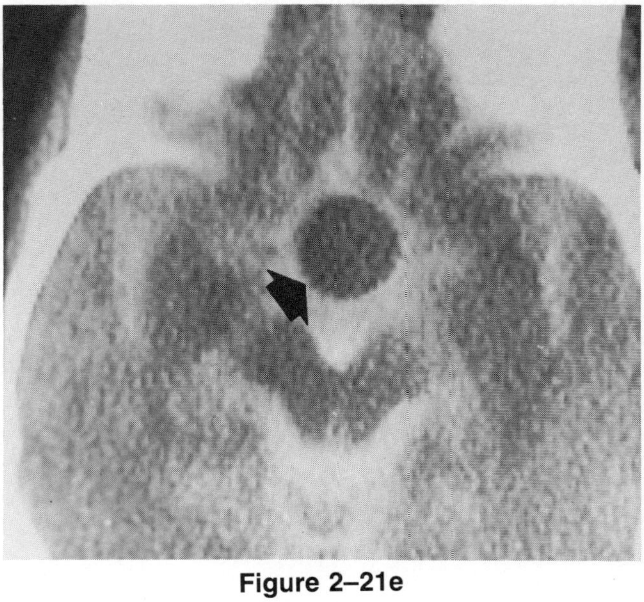

Figure 2–21e

GIANT ANEURYSM OF THE CAVERNOUS INTERNAL CAROTID ARTERY (Figure 2–22)

This 65 year old female presented with a left cavernous sinus syndrome—or paralysis of the left third, fourth, fifth, and sixth cranial nerves. The patient was blind in the left eye and complained of retro-orbital pain.

a. The preinfusion scan reveals a high density lesion with both peripheral and central calcification.

b. The postinfusion portion of the examination reveals a triangular area of enhancement anteriorly (X) as well as irregular enhancement of the mass.

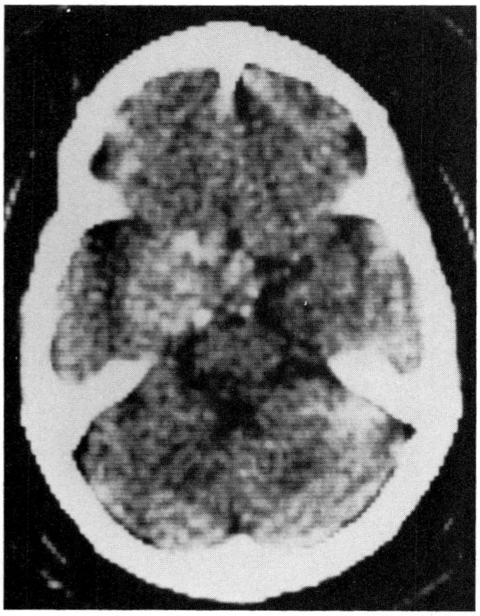

Figure 2–22a

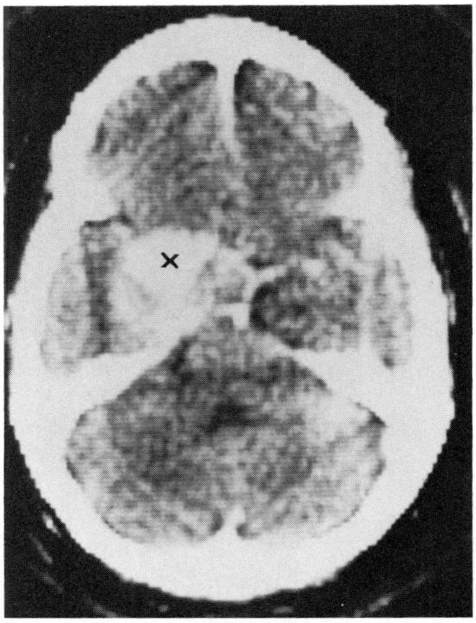

Figure 2–22b

c. Carotid angiography revealed a giant (larger than 2½ cm) aneurysm of the cavernous internal carotid artery (arrows). The aneurysm is partially thrombosed and there is only a small patent lumen remaining of the carotid artery (stars). The unthrombosed portion of the aneurysm (X) is the area of enhancement seen on the postinfusion portion of the examination.

The diagnosis is a giant partially thrombosed aneurysm. Differential diagnosis of CT scan also includes pituitary adenoma (unlikely) and medial sphenoid wing meningioma.

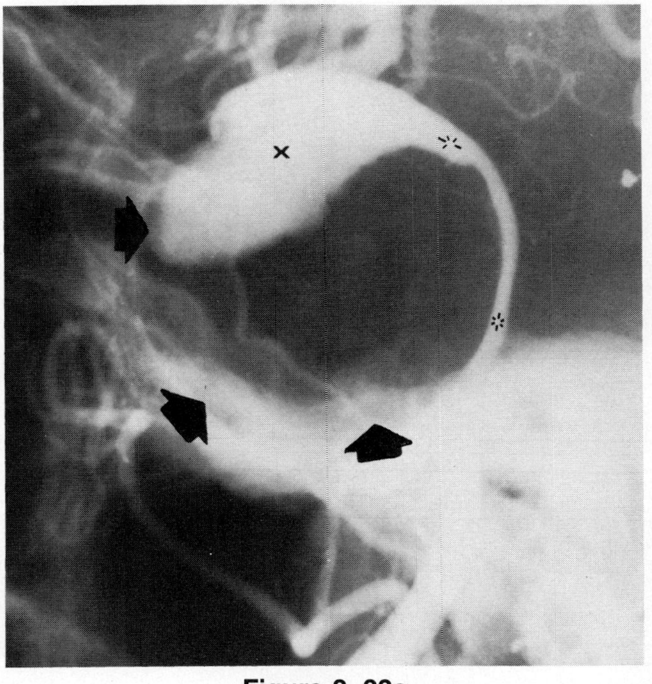

Figure 2–22c

ADULT AQUEDUCT STENOSIS (Figure 2–23)

a. The lateral view of the sella turcica reveals that the sella is enlarged, there is depression of the floor of the sella and thinning and posterior displacement of the dorsal sellae and posterior clinoids.

b. The metrizamide ventriculogram reveals total occlusion of the cerebral aqueduct (arrow). The lateral ventricles are dilated and the deformed, dilated anterior recesses of the third ventricle extend down into the sella turcica. This enlargement of the sella turcica is caused, over a prolonged period of time, by the transmitted pulsations of heartbeat and respiration.

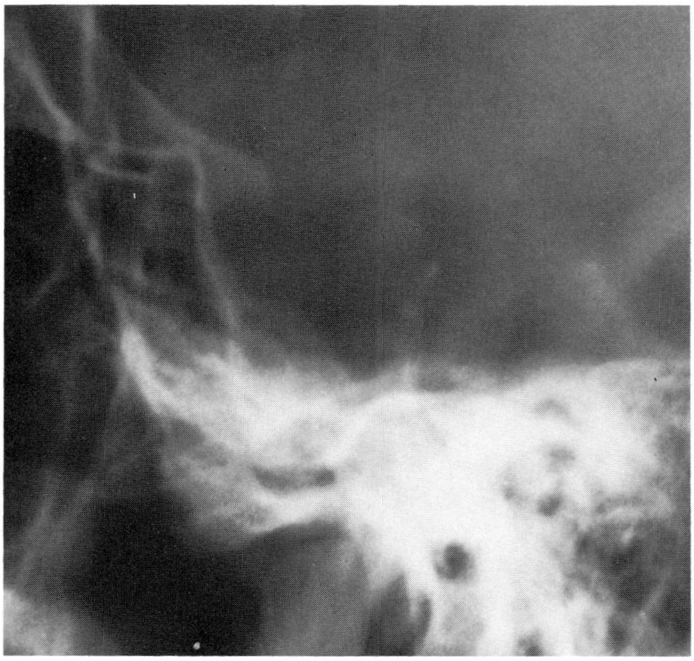

Figure 2–23a

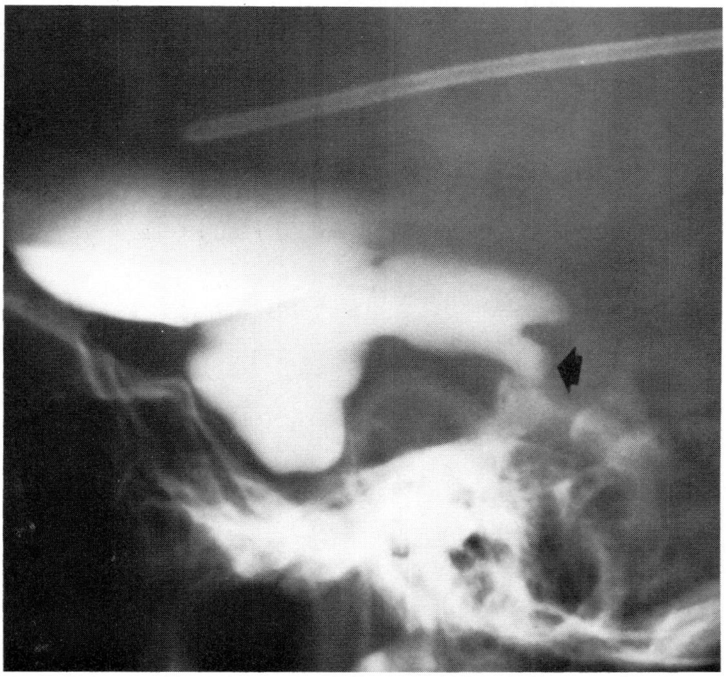

Figure 2–23b

Chronic hydrocephalus of any cause can lead to the development of these changes and can mimic an intrasellar lesion. Differential diagnosis also includes carotid artery aneurysm, parasellar meningioma, pituitary adenoma, or the nonspecific changes of chronic increased intracranial pressure.

PARTIALLY THROMBOSED ANEURYSM MIMICKING A CRANIOPHARYNGIOMA (Figure 2–24)

a. The axial view of the postinfusion examination reveals a multilobulated, peripherally calcified mass in the sella, extending into the suprasella cistern. There was little change from the preinfusion scan.

b. The midsagittal reconstruction view better demonstrates the mass, which can now be seen to contain both solid and peripheral areas of calcification. The mass is intrasellar, suprasellar, and subfrontal in position.

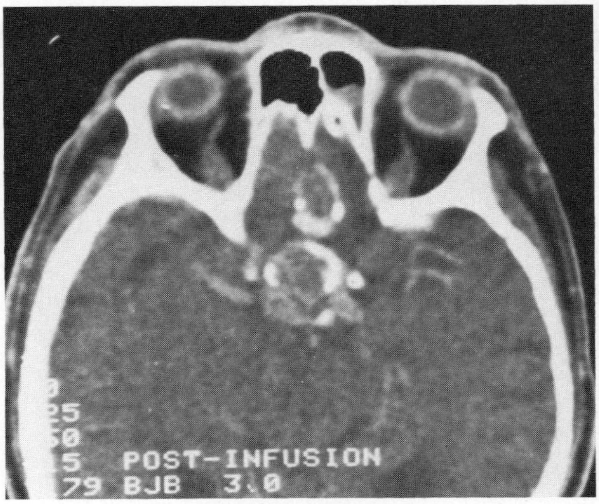

Figure 2–24a

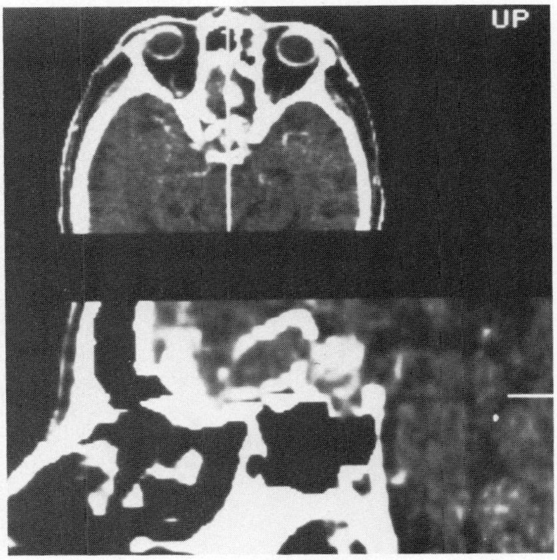

Figure 2–24b

c. The coronal reconstruction view shows the area of calcification within the sella turcica (C). Differential diagnosis includes craniopharyngioma, aneurysm, and teratoma.

d. Angiography confirms the presence of a partially thrombosed aneurysm (arrow).

The diagnosis was proved at surgery.

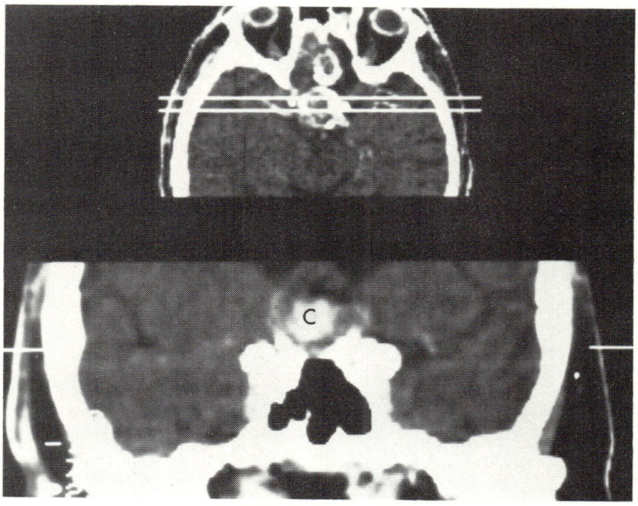

Figure 2–24c

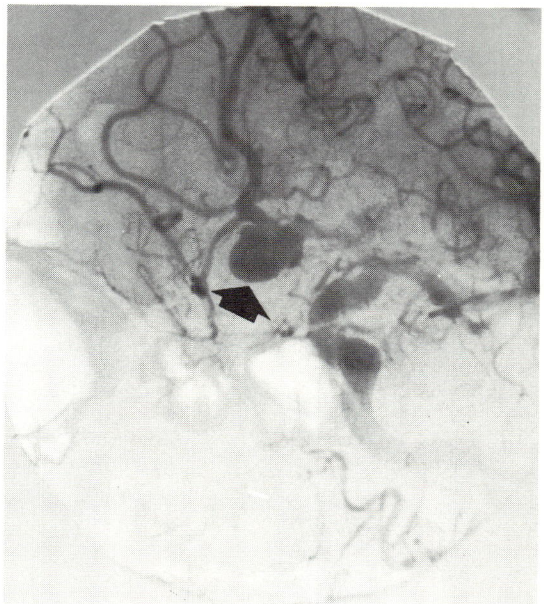

Figure 2–24d

Meningiomas

Meningiomas are quite readily diagnosed by computed tomography. Because of the psammous calcification, many are apparent on the preinfusion scan. Others are of low density prior to the infusion of contrast material. The position of the tumor is often a clue to the diagnosis of a meningioma. Meningiomas tend to occur in a few favored locations: parasagittal over the convexities, from the falx cerebri, from the greater wing of the sphenoid, from the tentorium, and in the parasellar regions. Meningiomas are also found in a variety of less common locations. The tentorial meningiomas may arise either supratentorially or infratentorially; we have seen several posterior fossa meningiomas presenting as masses in the cerebellopontine angle. After the infusion of contrast material, we most often see a very homogeneous blush of enhancement; this blush is reminiscent of the prolonged blush often observed on the arteriogram. Meningiomas usually arise from the dura, and their superficial position is helpful as a diagnostic clue. Low grade gliomas have also been noted to have a rather homogeneous blush following contrast enhancement. Meningiomas are at times surrounded by a very large amount of edema. This can be particularly apparent in the high convexity meningiomas; on the lower cuts the tumor itself may not be visualized, but we may see only the large amount of edema extending below the tumor. On the other hand, there may be no edema present in some patients with meningioma, apparently because the slow growth of the tumors results in pressure atrophy.

RIGHT PARASELLAR MENINGIOMA (Figure 2–25)

M. A. E. is a 48 year old woman who had suffered blurred vision for approximately 9 months prior to admission. She was found to have impairment of function of the II, III, and IV cranial nerves.

a. Cuts 1A and 1B show an area of increased density in the parasellar area along the medial edge of the greater wing of the sphenoid bone. The density is 44 to 64 u (arrow on 1A). After the infusion, there is dramatic homogeneous enhancement of a round tumor mass just behind the superior orbital fissure; density, 60 to 100 u. The findings are typical of a meningioma.

1A 11A 12A

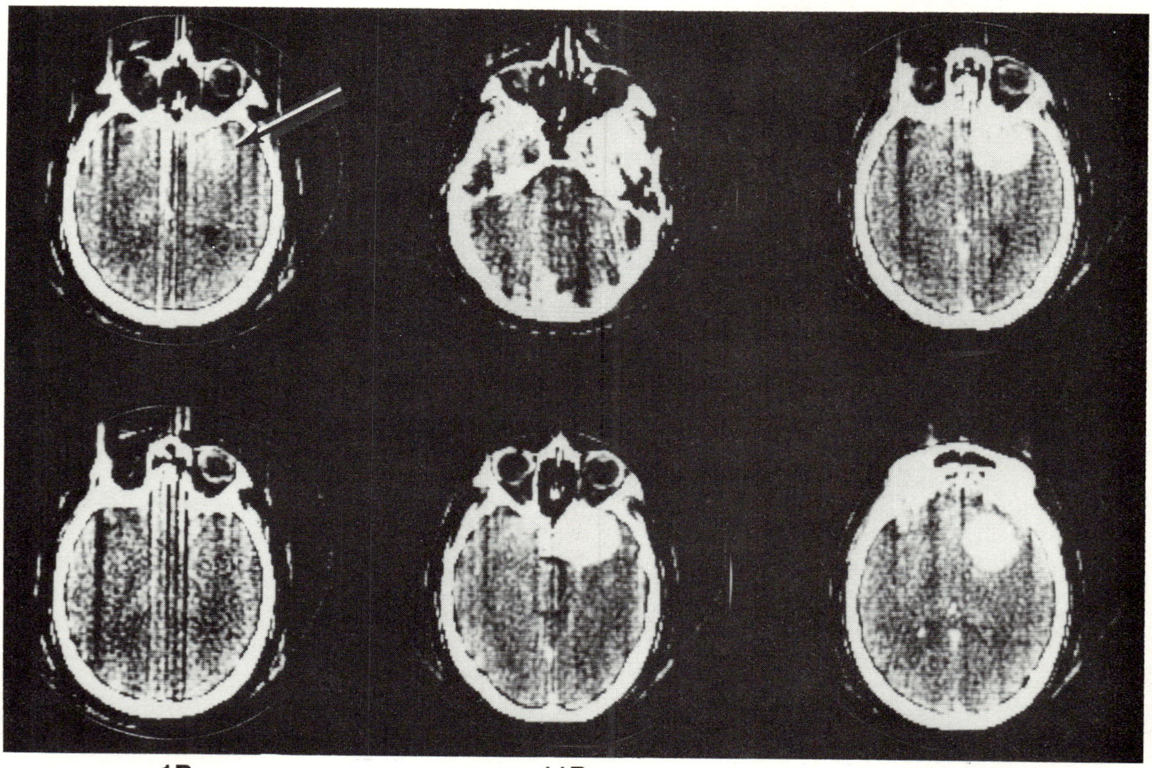

1B 11B 12B

Figure 2–25a

b. Anteroposterior late capillary phase of a right common carotid arteriogram reveals the large tumor blush just behind the right orbit (arrows).

c. The early arterial phase, lateral view, demonstrates enlargement of the middle meningeal artery (arrows) and a particularly large tortuous branch (small arrows) feeding the tumor. The internal carotid artery is encased and markedly narrowed by the tumor; only a small trickle of opacified blood is noted to reach the intracranial circulation (crossed arrow).

d. Later arterial phase reveals the typical sunburst blush of the meningioma.

Surgery revealed a meningotheliomatous meningioma.

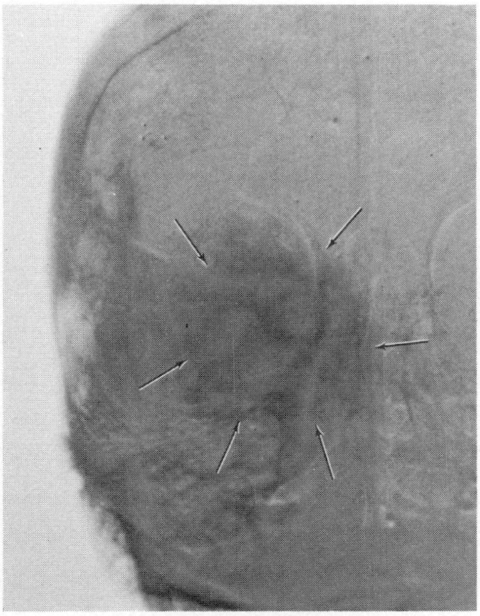

Figure 2–25b

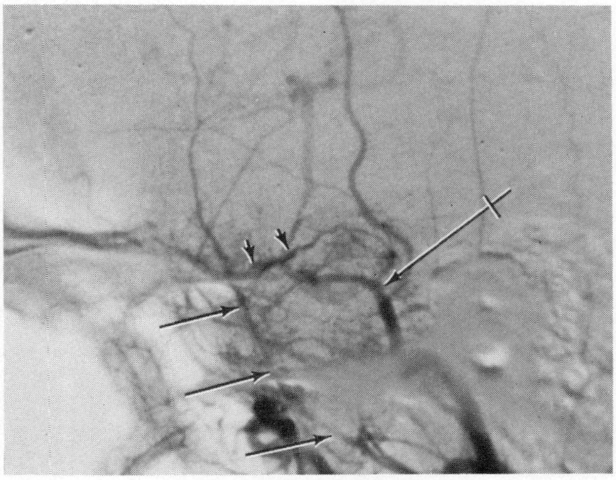

Figure 2–25c

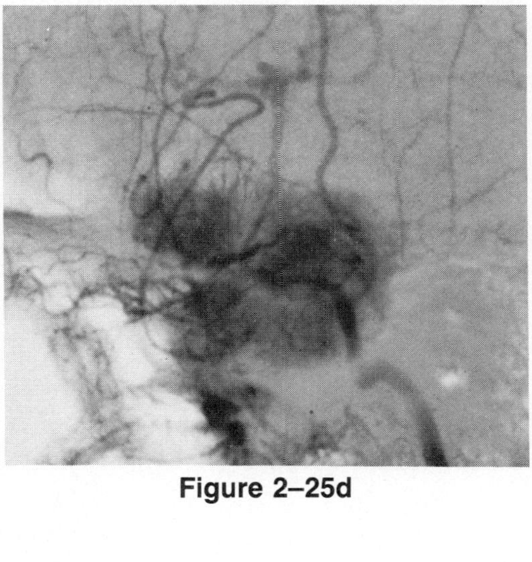

Figure 2–25d

LARGE RIGHT-SIDED MENINGIOMA (Figure 2–26)

R. M. is a 22 year old male with a bizarre affect, increasing headaches, and bilateral papilledema.

a to c. The right lateral (a), anterior (b), and posterior (c) views of the radionuclide scan reveal a large area of dense uptake of the radionuclide in the right temporal region adjacent to the cranial vault. The findings are consistent with a sphenoid wing meningioma.

d. The routine scan demonstrates a very large oval lucent area on the right side. The mass has a well defined border. There is a marked shift toward the left side. Density, 16 to 40 u.

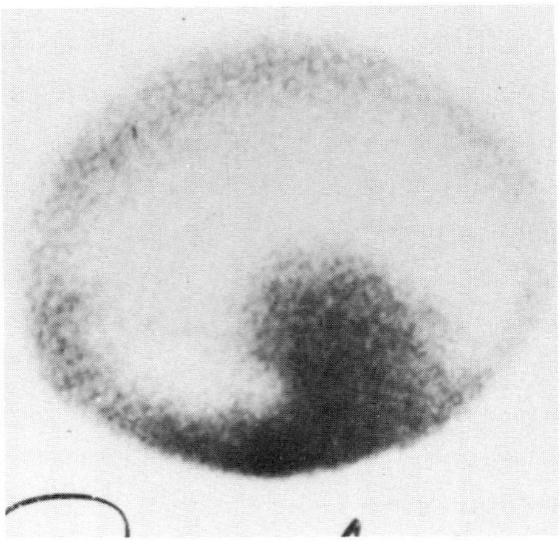

Figure 2–26a

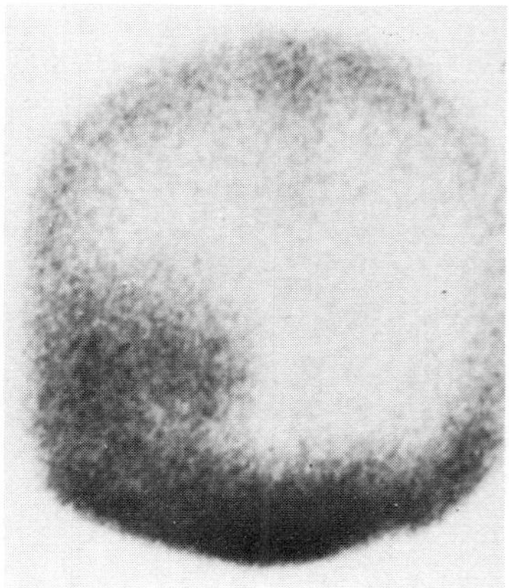

Figure 2–26b

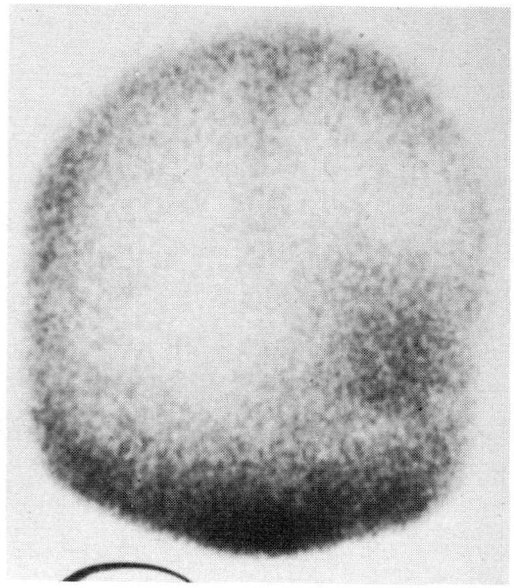

Figure 2–26c

1A 2A 3A

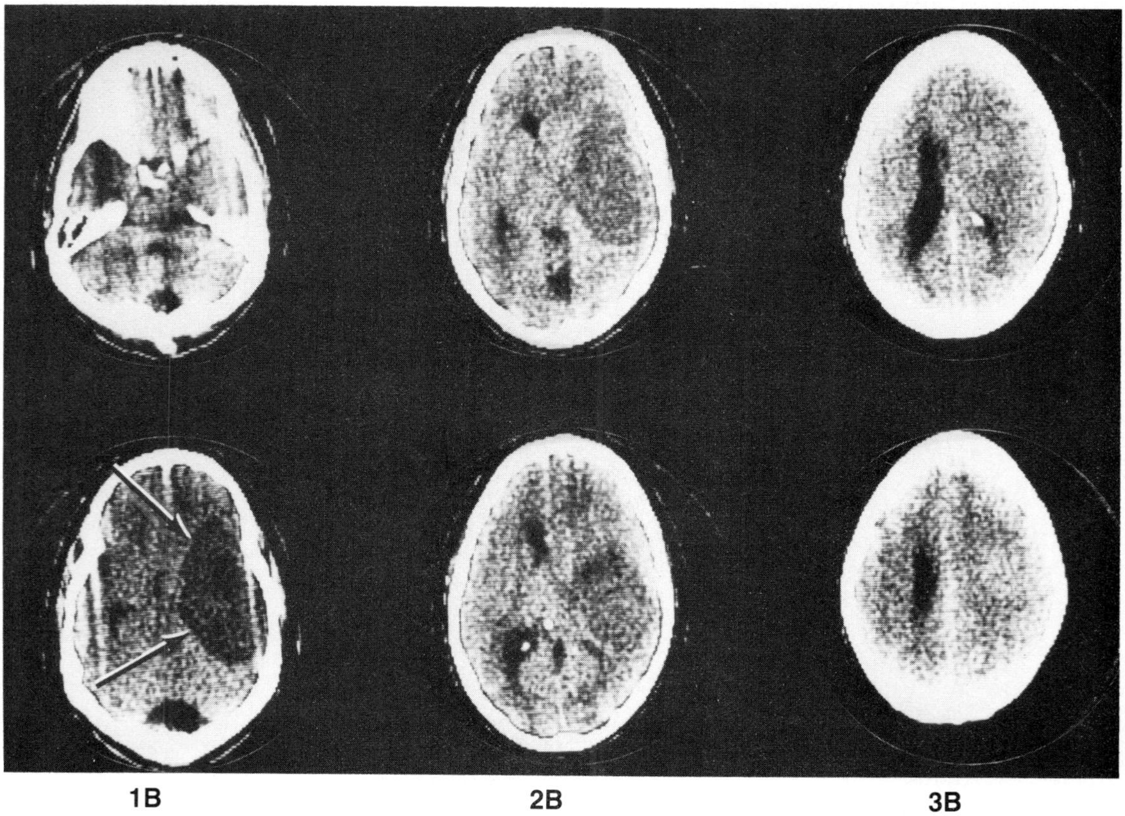

1B 2B 3B

Figure 2–26d

e. Contrast enhancement reveals spectacular enhancement of the lesion. Density, 26 to 84 u.

f. In the anteroposterior arterial phase, marked elevation of the entire middle cerebral artery group (arrows) is seen. In addition, the middle cerebral artery branches are displaced away from the inner table of the skull by an extra-axial mass lesion (small arrows). There is moderate proximal and distal shift of the anterior cerebral artery.

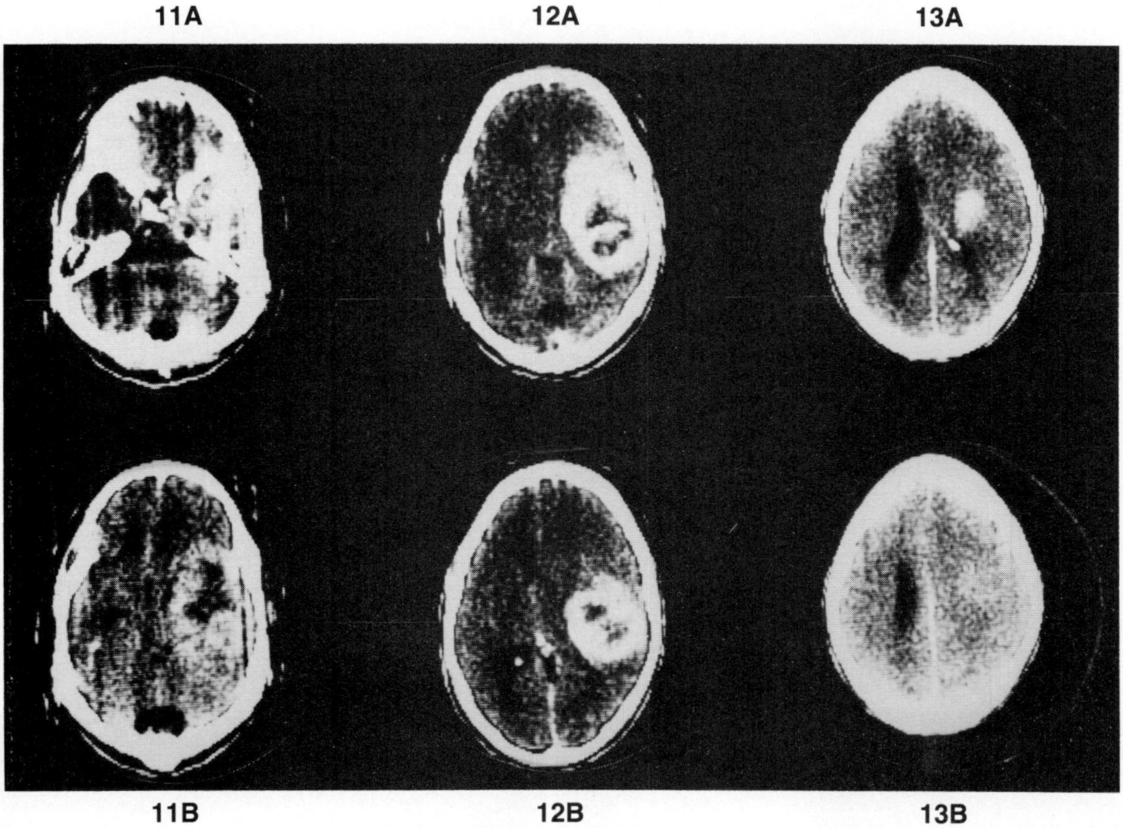

Figure 2–26e

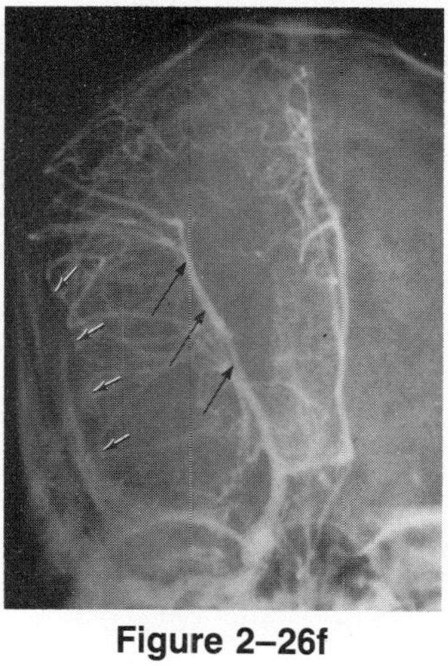

Figure 2–26f

g. The anteroposterior venous phase discloses a greater shift of the internal cerebral vein.

h. The lateral view reveals such marked elevation of the middle cerebral artery group that it appears as if only the anterior cerebral artery is filling. There is stretching of the poorly filled posterior cerebral artery (lower two arrows) and straightening of the anterior choroidal artery (upper arrow).

i. The late arterial phase shows a mass of fine irregular vessels filling from the external carotid circulation in a sunburst pattern typical of meningioma.

Total surgical removal was possible. Note that the CT scan appearance is very unusual for a meningioma.

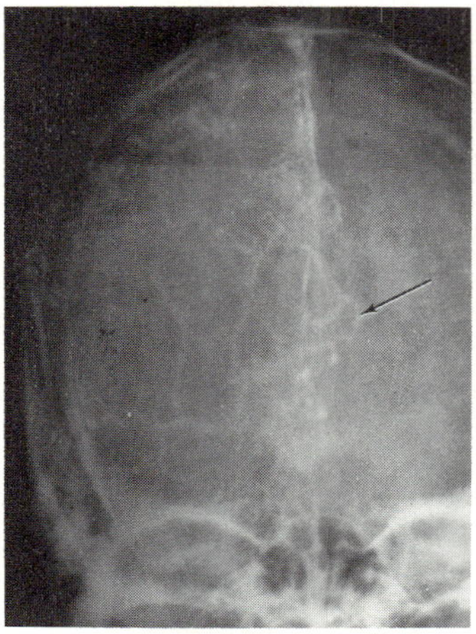

Figure 2–26g

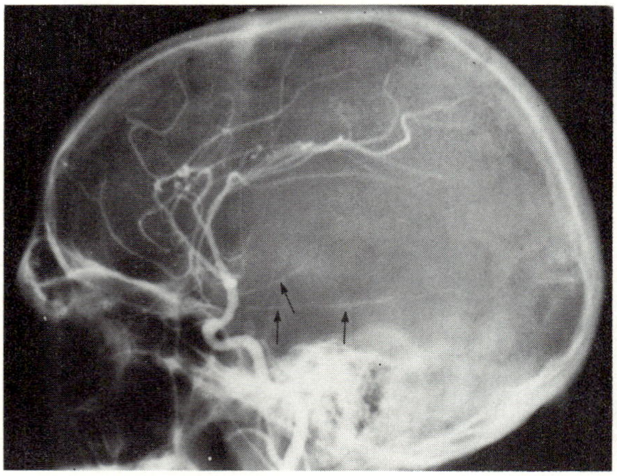

Figure 2–26h

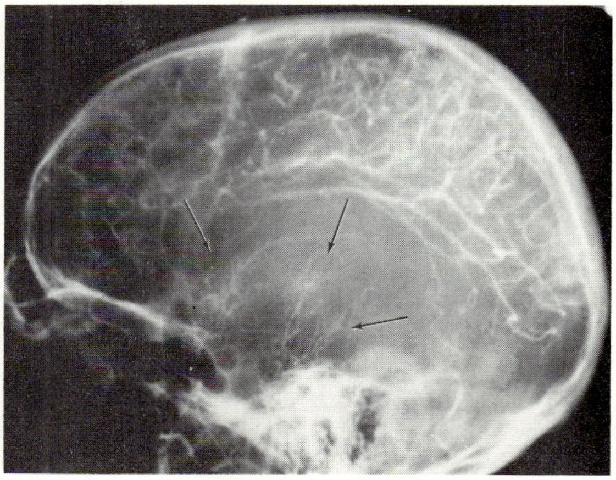

Figure 2–26i

LEFT FRONTAL MENINGIOMA (Figure 2–27)

W. M. is a 68 year old male with a history of confusion and an abnormal brain scan (not available).

a. The routine scan reveals an abnormal area of increased density, 36 to 56 u, in the left frontal region. The mass is broad based and closely applied to the inner table of the cranial vault, extending into the frontal lobe on the

1B 2B

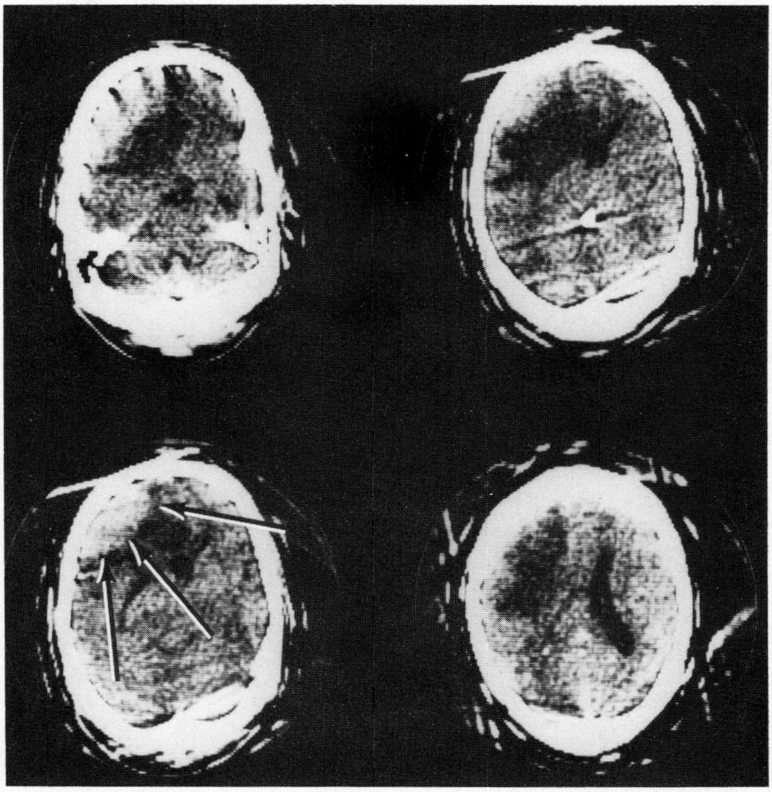

2A 3A

Figure 2–27a

11B

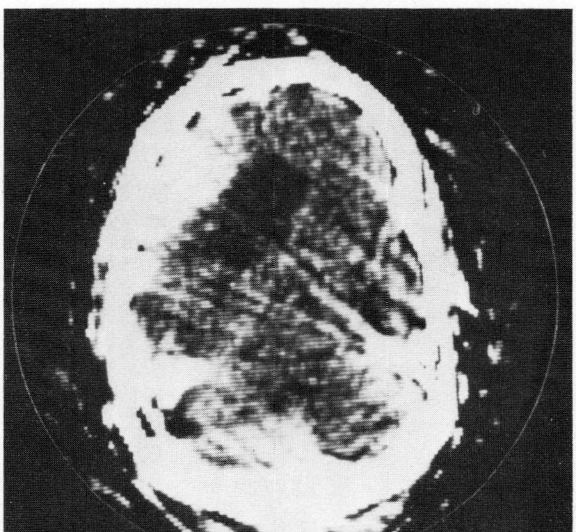

Figure 2–27b

left side and creating a left to right shift. The arrows outline the tumor on cut 2A; note that there is a large amount of surrounding edema.

b. Following the infusion of contrast material, the tumor has increased in density to 60 to 80 u. The enhancement is homogeneous, and the tumor has the appearance of a left frontal meningioma.

c to e. The arterial views reveal enlargement of the middle meningeal artery (arrows) and posterior displacement of the anterior cerebral artery. There is a marked and prolonged blush of the frontal tumor. Note the rather uncommon finding of multiple early draining veins (arrows on e) in this left frontal meningioma.

f. The AP view demonstrates the "round" shift of the anterior cerebral artery so typical of frontal lesions.

Surgery revealed a meningioma.

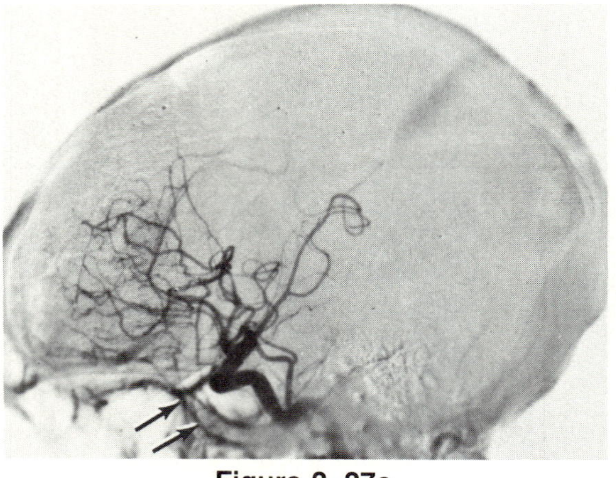

Figure 2–27c

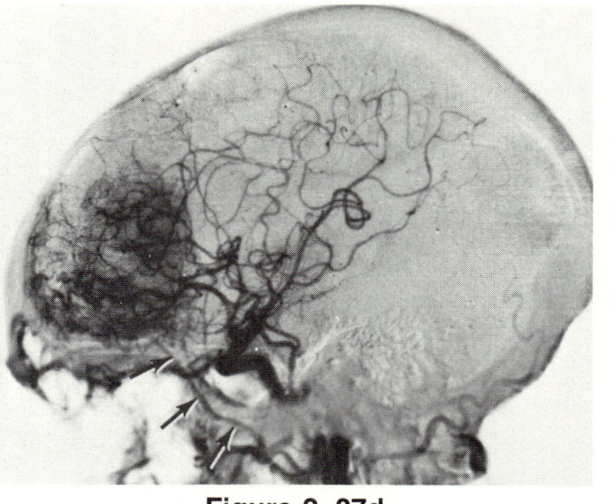

Figure 2–27d

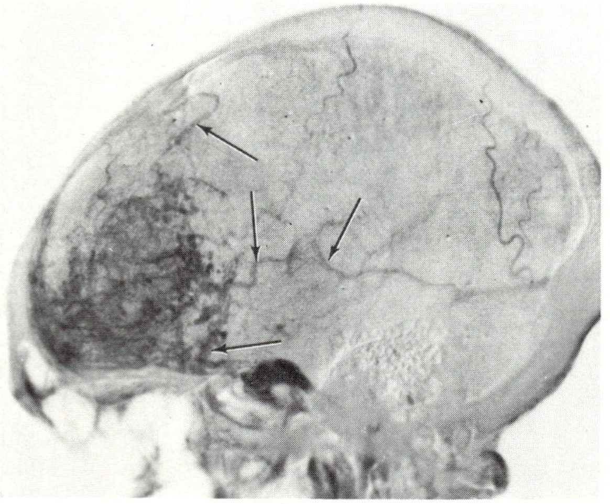

Figure 2–27e

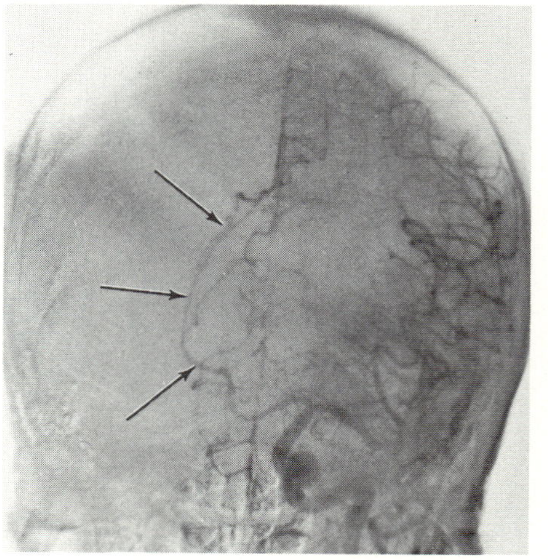

Figure 2–27f

TENTORIAL MENINGIOMA (Figure 2–28)

This 28 year old female presented with a history of headache and decreased hearing on the left side. The corneal reflex was decreased on the left side.

a and b. The preinfusion scan reveals a higher than normal brain density mass that extends from the medial petrous region superiorly through the tentorial notch into the parasellar region (arrows). The third ventricle is displaced to the contralateral side.

c and d. The postinfusion portion of the examination reveals homogeneous enhancement of the tumor. The appearance is quite typical of clivus or tentorial edge meningioma.

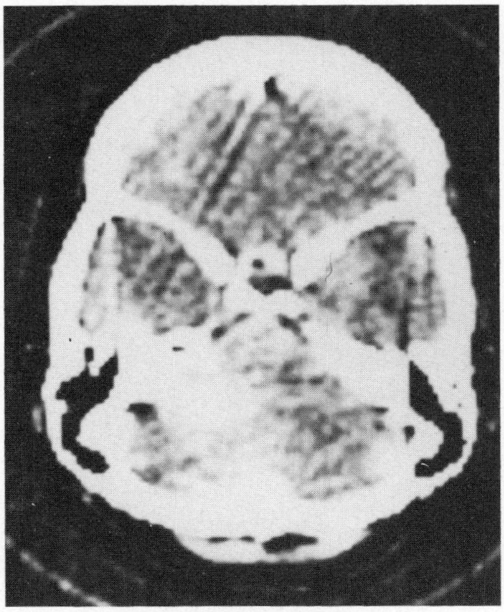

Figure 2–28a

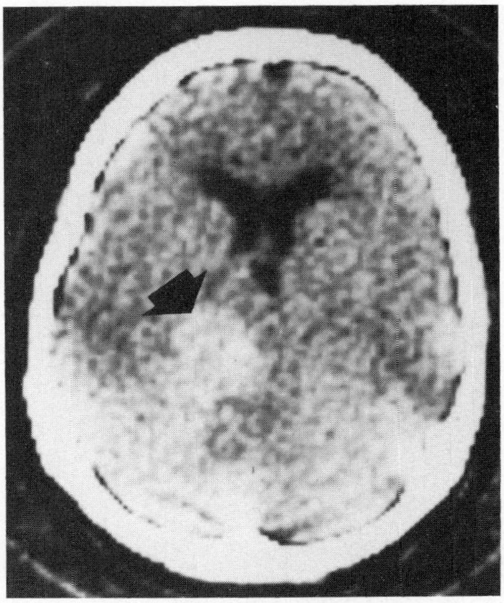

Figure 2–28b

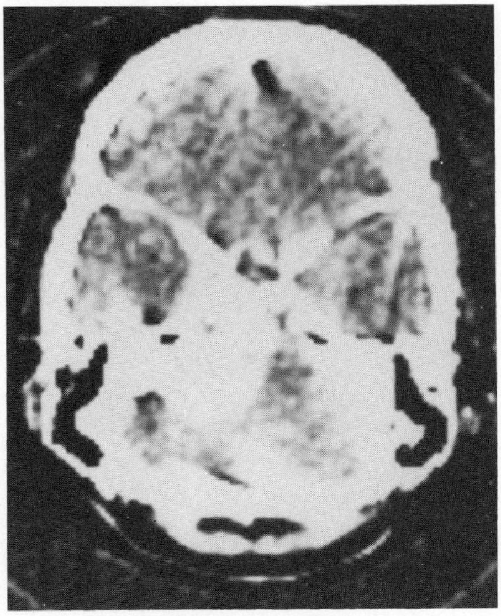

Figure 2–28c

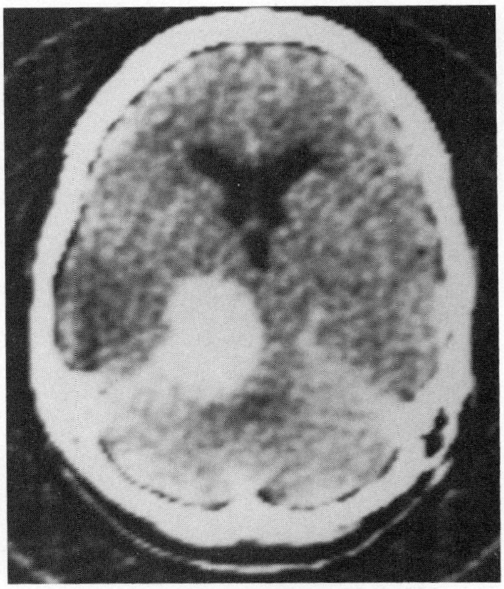

Figure 2–28d

e. The lateral view of the carotid angiogram reveals enlargement of the tentorial artery (arrow), which courses posterolaterally and then branches in a tree-like fashion to supply the meningioma.

f. The AP view again demonstrates this enlarged tentorial artery (T) which courses posterolaterally to supply the tumor. The ophthalmic artery courses anterolaterally and projects below the tentorial artery (O).

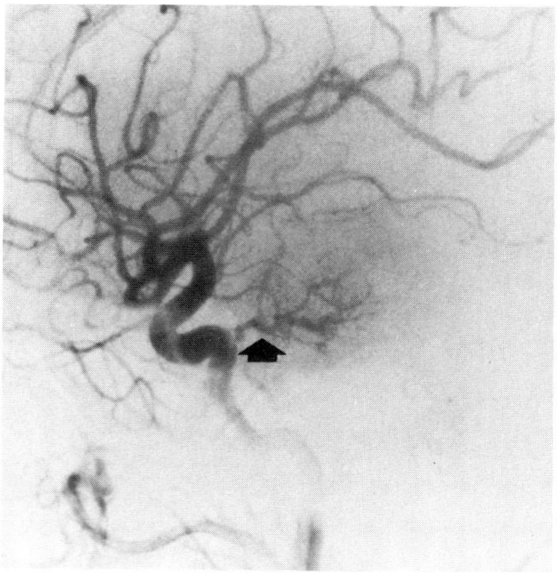

Figure 2–28e

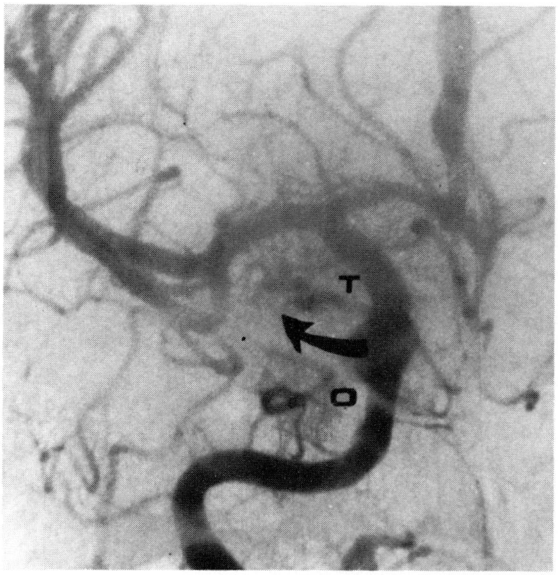

Figure 2–28f

MENINGIOMA WITH EXTRACRANIAL METASTASES (Figure 2–29)

R. G. is a 57 year old female who presented initially 8 years prior to the present admission with headaches, papilledema, and right homonymous hemianopsia. The work-up revealed a left occipital meningioma, which was subsequently resected. Although extracranial metastases developed, she had no further signs of intracranial involvement until the present. She returned at this time with headaches and almost total blindness.

a and b. Posteroanterior and lateral views of the chest reveal a large lobulated mass posteriorly in the left side and a smaller, slightly lobulated mass just anterior to the large mass. These are extracranial metastases from the meningioma. In addition, the patient had diffuse bony involvement with metastatic meningioma. The systemic metastases developed several years after the initial diagnosis of intracranial meningioma.

c and d. Right lateral (c) and posterior (d) views show a large area of uptake of the radionuclide in the right occipital pole at the junction between the superior sagittal and transverse sinuses. Postsurgical changes are noted on the left side.

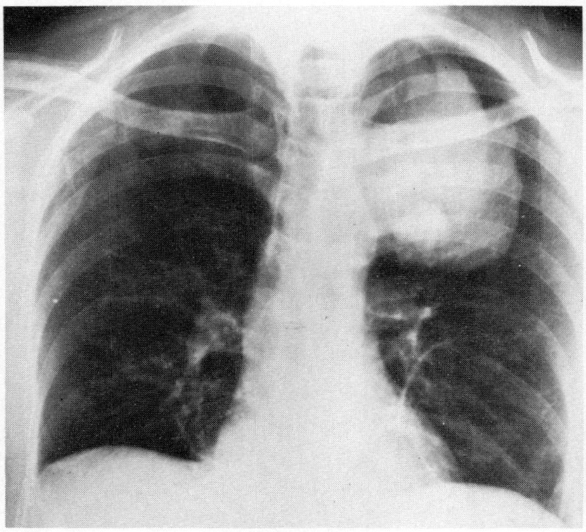

Figure 2–29a

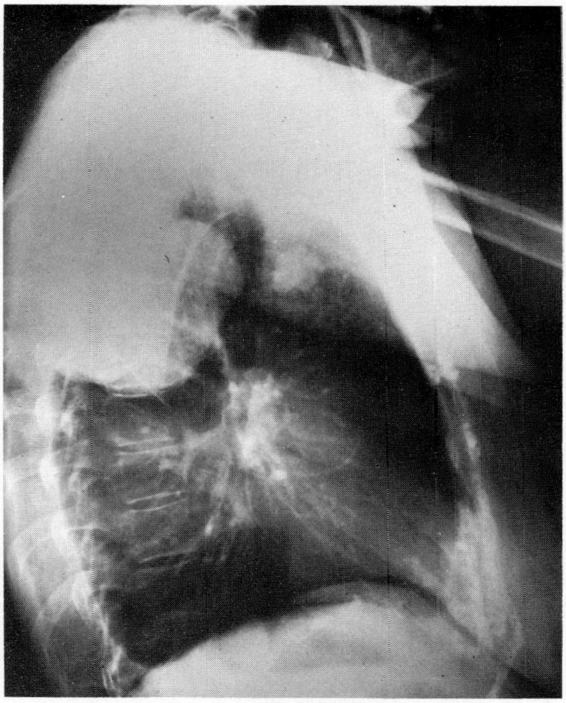

Figure 2–29b

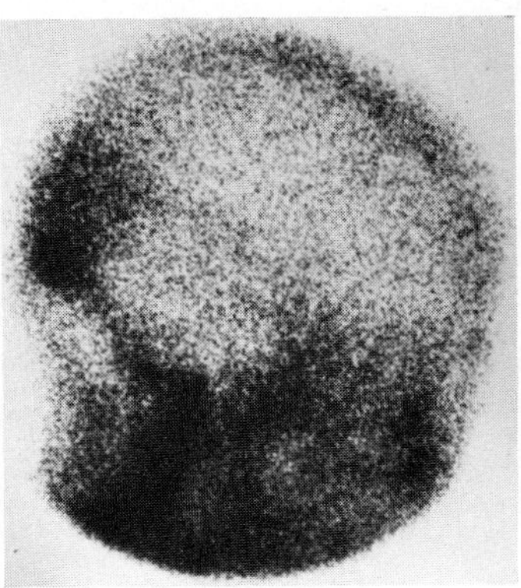

Figure 2–29c

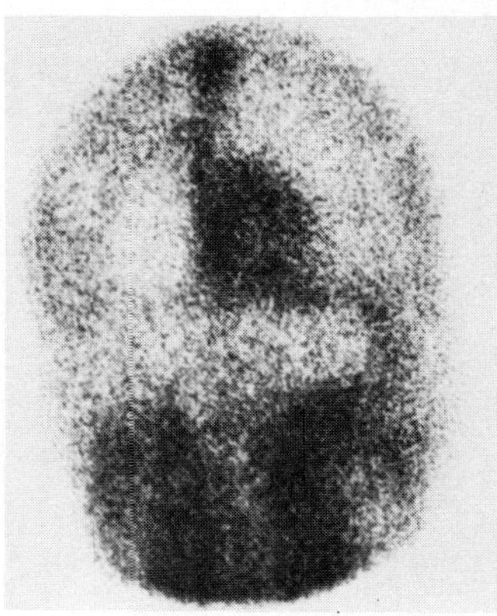

Figure 2–29d

2A 3A

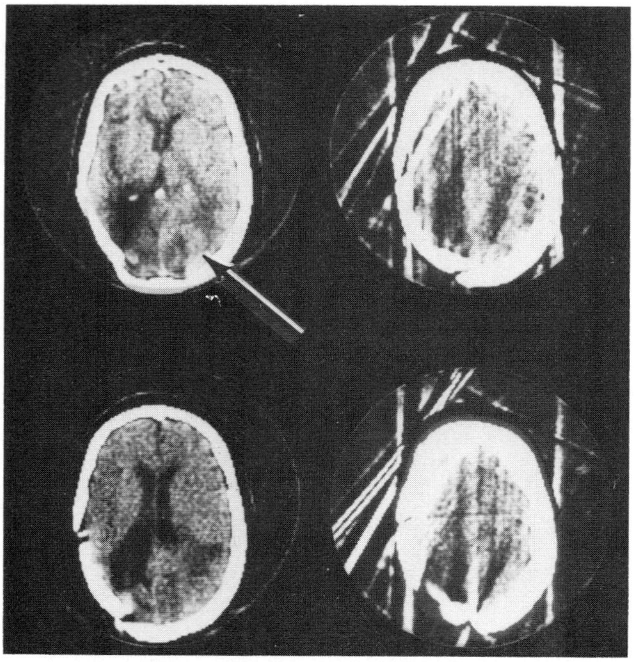

2B **Figure 2–29e** 3B

e. Routine CT scan reveals an irregular area in the left cranial vault from the previous surgery. There is an area of postsurgical porencephaly noted in the left parieto-occipital region. In the right occipital pole is a poorly defined area of increased density, 34 to 68 u, surrounded by an area of edema (arrow on 2A). There is mass effect, with forward and medial displacement of the choroid plexus and calcification on the right side (see 2A).

f. After contrast enhancement, the tumor increased in density to 48 to 94 u. The blush appeared to be both homogeneous and in a ring. The ring of enhancement is less common with meningioma.

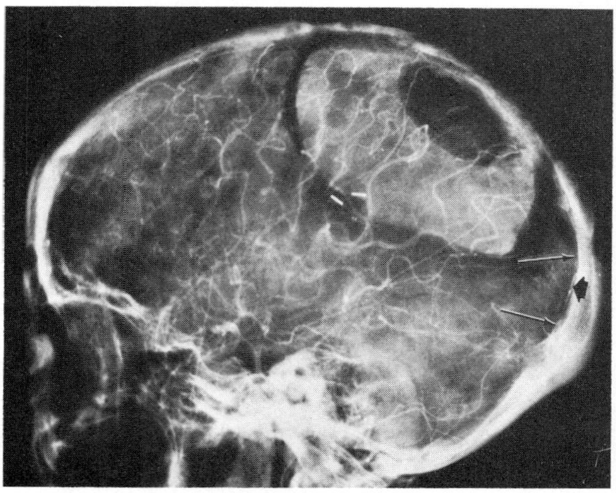

Figure 2–29g

11A 12A

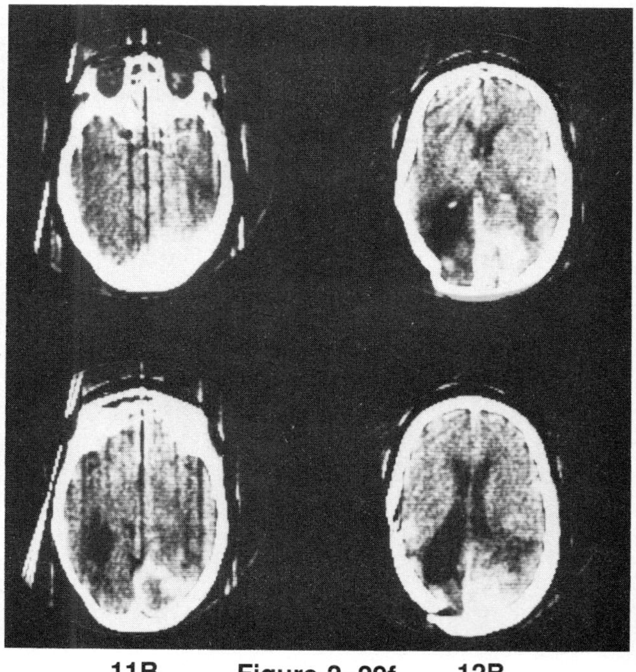

11B **Figure 2–29f** 12B

g. Late arterial phase of the right brachial arteriogram reveals an enlarged posterior meningeal artery (arrows) and spreading of the vessels in the right parietal and occipital lobes.

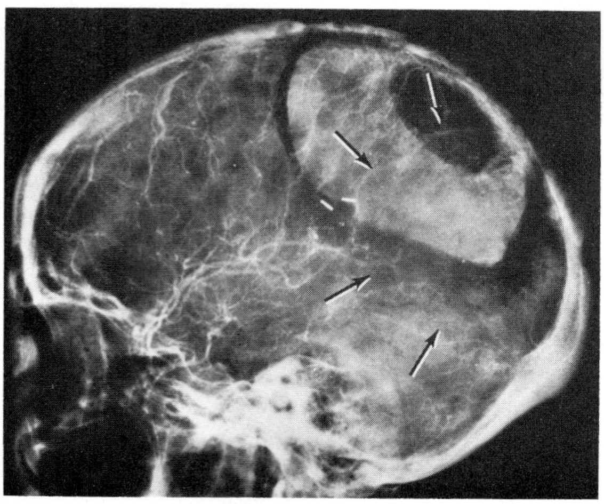

Figure 2–29h

h. The venous phase discloses a relatively avascular area in the right occipital pole, but no evidence of the "cloud-like" blush seen so commonly with meningioma. The unusual appearance of the bone flap is secondary to aseptic necrosis of the bone following surgery.

A second meningioma, similar in histologic appearance to the initial tumor, was removed at the time of surgery.

CEREBELLOPONTINE ANGLE MENINGIOMA (Figure 2–30)

L. M., a 48 year old woman, presented with dizziness of long standing and a recent onset of instability. Physical examination revealed a mild decreased corneal reflex on the left side. The audiogram was normal bilaterally.

a. Internal auditory canal tomograms are normal. There is a question of faint calcifications (long arrow) superior to the canal (short arrows).

b and c. The posterior (b) and left lateral (c) views of the radionuclide scan reveal a large cerebellopontine angle mass.

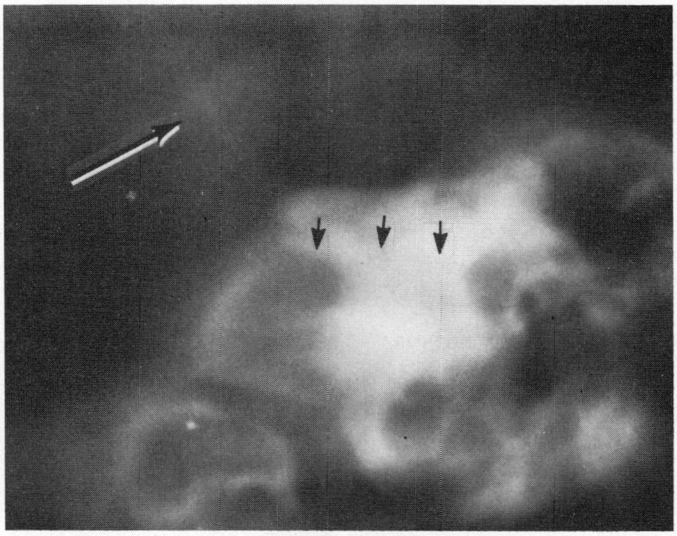

Figure 2–30a

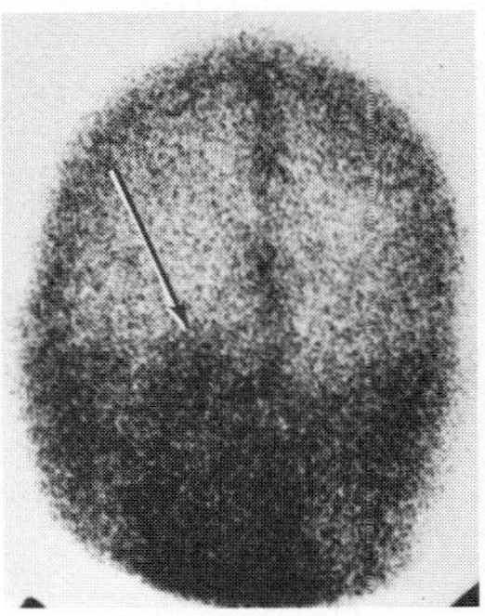

Figure 2–30b

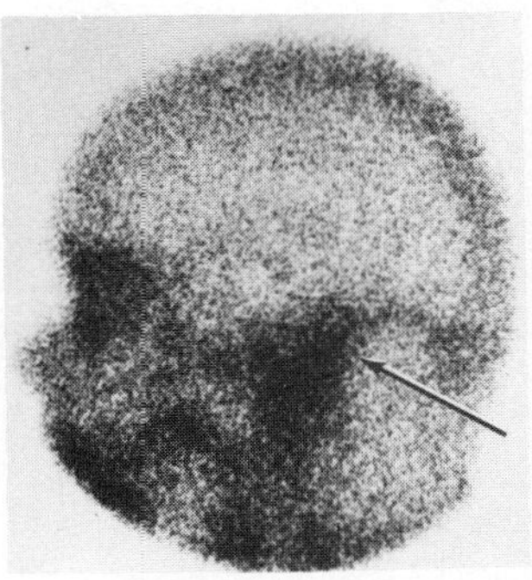

Figure 2–30c

d. The routine computed tomogram shows an abnormal area of increased density, 36 to 62 u, in the region of the left cerebellopontine angle. An area of surrounding edema and slight displacement of the fourth ventricle (arrow) from left to right is seen. Mild obstructive hydrocephalus is also present.

e. Contrast enhancement reveals spectacular enhancement of the tumor, which increased in density to 90 to 130 u. The view with electronic enhancement shows the tumor to better advantage.

At surgery, gross total removal of a left cerebellopontine angle meningioma was performed.

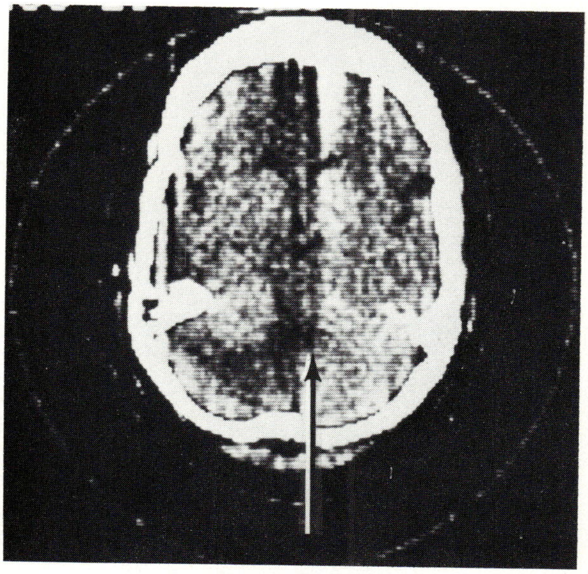

Figure 2–30d

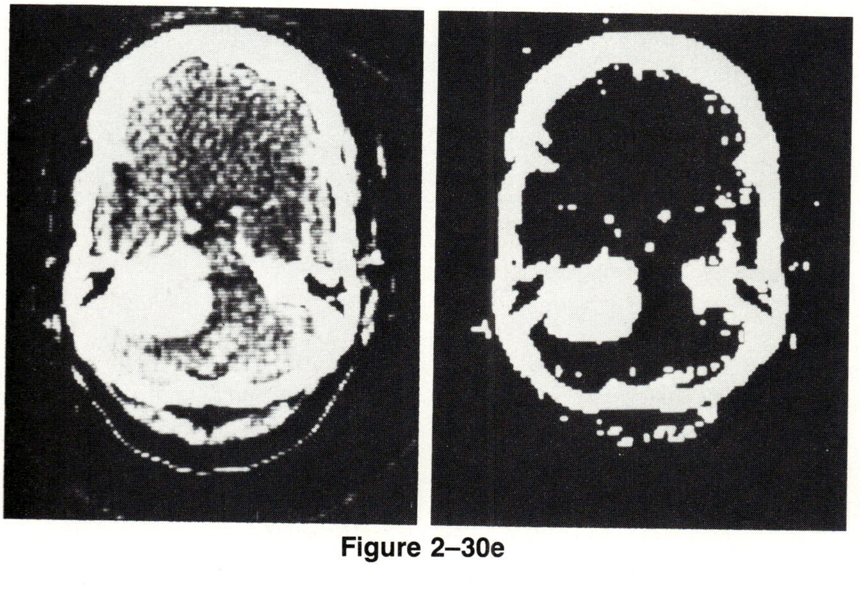

Figure 2–30e

TENTORIAL MENINGIOMA (Figure 2–31)

S. K. is a 52 year old female who presented with mild progressive hearing loss on the left side. Physical examination revealed a decreased corneal reflex on the left side. There was mild hearing loss; the facial nerve was intact. Internal auditory canal tomograms were normal.

a and b. Left lateral (a) and posterior (b) views reveal a large area of increased uptake of the radionuclide in the left cerebellopontine angle. The abnormal uptake seems to extend up through the tentorial notch (see arrows); this is felt to be distinctly unusual for an acoustic neurinoma.

c and d. The computed tomogram shows an area of increased density in the left cerebellopontine angle measuring 30 to 50 u. Following contrast enhancement the mass increased in density to 80 to 130 u. The mass is bilobed and readily identified in the region of the left cerebellopontine angle and extending forward through the tentorial notch. There is, in addition, mild displacement of the posterior aspect of the third ventricle from left to right (arrow). The fourth ventricle is noted to be displaced both posteriorly and to the right (crossed arrow). There is no hydrocephalus.

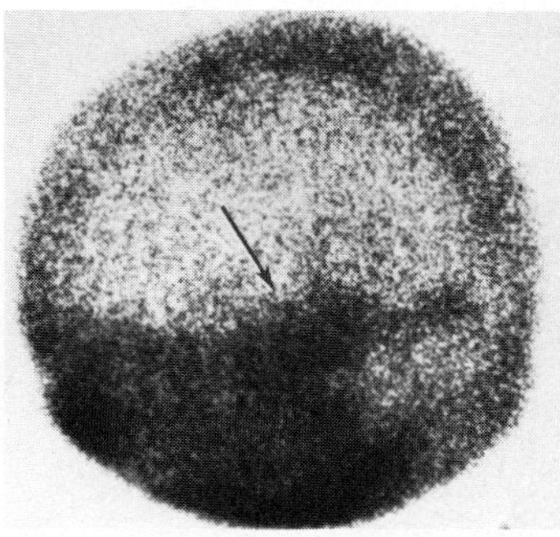

Figure 2–31a

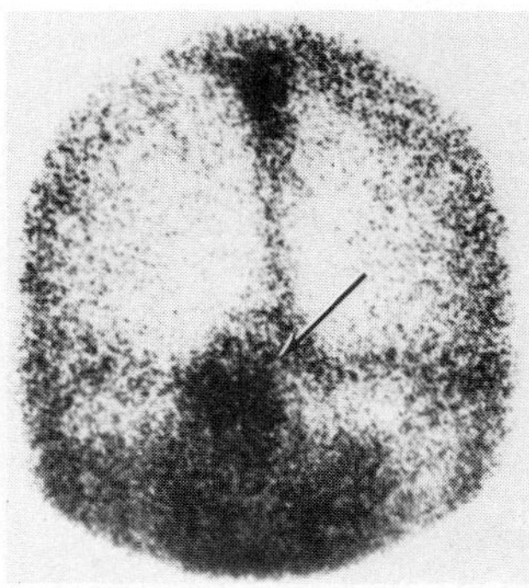

Figure 2–31b

1A

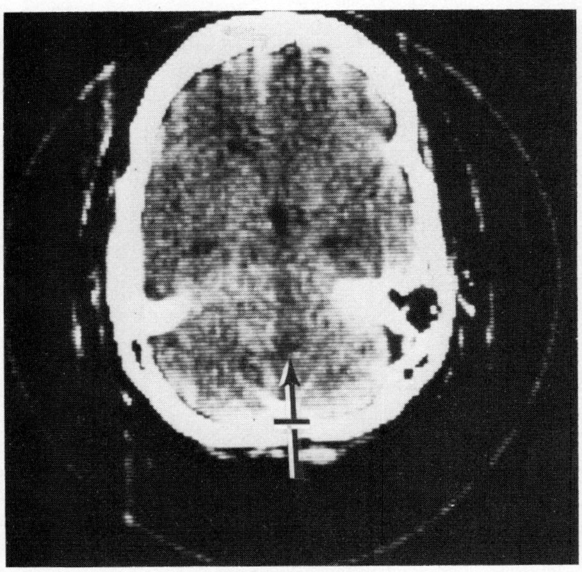

Figure 2–31c

11A

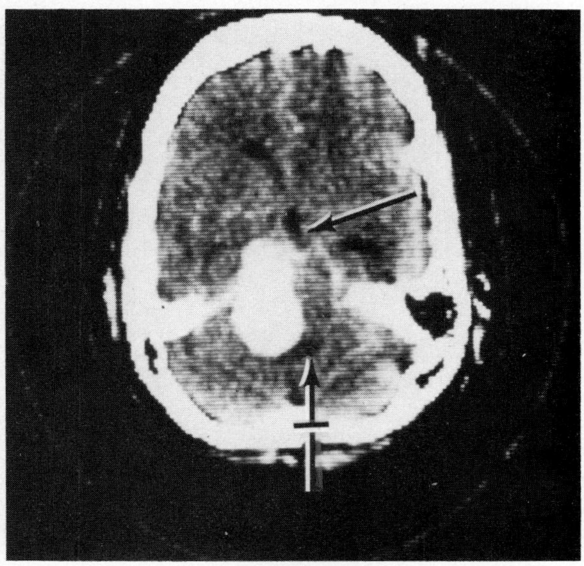

Figure 2–31d

e. Lateral arterial phase of the left brachial arteriogram demonstrates elevation of the left posterior cerebral (upper small arrows) and superior cerebellar arteries (arrows). The right side follows a normal course (crossed arrows).

f. The anteroposterior arterial phase reveals displacement of the basilar artery from left to right. Again noted is the elevation and medial displacement of the left posterior cerebral and superior cerebellar arteries (arrows). There is a very faint tumor stain noted just above the left internal auditory canal (long arrow). A left carotid arteriogram did not reveal an enlarged tentorial artery as is often seen with posterior fossa tentorial meningiomas.

Surgery revealed a meningioma that appeared to arise from the clivus and to extend well up through the tentorial notch and under Meckel's cave. The extent of the tumor was such that a total excision was impossible.

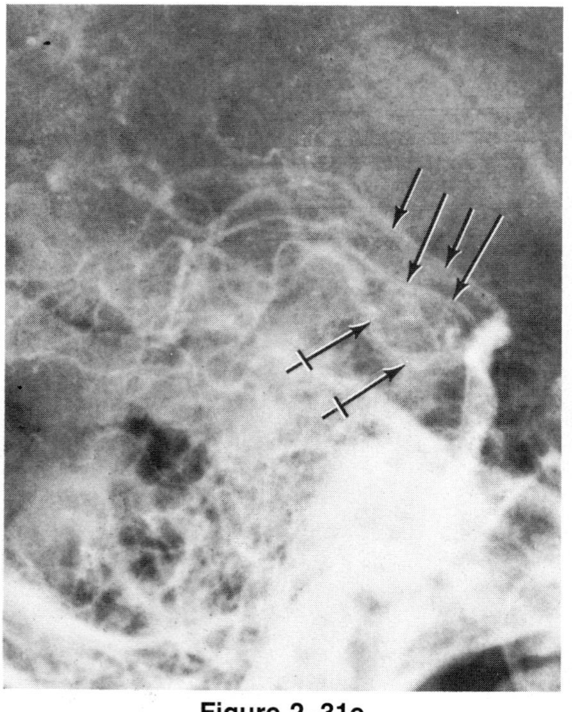

Figure 2–31e

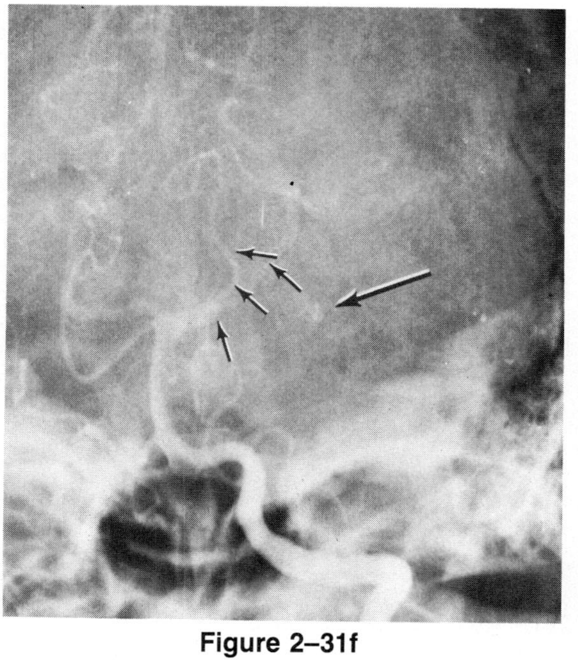

Figure 2–31f

RIGHT SPHENOID WING MENINGIOMA (Figure 2–32)

W. M. is a 58 year old man who was hospitalized at a mental institution for 2 months prior to admission. He was found to have an abnormal brain scan and was sent to us for diagnosis and treatment. His skull series was normal.

a and b. Anterior (a) and right lateral (b) views of the radionuclide scan reveal a large dense area of increased uptake in the region of the right sphenoid wing. The findings are typical of a meningioma.

c. The routine CT scan discloses an abnormal area of increased density on the right side that was broad based superficially at the level of the greater wing of the sphenoid and was surrounded by an area of edema. (Unfortunately, for technical reasons the density could not be obtained.) There was mild shift to the left. Following contrast enhancement, the tumor increased to a density of 50 to 110 u. The blush was homogeneous,

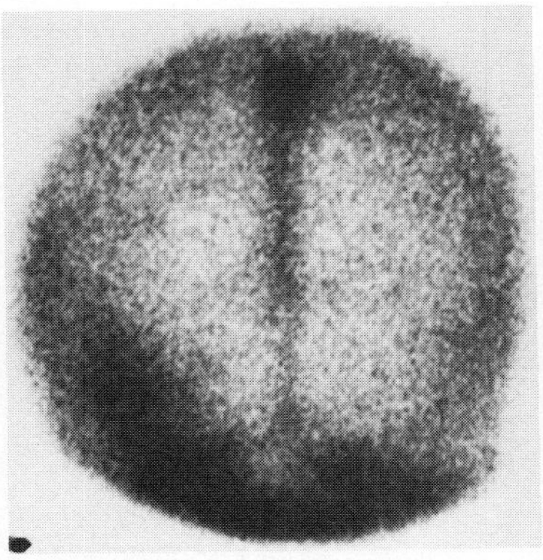

Figure 2–32a

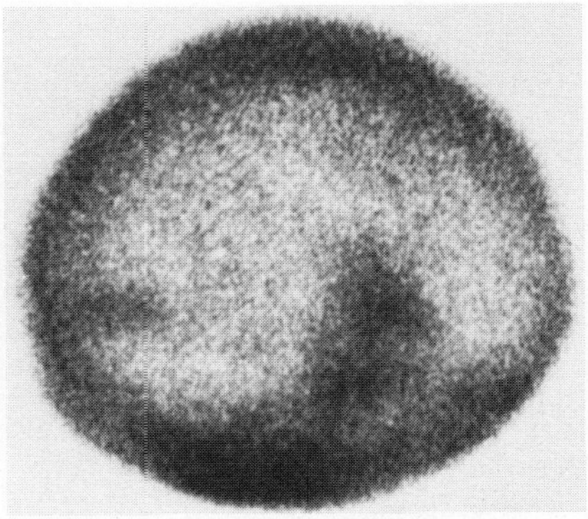

Figure 2–32b

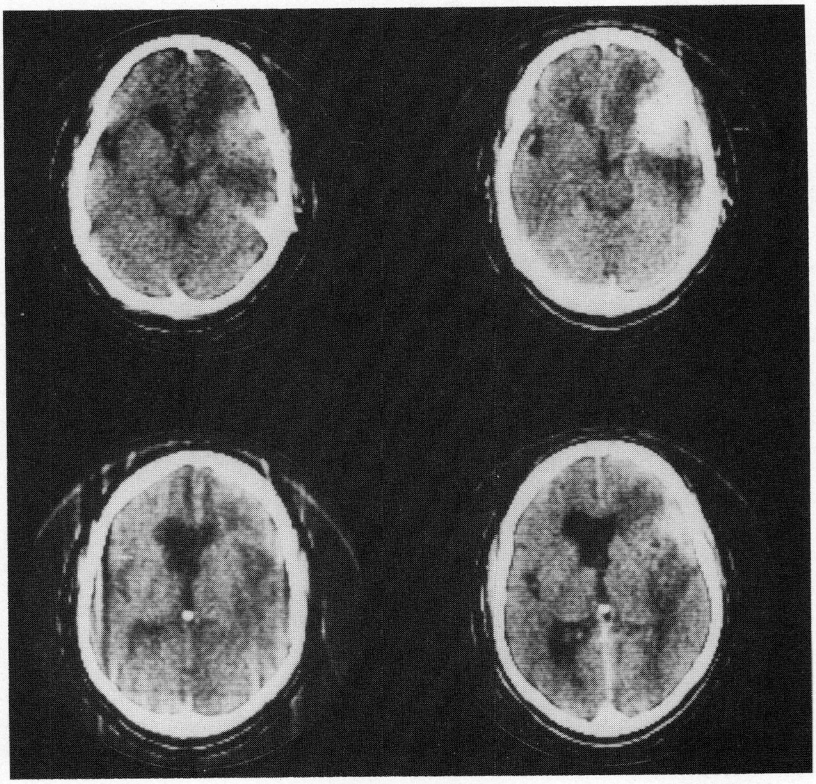

Figure 2–32c

and this was felt to be a right sphenoid wing meningioma.

d and e. Selective right internal carotid arteriogram shows marked elevation of the middle cerebral artery vessels and displacement of the middle cerebral artery vessels away from the inner table of the skull. There appears to be draping of the branches of the middle cerebral artery over a large extra-axial mass lesion.

f and g. Common carotid arteriogram reveals the typical tortuous irregular vessels in a sunburst pattern arising from the middle meningeal artery (wide arrows) and feeding the meningioma. The faint blush is apparent on the late arterial view (arrows).

Surgery revealed a right sphenoid wing meningioma extending into the sylvian fissure.

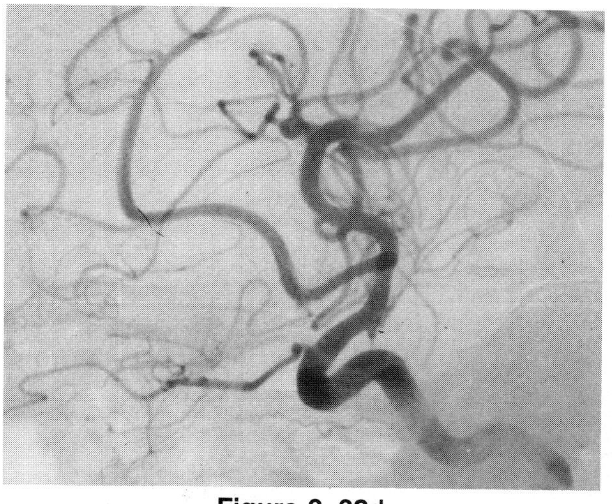

Figure 2–32d

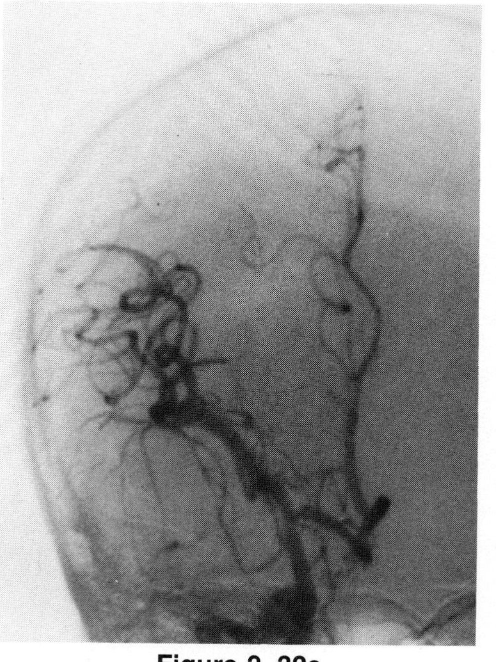

Figure 2–32e

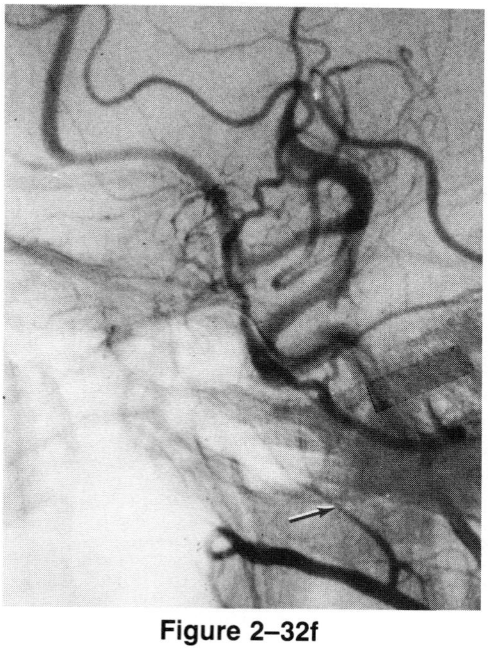

Figure 2–32f

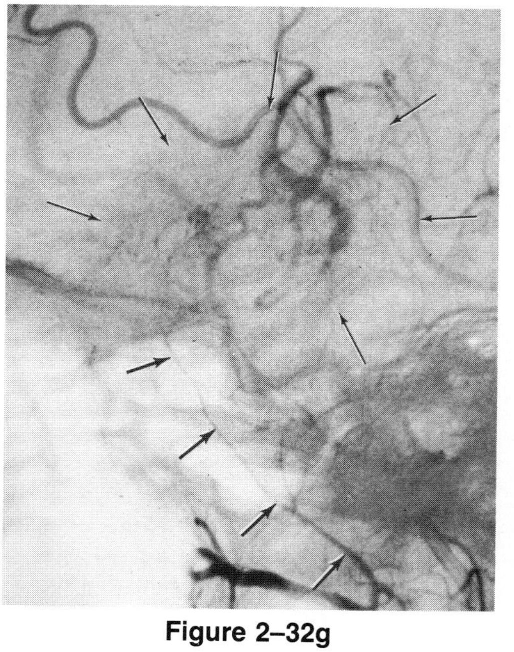

Figure 2–32g

ANTERIOR FALX MENINGIOMA (Figure 2–33)

M. T. is a 57 year old female with a 1-month history of involuntary movements of her right leg, preceded by weakness in the right leg. These "movements" spread up her body to involve her arm and were followed by short periods of unconsciousness. Physical examination revealed slight weakness of dorsiflexion of the right foot. Arteriography was within normal limits. Pneumoencephalography was normal.

The routine CT scan (top row) revealed very slight posterior displacement of the anterior tip of the left frontal horn. A small area of edema was noted in the left posterior frontal region (arrow on 3A). The tumor measured 34 to 52 u and could be faintly seen on cut 3B just medial to the area of edema. After the infusion of contrast material, the small anterior falx meningioma is readily apparent. The density increased to 52 to 76 u.

2B 3A 3B

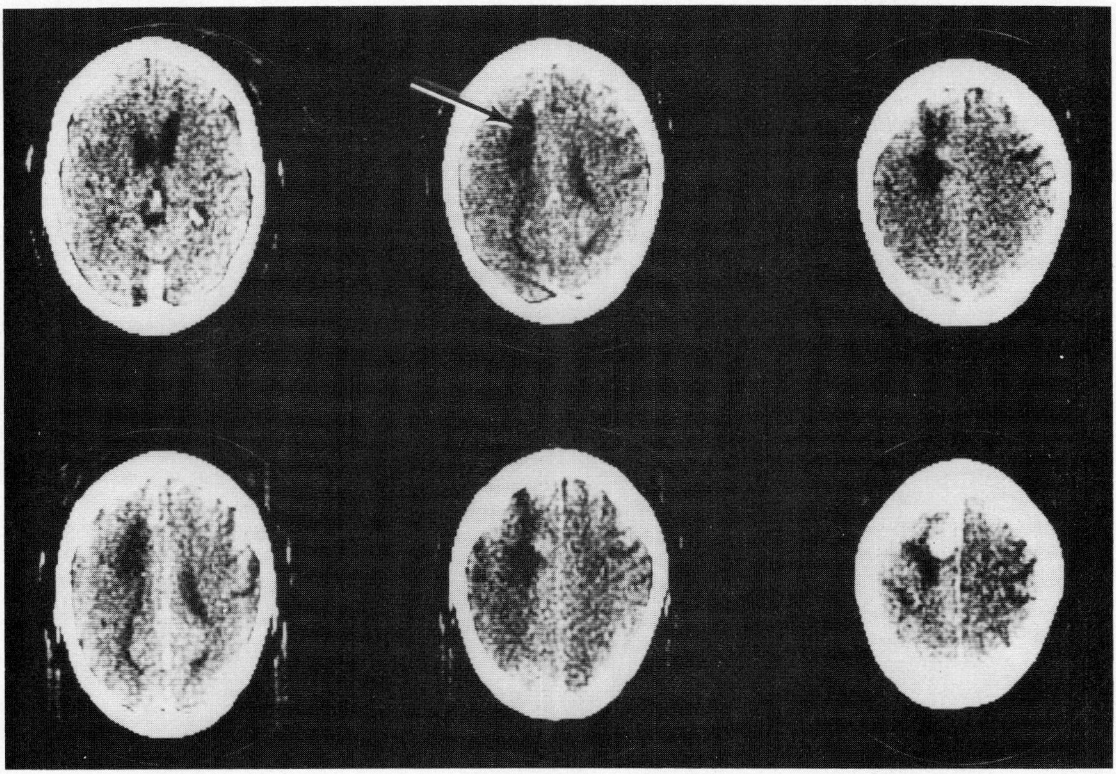

13A 13B 14A

Figure 2–33

LARGE FALX MENINGIOMA (Figure 2–34)

M. G. is a 73 year old woman with a history of a gradually progressive left hemiparesis of many years' duration.

a and b. Posteroanterior and lateral views of the skull reveal a very large densely calcified mass in the right parietal parasagittal region.

c. The routine CT scan shows a large dense mass in the right parietal region consistent with a large, densely calcified meningioma; density, 200 to 600 u. The tumor appears to arise from the falx and to extend laterally into the parietal lobe. There is almost no shift of the lateral ventricles, probably because the indolent nature of the tumor had produced pressure atrophy of the surrounding brain tissue. There was very slight enhancement after contrast infusion.

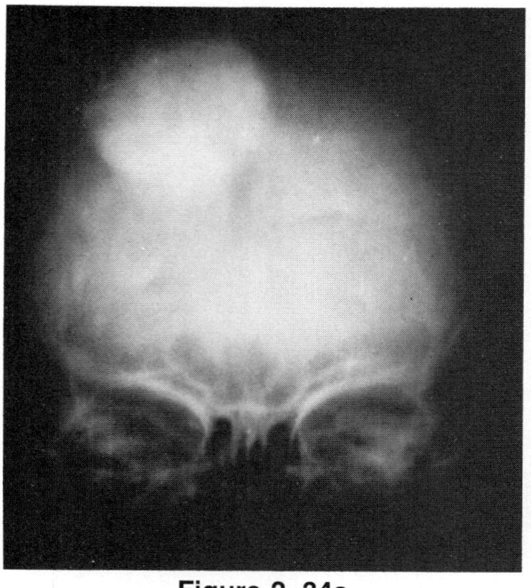

Figure 2–34a

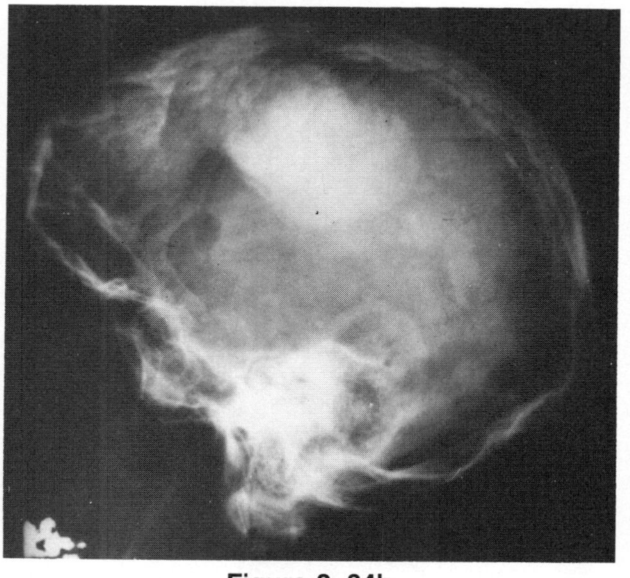

Figure 2–34b

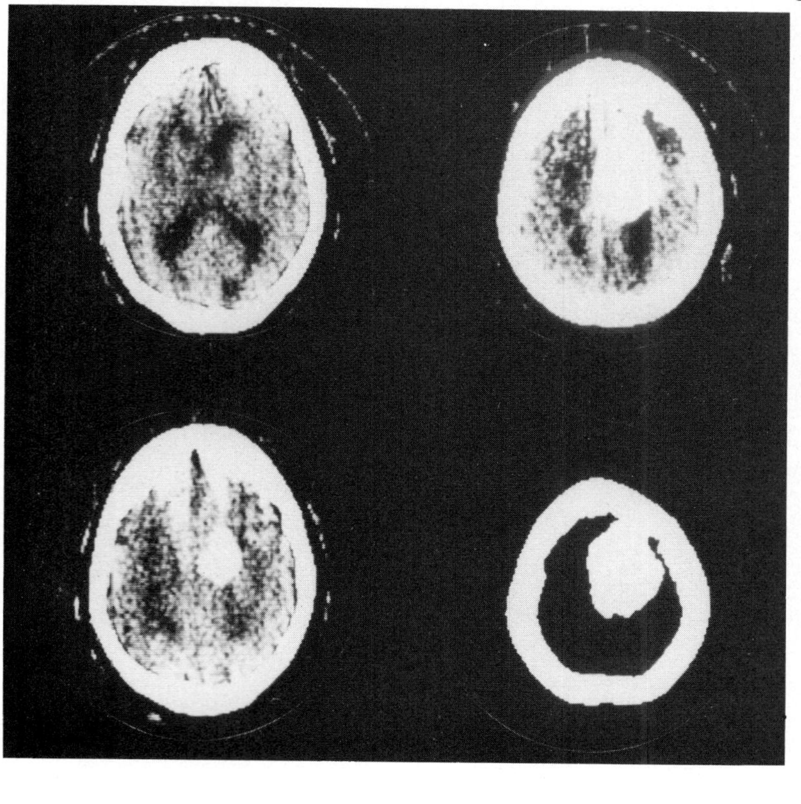

Figure 2–34c

PARASAGITTAL CONVEXITY MENINGIOMA (Figure 2–35)

G. D., a 42 year old male, had a recent onset of focal seizures that consisted of twitching of the right foot. These seizures were followed by weakness in the right foot that lasted several hours after the seizure episode.

The routine CT scan (left) reveals the area of edema high in the convexity region on the left side. This finding is quite typical of convexity meningioma. The tumor in this case is isodense with the brain, and is in the parasagittal region medial to the surrounding edema. Arrows point to the meningioma. After contrast infusion (right), there is marked enhancement of the meningioma, which is now readily apparent. Density, 70 to 100 u. Note that the blush is homogeneous, a finding that is frequently seen with the meningiomas.

Surgery revealed a left parasagittal meningioma.

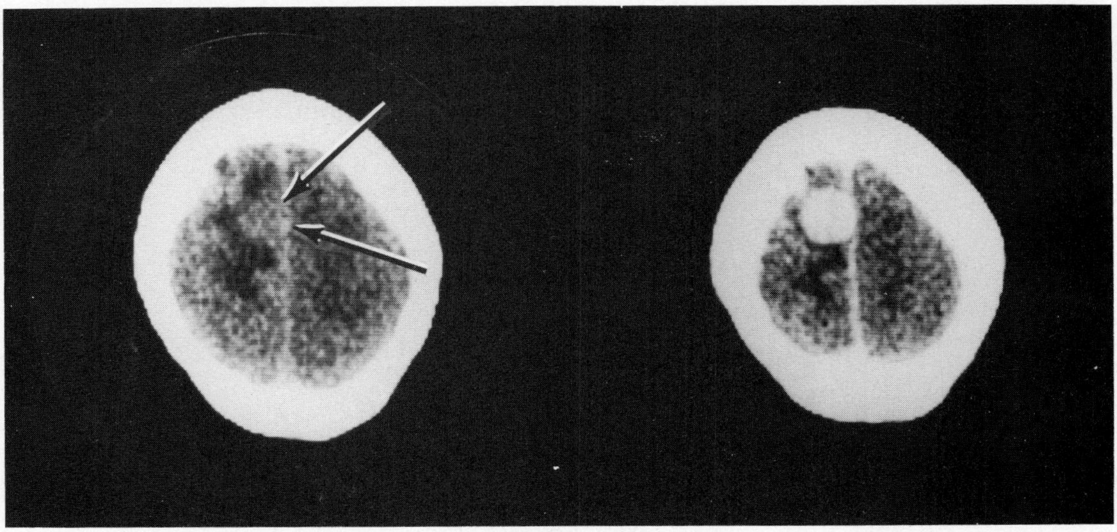

Figure 2–35

Acoustic Neurinomas

Patients having eighth nerve neurinomas usually present with a history of progressive hearing loss on the affected side. Patients with neurofibromatosis have an increased incidence of acoustic neurinomas. There is also a familial form of acoustic neurinoma.

Computed tomography has revolutionized the approach to the diagnosis of acoustic neurinoma. With third and fourth generation scanners, CT may be the only study necessary. The size of the internal auditory canal is evaluated by 5-mm cuts viewed at window width and window lengths which are optimal for visualization of the bony structures. For small, purely intracanalicular, acoustic neurinomas the preinfusion scan may be normal. Most acoustic tumors are isodense with the normal brain tissue. With larger tumors, the fourth ventricle may be shifted to the contralateral side. Since these tumors may be bilateral, the fourth may be in normal position, even in an abnormal case. Following the infusion of contrast material, there is usually homogeneous enhancement of the tumor. Occasionally, these tumors may be cystic or even multicystic, so low density areas are visible on the preinfusion scan. In those cases, cystic areas are present within the homogeneously enhancing mass. The mass is broadly based against the internal auditory canal. Meningiomas can have a similar appearance but usually arise from the tentorium or clivus.

For small tumors or purely intracanalicular tumors (Figure 2–39), air cisternography or metrizamide cisternography followed by CT can demonstrate the abnormality.

RIGHT ACOUSTIC NEURINOMA (Figure 2–36)

M. P. is a male who presented with right-sided hearing loss.

a and b. The tomograms of the internal auditory canals reveal a normal appearing left side, with flaring of the porus acusticus of the right internal auditory canal. The arrows outline the upper margins of the internal auditory canals bilaterally.

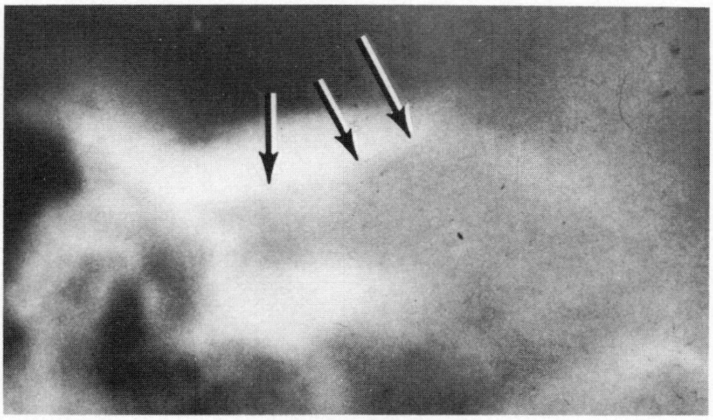

Figure 2–36a

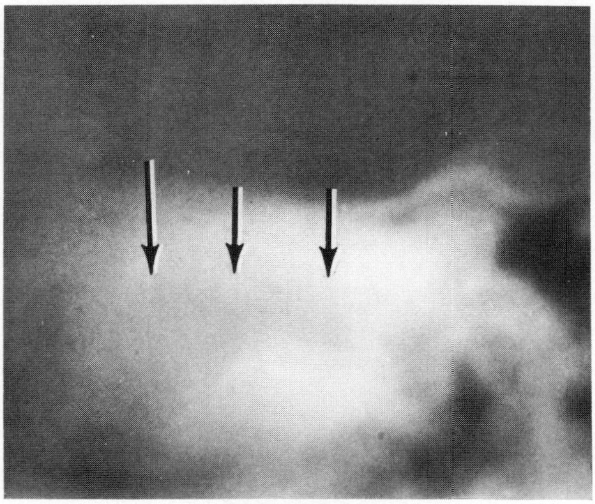

Figure 2–36b

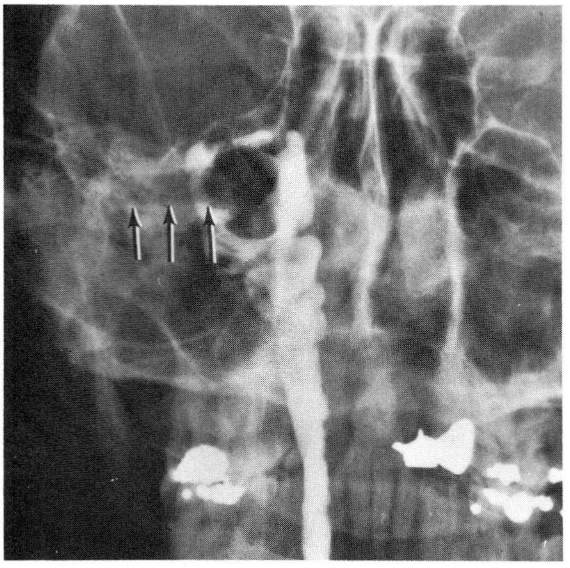

Figure 2–36c

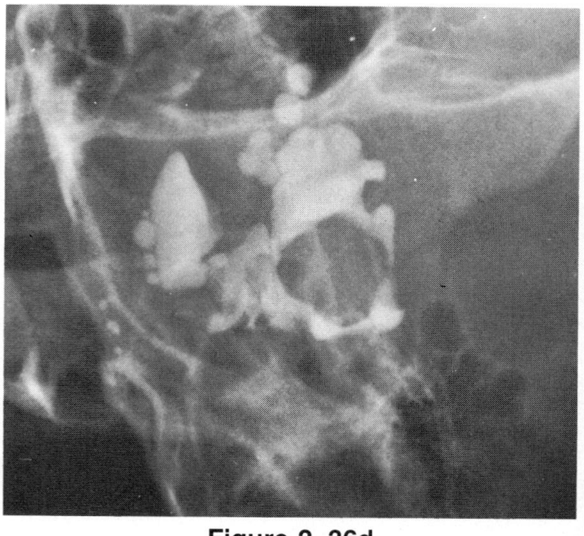

Figure 2–36d

c and d. A Pantopaque cisternogram discloses a slightly irregular rounded tumor mass at the porus acusticus of the right internal auditory canal. The anteroposterior view in the right lateral decubitus position (c) and the prone oblique view (d) demonstrate the tumor very well. The arrows mark the internal auditory canal on (c), and the tumor is noted to be outlined by the pool of Pantopaque.

e. Cut 1A, prior to the infusion, appears within normal limits. Cut 11A, obtained after the infusion of contrast, reveals enhancement of a small round area adjacent to the right internal auditory canal, consistent with an acoustic neurinoma. The fourth ventricle is in the midline (crossed arrow).

Note: We no longer do Pantopaque cisternograms in patients with hearing loss and the typical computed tomographic findings.

1A

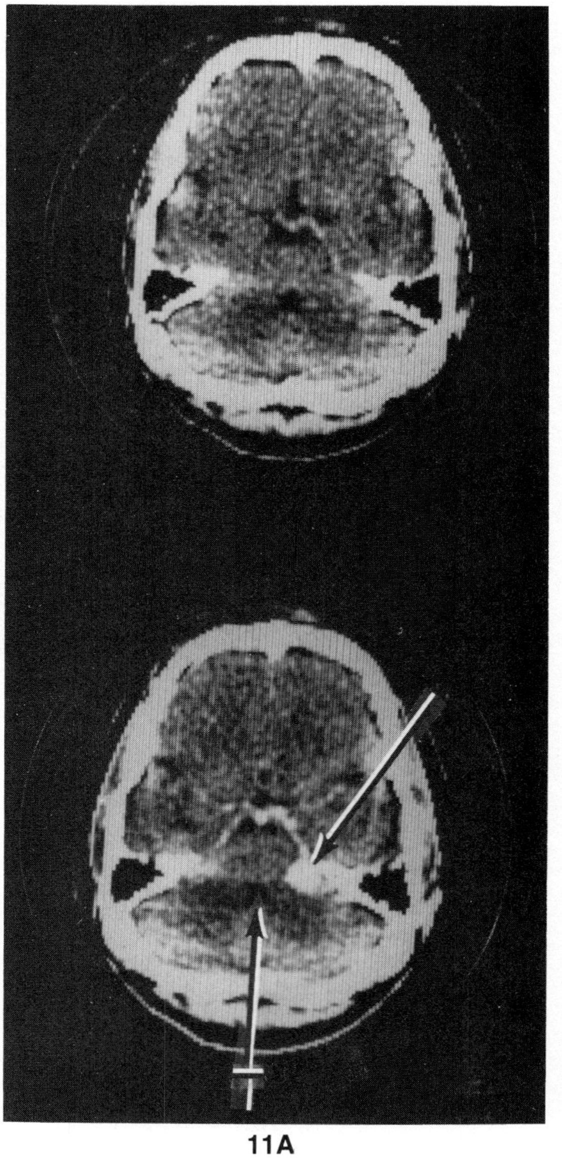

11A

Figure 2–36e

AIR CISTERNOGRAM (Figure 2–37)

This 56 year old male presented with deafness in the right ear.

a. The initial film of the air cisternogram reveals that there is air in the cerebellopontine angle cistern. The internal auditory canal is poorly visualized (arrow) at this setting.

b. The patient is placed so that the side of interest is superior in position. This causes the air to enter into the internal auditory canal in the normal patient. In this patient, a small soft tissue mass extends out of the canal and into the cerebellopontine angle cistern. This is consistent with a small acoustic neurinoma. It was not surgically proved.

Metrizamide cisternography can also be used for diagnosis of an extra-axial mass such as an acoustic neurinoma.

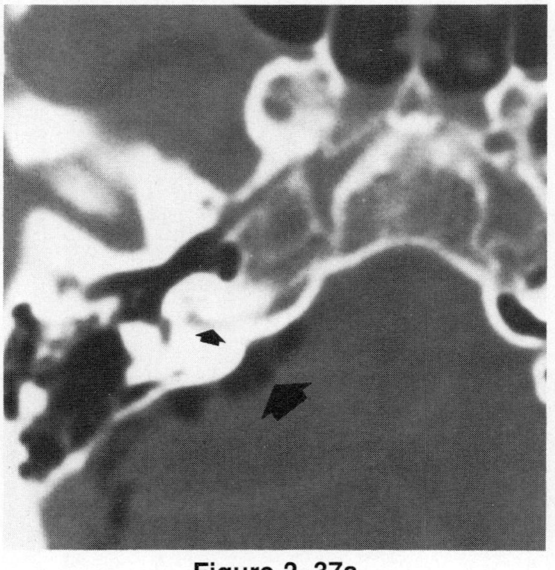

Figure 2–37a

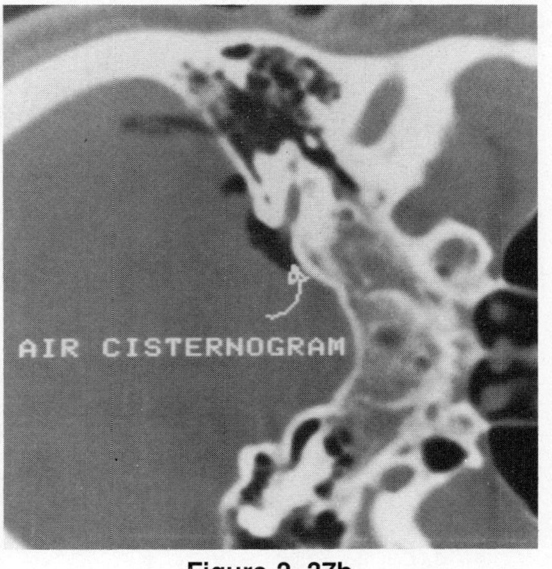

Figure 2–37b

LEFT ACOUSTIC NEURINOMA (Figure 2–38)

G. B. is a 31 year old female who presented with a history of progressive hearing loss in the left ear. The hearing loss had been rather insidious in onset.

a and b. Tomograms of the internal auditory canals bilaterally reveal a normal right internal auditory canal (a) and flaring of the left internal auditory canal and shortening of the posterior margin of the canal (arrows in b). There is no evidence of calcification and the findings are consistent with a left acoustic neurinoma.

c. The routine CT scan shows the internal auditory canals well (small arrows). There is an area of lucency just posterior to the anticipated position of the internal auditory canal. This represents a small cystic component of the tumor. The area of the tumor measures 20 to 30 u.

d. After the infusion of contrast, the acoustic neurinoma is noted to enhance markedly. The density is 54 to 76 u. Note that the tumor is rounded and rests just adjacent to the porus acusticus. The sigmoid sinus may enhance in this area and should not be mistaken for an acoustic tumor.

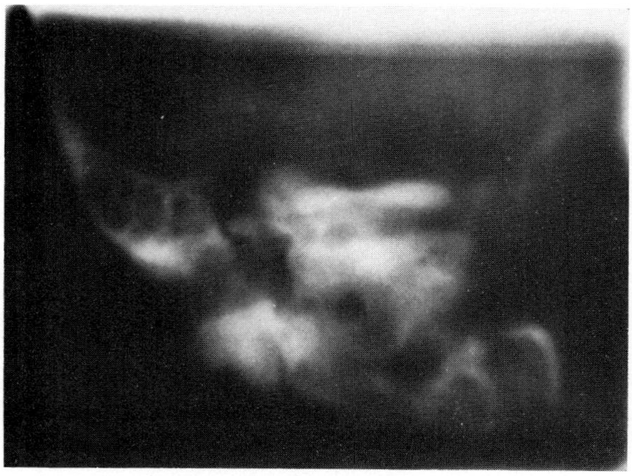

Figure 2–38a

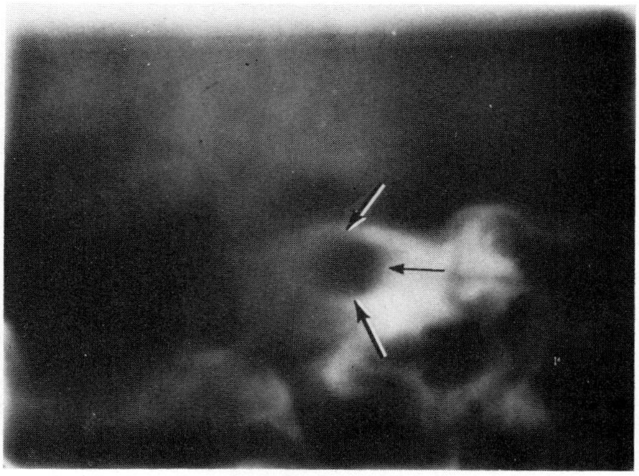

Figure 2–38b

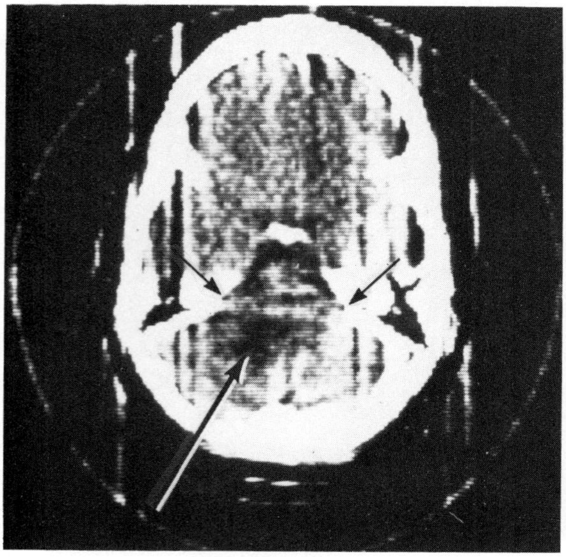

Figure 2–38c

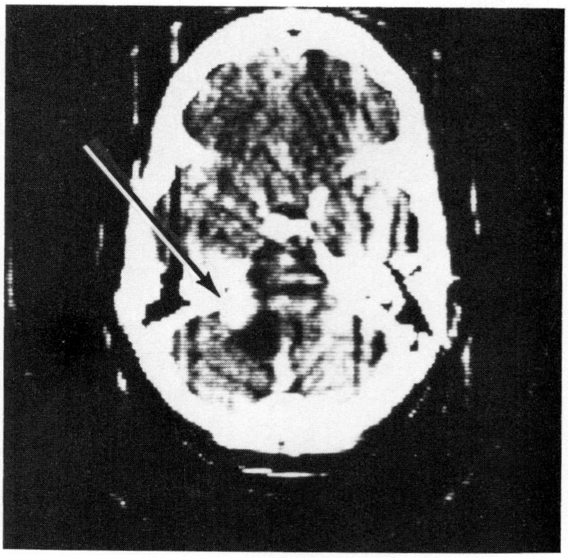

Figure 2–38d

LEFT ACOUSTIC NEURINOMA (Figure 2–39)

C. V. is a 65 year old female with a 1-year history of progressive hearing loss on the left side. Physical examination revealed a mild left facial palsy and a decreased corneal reflex on the left side in addition to the hearing loss on that side. Her past history was significant in that tomographic studies of the internal auditory canals obtained 1 year prior to this study revealed mild enlargement of the left internal auditory canal.

1A 2A

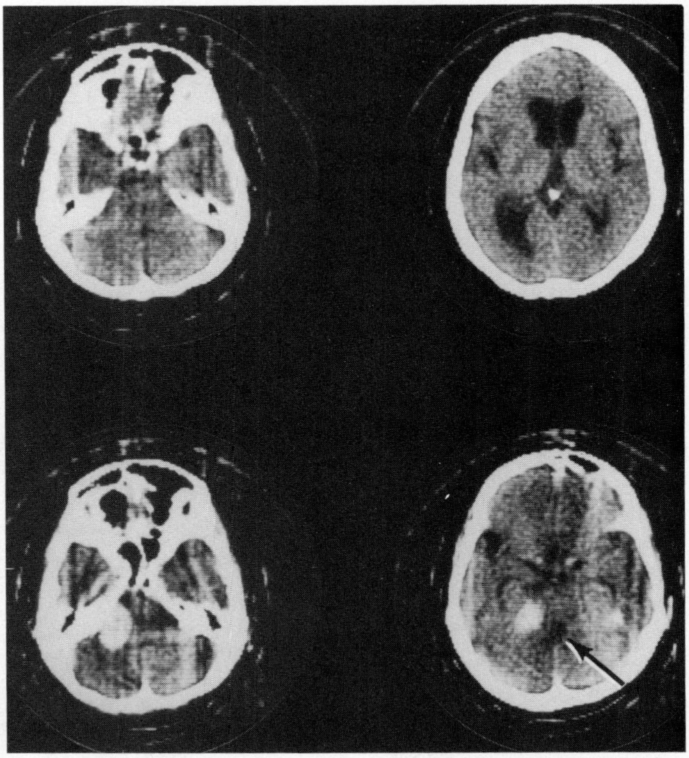

11B 11A

Figure 2–39a

a. The initial CT scan cuts through the level of the internal auditory canals appear unremarkable. The area of the tumor is isodense with the brain and measures 20 to 46 u on cut 1A. On cut 2A a mild symmetrical hydrocephalus is noted. Cuts 11A and 11B, obtained post infusion, reveal marked enhancement of the oval-shaped tumor, which appears to "hug" the internal auditory canal on the left side. The density increased to 56 to 110 u. The mild hydrocephalus is presumably secondary to mild obstruction at the level of the sylvian aqueduct. Note that the fourth ventricle appears to lie in the midline on cut 11B (arrow).

b. Cut 11A with electronic enhancement illustrates the surgically proved left acoustic neurinoma quite well (arrow).

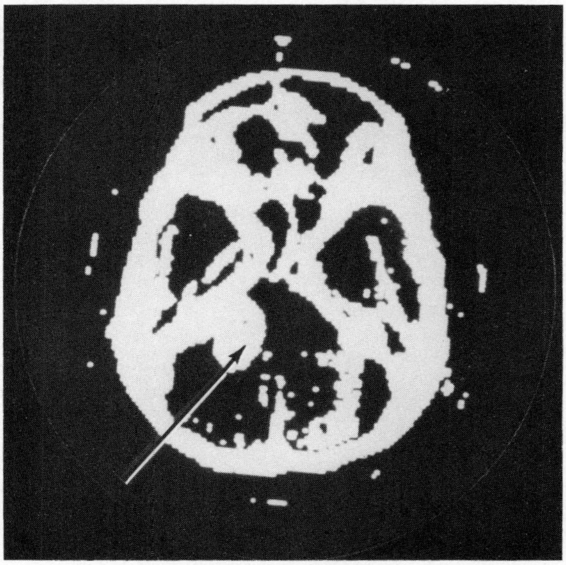

Figure 2–39b

LEFT ACOUSTIC NEURINOMA (Figure 2–40)

M. K. is a 62 year old female with left-sided hearing loss.

The preinfusion study, cut 1A, appears normal; density, 26 to 40 u. The postinfusion study, cut 11B, reveals a left acoustic neurinoma, density 48 to 78 u (arrow). Cuts 11A and 11B with electronic enhancement illustrate the tumor to better advantage.

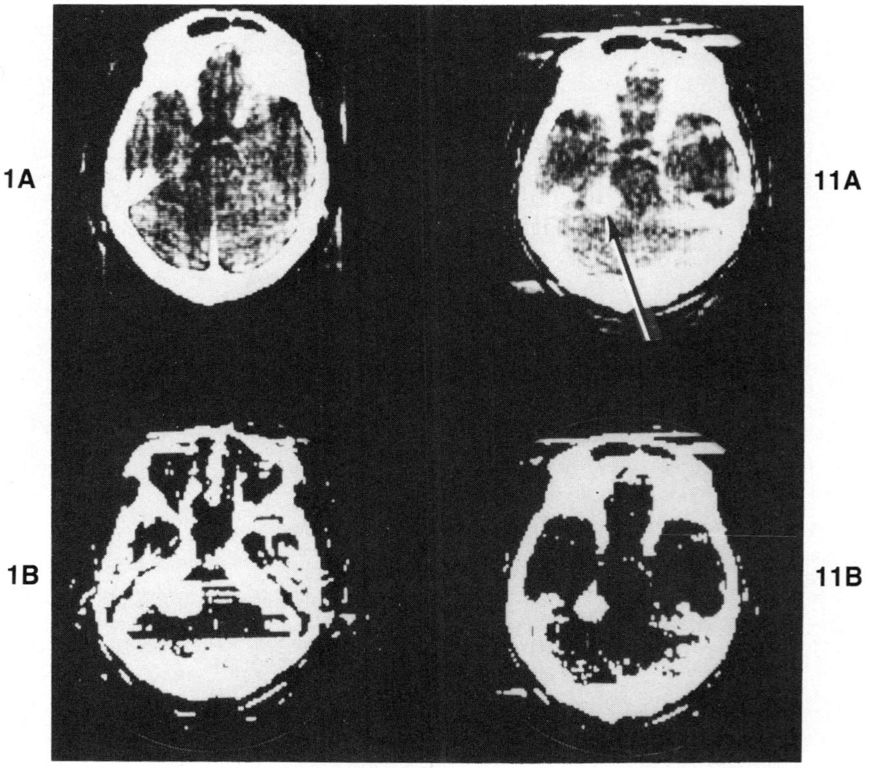

Figure 2–40

BILATERAL ACOUSTIC NEURINOMAS (Figure 2–41)

L. L. is a 23 year old male with bilateral hearing loss. There is no history of neurofibromatosis.

a. The preinfusion study reveals that the fourth ventricle (arrow) is shifted to the left. The density adjacent to the right petrous bone measures 28 to 46 u.

b. Cut 11A shows marked enhancement of the right acoustic neurinoma to a density of 60 to 110 u. A small left acoustic neurinoma is also present. Note also the enhancement of the lateral sinus on the left side (arrow) just at the level of its junction with the sigmoid sinus.

1A

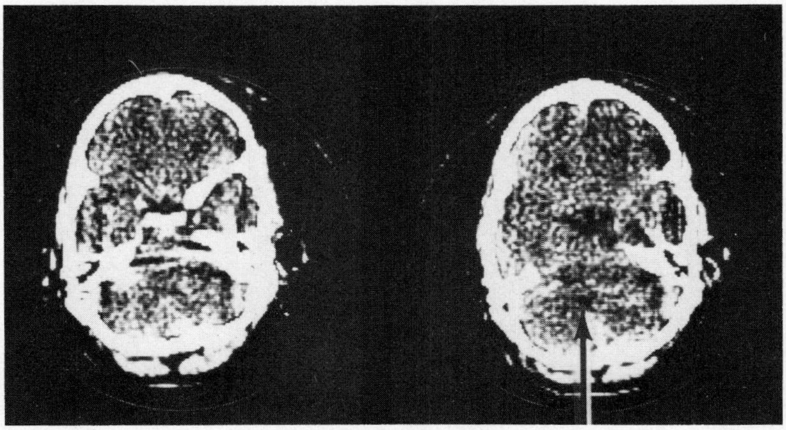

1B

Figure 2–41a

11A

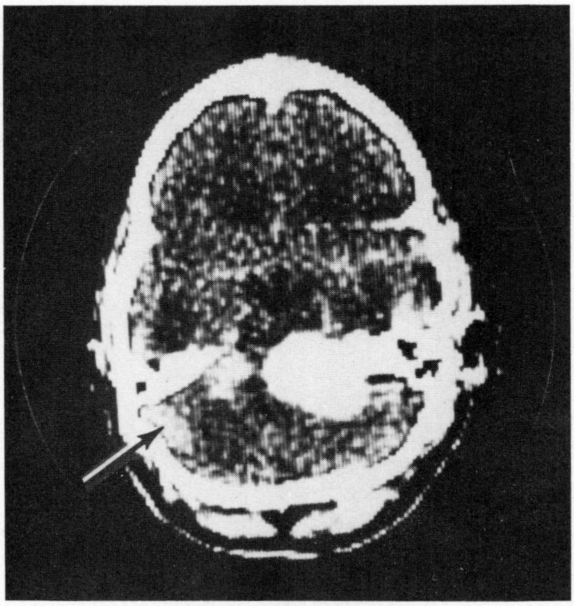

Figure 2–41b

LEFT ACOUSTIC NEURINOMA AND FALX MENINGIOMA (Figure 2–42)

M. S. is a 24 year old female with a history of hearing loss on the left side.

a. Cut 1A appears normal.

b. Cut 11A reveals a small left acoustic neurinoma.

c. Cut 3A appears unremarkable.

d. Cut 13A reveals a small unsuspected meningioma (surgically confirmed) that appears to arise from the falx cerebri and extend to the left side.

Interestingly, M. S. is the older sib of R. S. (see p. 107). A third female sibling had bilateral acoustic neurinomas, and a fourth female sib had a unilateral acoustic neurinoma. Family history revealed that the mother had died at age 28 following several years of "staggering gait" (?ataxia) and hearing loss on one side.

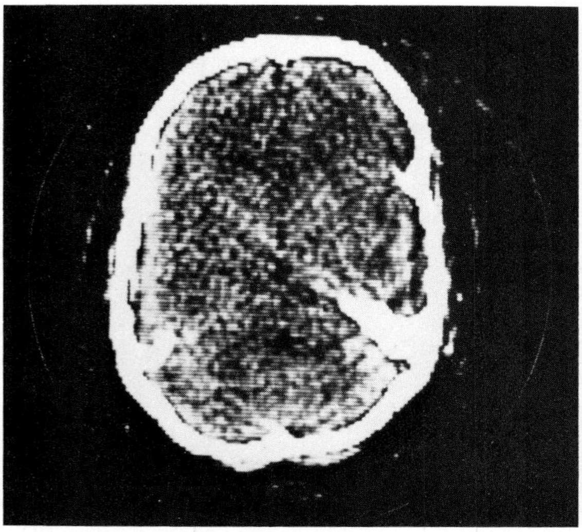

Figure 2–42a

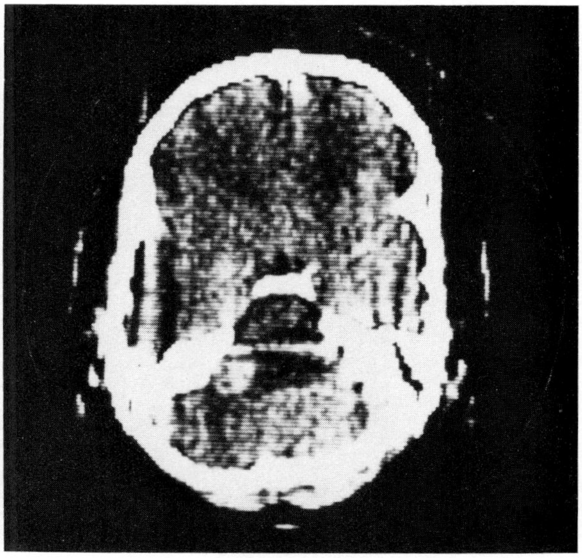

Figure 2–42b

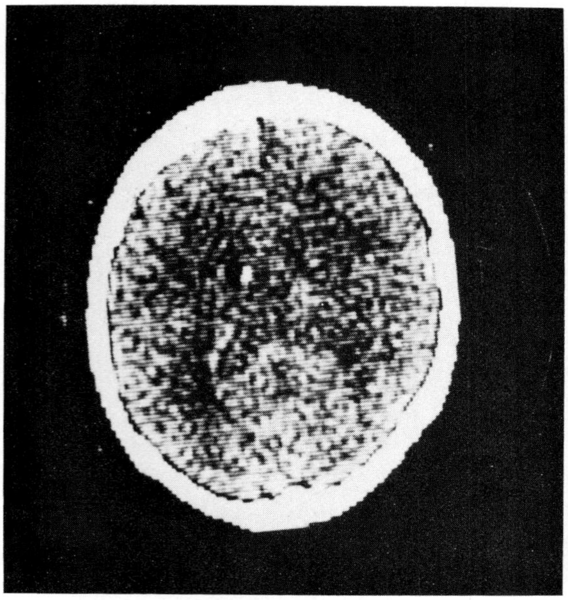

Figure 2–42c

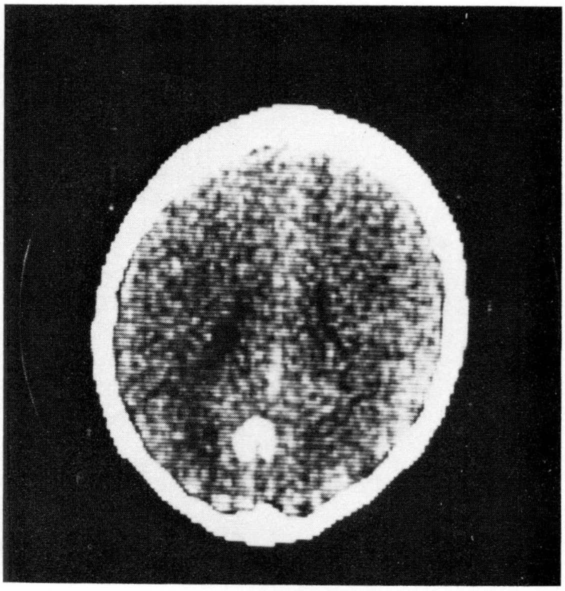

Figure 2–42d

RIGHT ACOUSTIC NEURINOMA (Figure 2–43)

R. S. is a 16 year old male with right-sided hearing loss.

Cut 1A reveals a density in the area of the tumor of 32 to 46 u. Cut 11A shows marked enhancement of a large right acoustic neurinoma, density 50 to 86 u. The fourth ventricle is displaced to the left side and compressed along the right side as well (arrow).

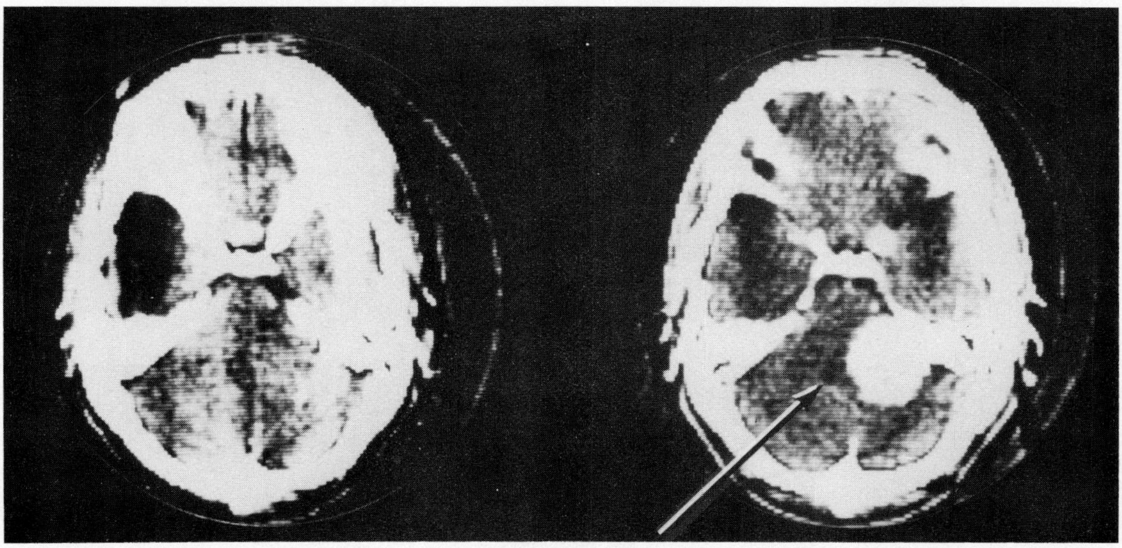

Figure 2–43

Posterior Fossa Tumors

CEREBELLAR ASTROCYTOMA (?GANGLIONEUROMA) (Figure 2–44)

S. D. is a 6 year old male who presented with multiple cranial nerve palsies. He appeared markedy wasted and listless. Routine skull films revealed widening of the coronal sutures.

a and b. The radionuclide scan reveals a definite mass lesion in the right cerebellum. This is best seen on the posterior (a) view, but can also be identified on the right lateral (b) view.

c. The routine CT scan shows a small linear calcification in the cerebellum just to the right of the midline, which is best seen on cut 1A. Surrounding the calcification there appear to be bilateral areas of lucency (arrows on 1A and 11A). The fourth ventricle could never be identified with certainty. There is mild to moderate obstructive hydrocephalus.

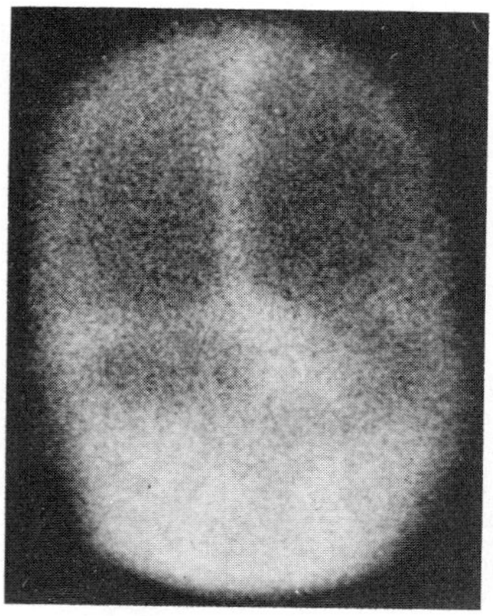

Figure 2–44a

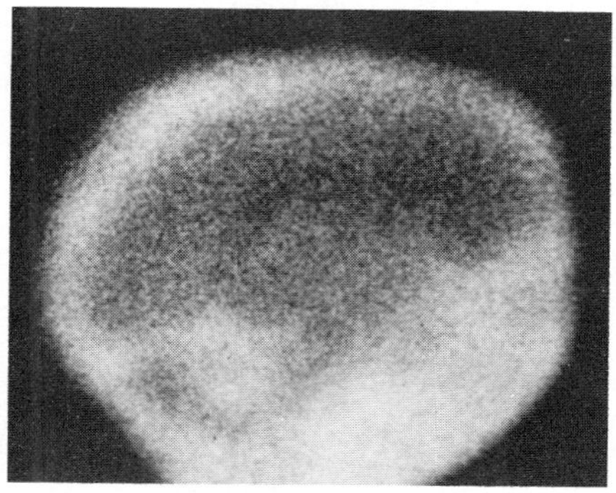

Figure 2–44b

1A 2A

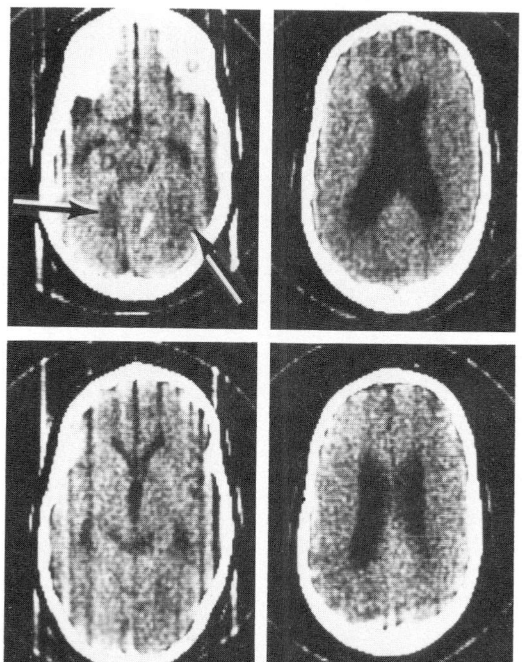

1B 2B

Figure 2–44c

11A

11B

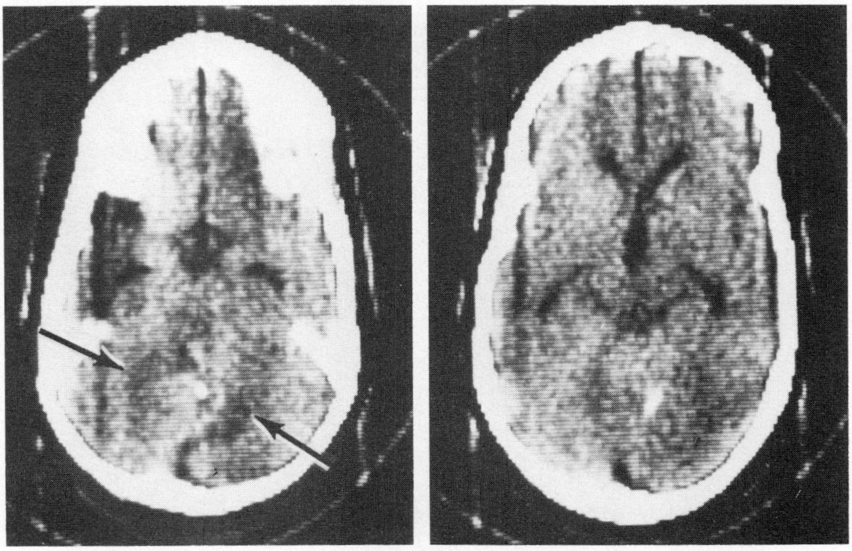

Figure 2–44d

d. Following contrast enhancement, no definite tumor mass could be identified.

e and f. Following a shunt procedure, a Pantopaque ventriculogram reveals that the fourth ventricle appears intact but displaced to the left of the midline.

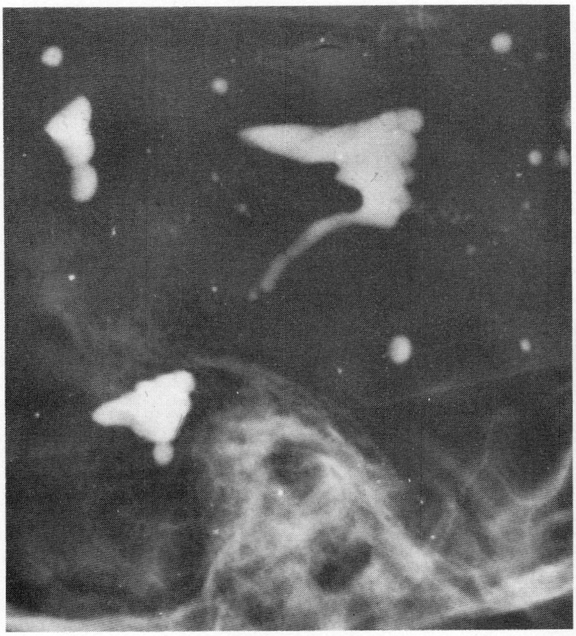

Figure 2–44e

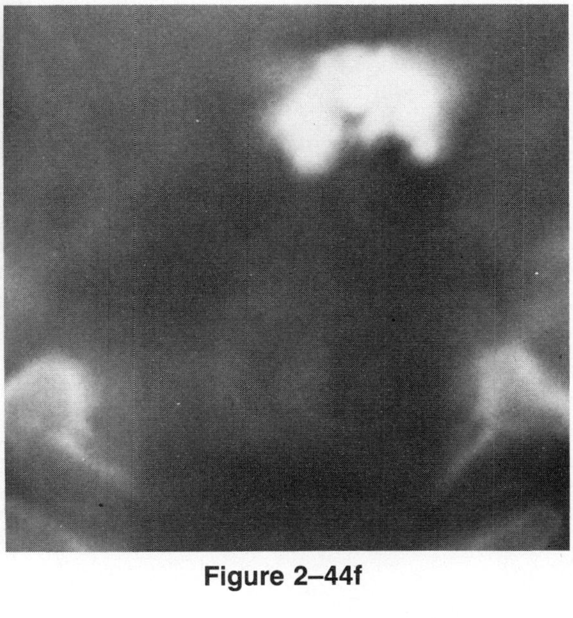

Figure 2–44f

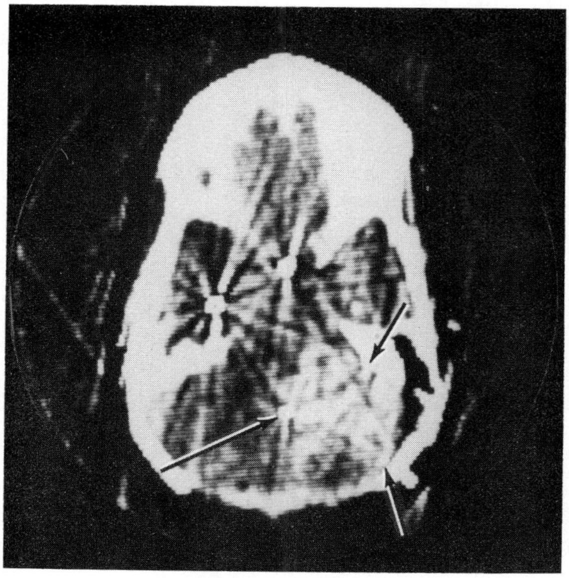

Figure 2–44g

Surgery disclosed a multicystic tumor arising from the right cerebellar tonsil. It appeared to be an astrocytoma; however, histologically it was a ganglioneurinoma.

g. Six months later, the postinfusion scan reveals a large, solid-appearing area of recurrent tumor occupying the entire right cerebellar hemisphere.

MEDULLOBLASTOMA (Figure 2–45)

L. P. is a 13 year old male who presented with nausea, vomiting, and cerebellar ataxia.

a. The routine CT scan shows an area of increased density in the typical midline position in the posterior fossa that measured from 28 to 50 u. There was moderate obstructive hydrocephalus (not shown).

b. Following the infusion of contrast material, this area has increased in density to 38 to 82 u. The mass is surrounded by an area of edema bilaterally, but more on the right than on the left side. At surgery, a medulloblastoma was removed.

c. The postoperative study reveals the craniectomy in the occipital bone. The fourth ventricle is displaced anteriorly and to the left (arrow). There is a remaining area of increased density noted on cut 1A as well as some surrounding edema; however, this area did not enhance with contrast infusion and may be a postoperative change. Additional follow-up scans are essential for complete study.

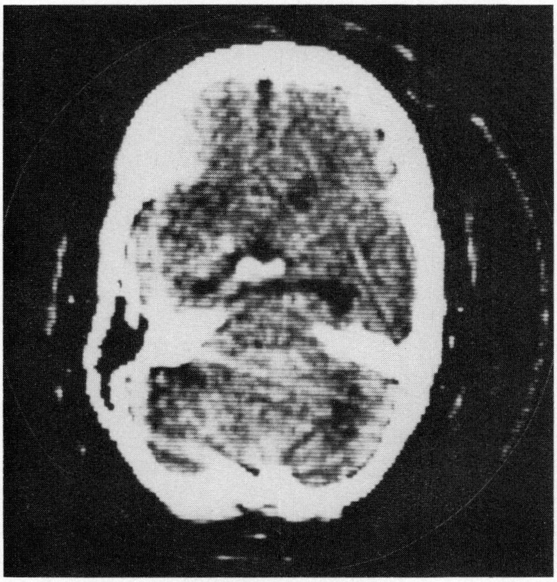

Figure 2–45a

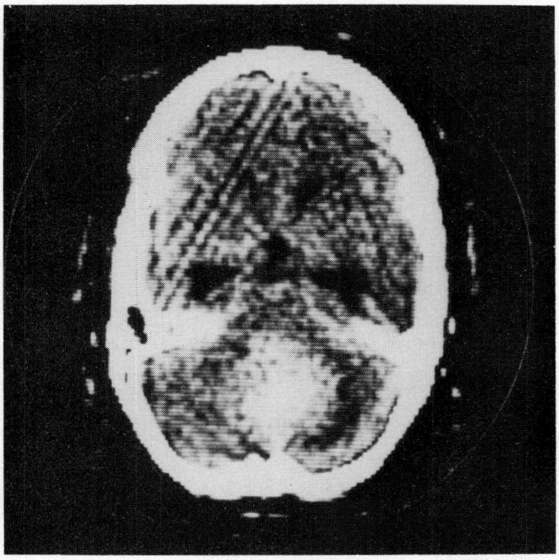

Figure 2–45b

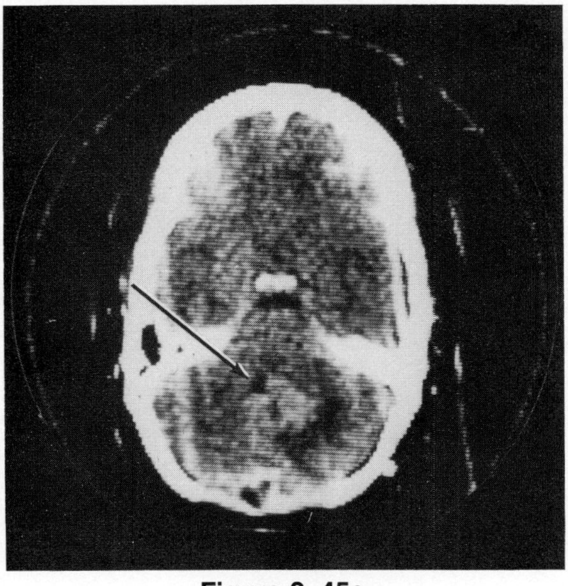

Figure 2–45c

MEDULLOBLASTOMA (Figure 2–46)

B. L. is a 12 year old male with known neurofibromatosis who had had a previous enucleation of the left eye for an optic glioma. He presented at this time with severe neck pain and weakness of the arms.

a. The posterior view of the radionuclide scan shows a small area of increased activity in the midline below the level of the transverse sinuses (arrow).

b and c. The routine CT scan reveals mild obstructive hydrocephalus. A shunt procedure had been performed in anticipation of the posterior fossa surgery, and the starburst computer artifact can be seen on cut 1A. The artifact obscures the midline tumor on the preinfusion study.

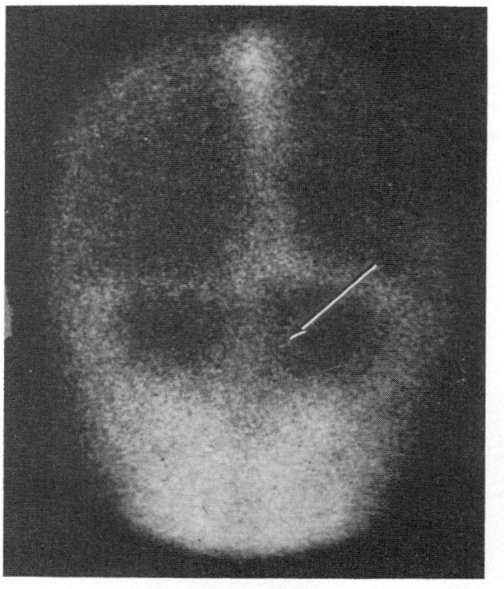

Figure 2–46a

1A

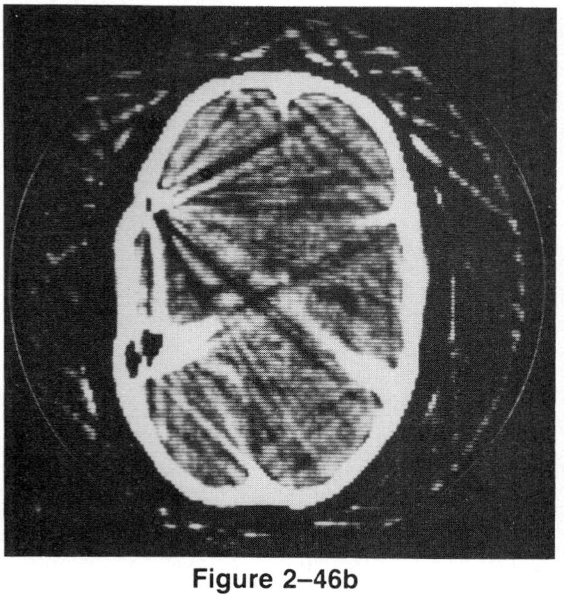

Figure 2–46b

2A

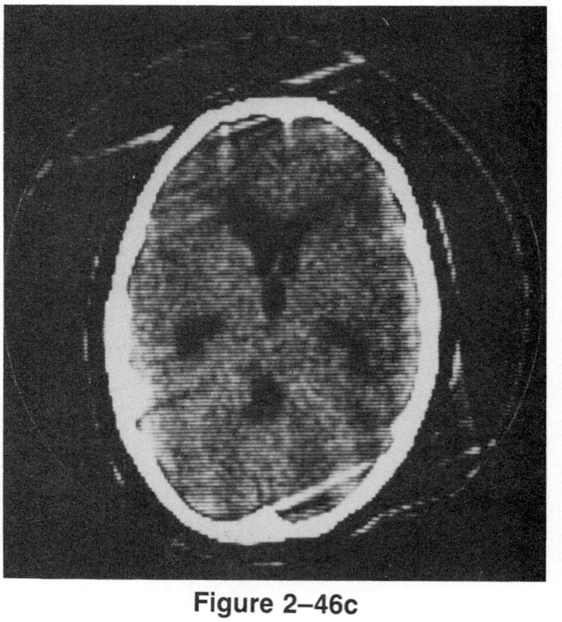

Figure 2–46c

11A 11B

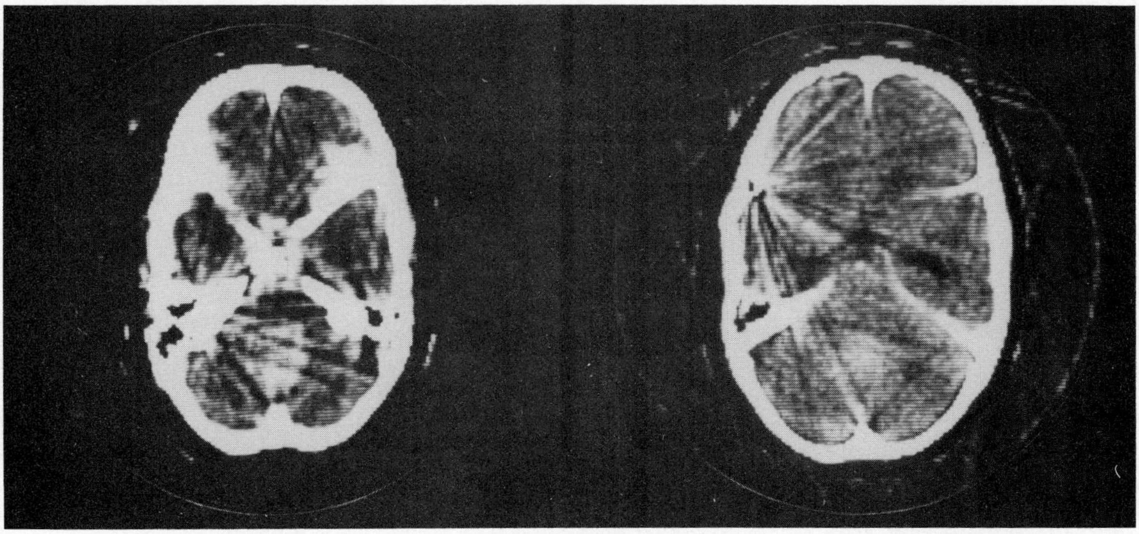

Figure 2–46d

d. Following contrast enhancement, a round, solid-appearing mass is seen in the midline in the posterior fossa. The appearance is typical of a medulloblastoma.

At surgery, a medulloblastoma (? medullary astrocytoma) was partially removed. The tumor was found to extend far inferiorly into the upper cervical cord.

PONTINE GLIOMA (Figure 2–47)

L. B. is a 17 year old, markedly obese female who presented with a 6-month history of amenorrhea and recent onset of diplopia, polydipsia, and polyurea. Physical examination revealed marked obesity and a left sixth nerve palsy. She was noted to have mild weakness of the right arm.

a and b. The posterior (a) and left lateral (b) views of the radionuclide scan reveal a questionable area of increased uptake in the midline in the posterior fossa.

c. The routine CT scan discloses an area of increased density in the pons just to the left of the midline (arrow) that measured 34 to 50 u.

d and e. Following the infusion of contrast material, this area has increased to a density of 46 to 70

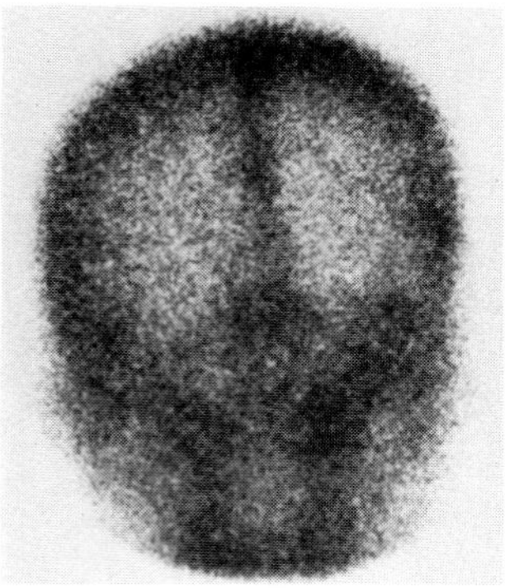

Figure 2–47a

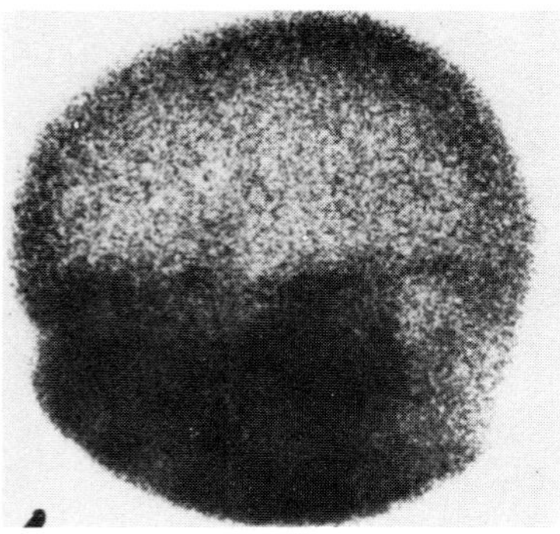

Figure 2–47b

11A

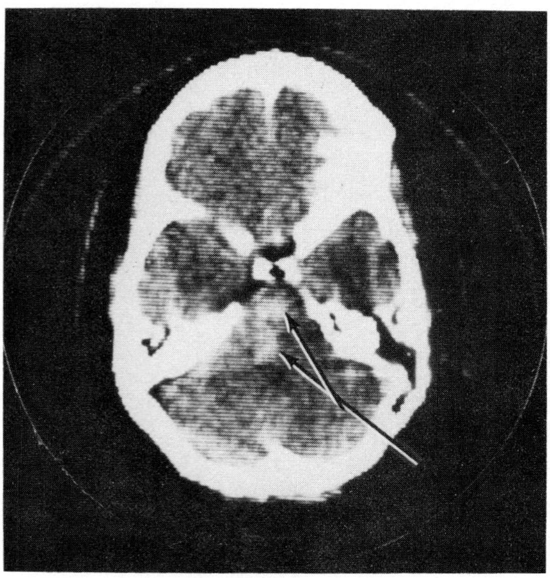

Figure 2–47d

1A

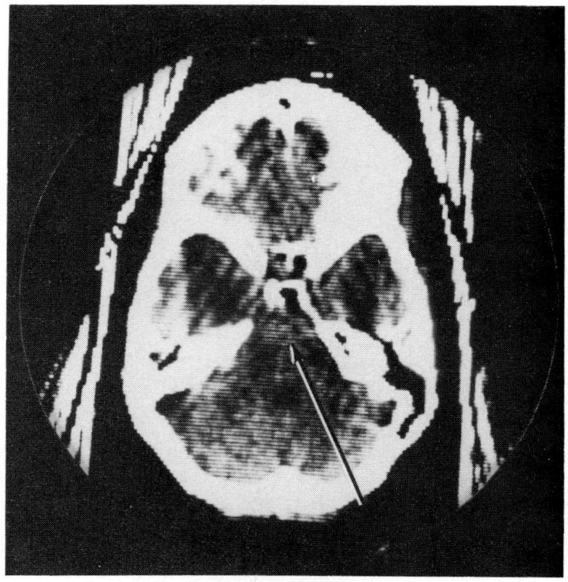

Figure 2–47c

11A

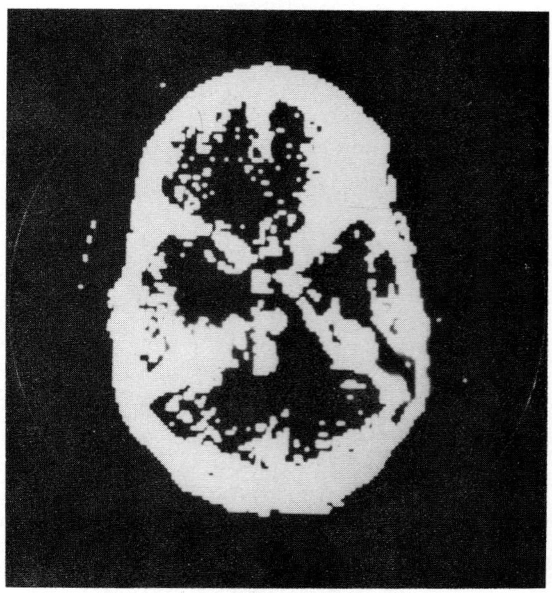

Figure 2–47e

u. The mass is noted to have a bilobed appearance, to be in the midline and just to the left of the midline anteriorly, and to extend farther to the left in its more posterior extent (arrows). Cut 11A with electronic enhancement reveals the bilobed area of enhancement to better advantage.

f. The anteroposterior arterial view of the left vertebral arteriogram shows elevation of the left superior cerebellar artery, but is otherwise unremarkable (arrows).

g. On the lateral arterial view of the left vertebral arteriogram, the basilar artery is closely applied to the clivus in its mid-portion. The posterior inferior cerebellar artery appears in normal position. The left superior cerebellar artery is elevated and overlaps the posterior cerebral arteries (upper two arrows); the right superior cerebellar artery is in normal position (three arrows).

h. The venous phase reveals straightening of the precentral cerebellar vein (arrows). This view is normally convex anteriorly. Ventriculography (not shown) reveals minimal backward displacement of the fourth ventricle.

The diagnosis was thought to be a pontine glioma, and radiotherapy was given.

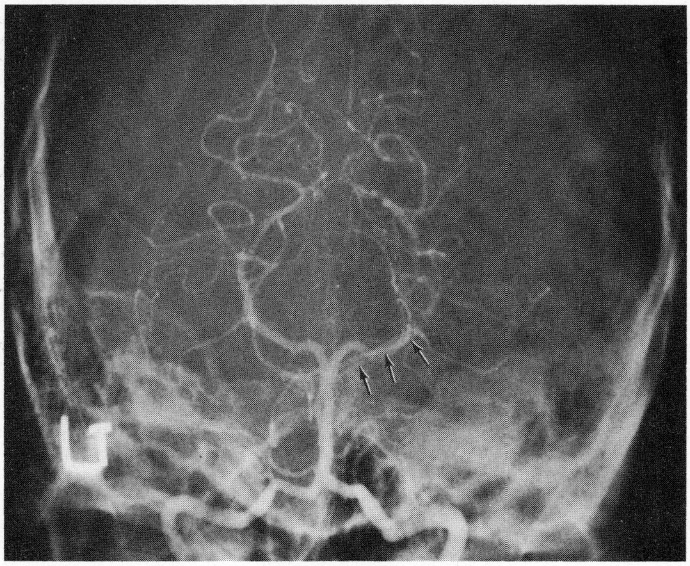

Figure 2–47f

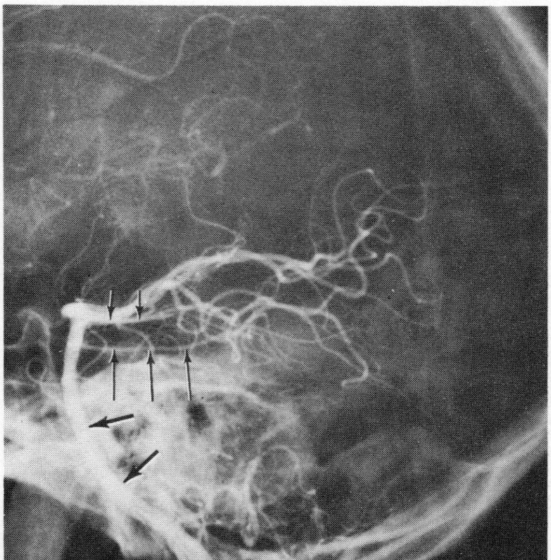

Figure 2–47g

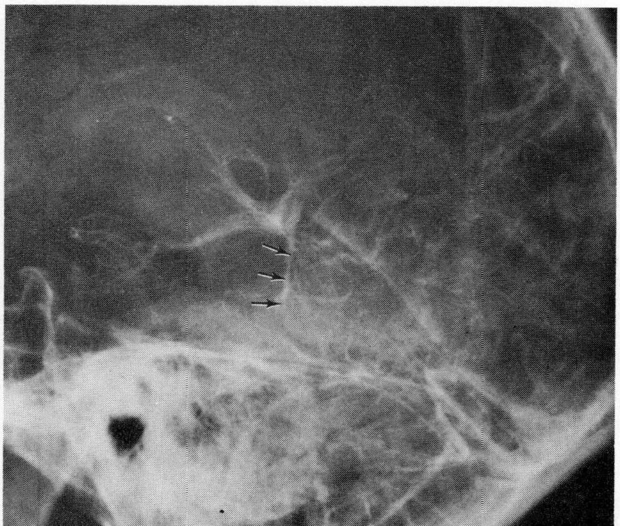

Figure 2–47h

PONTINE GLIOMA (Figure 2–48)

C. D. is an 11 year old female who presented with diplopia and mild ataxia.

a to c. A left brachial arteriogram shows questionable elevation of the superior cerebellar arteries, but no gross vascular displacements.

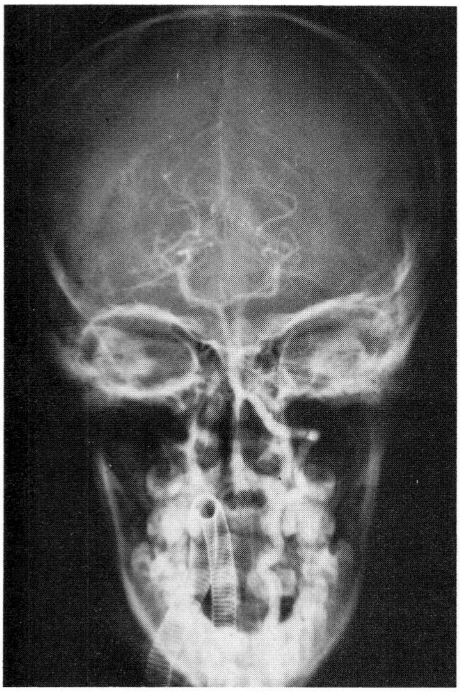

Figure 2–48a

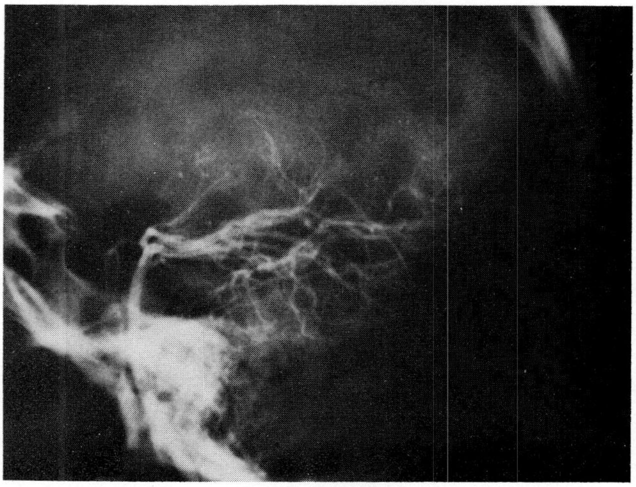

Figure 2–48b

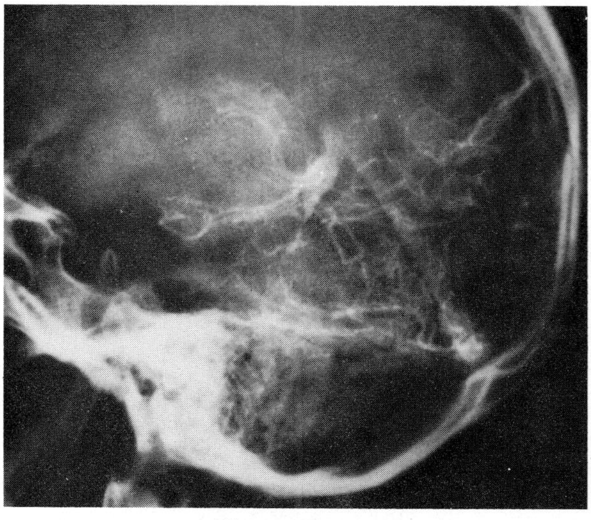

Figure 2–48c

d. The routine CT scan at the time of arteriography (upper row) reveals no evidence of hydrocephalus. The fourth ventricle is questionably displaced posteriorly (arrow).

The patient returned two months later with diplopia and bilateral facial nerve palsies. A right hemiparesis, a tenth nerve palsy, and slight ataxia were also noted.

d. (lower row). Routine CT scan at this time reveals definite enlargement of the pons. The fourth ventricle is flattened and displaced posteriorly (arrow on 1A). There is now mild obstructive hydrocephalus.

e and f. A Pantopaque ventriculogram following a shunting procedure reveals flattening and upward displacement of the fourth ventricle (arrows on e) and marked posterior displacement of the fourth ventricle (arrow on f) secondary to enlargement of the pons.

1A **2A**

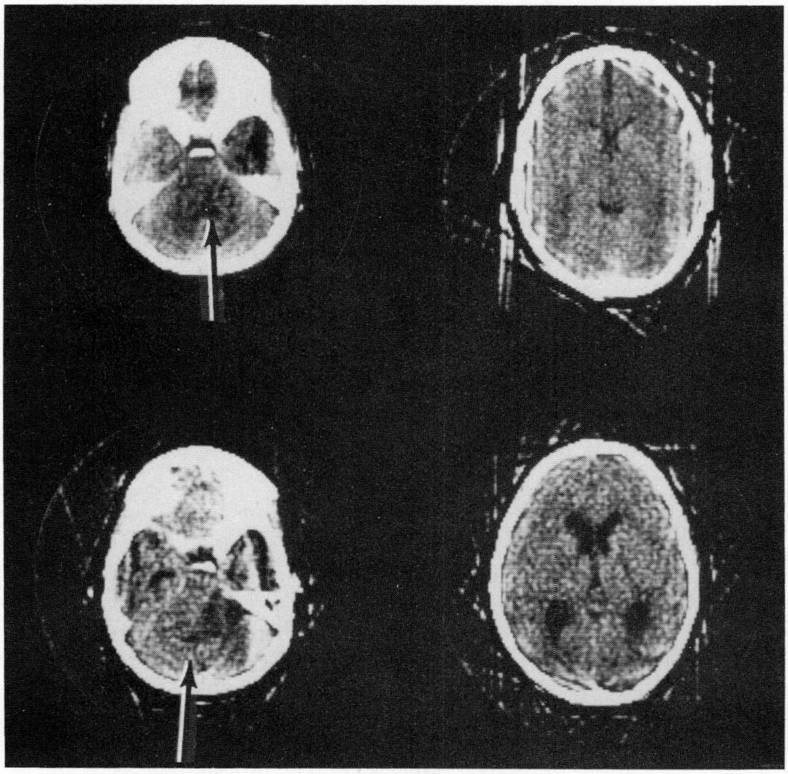

1A **Figure 2–48d** **2A**

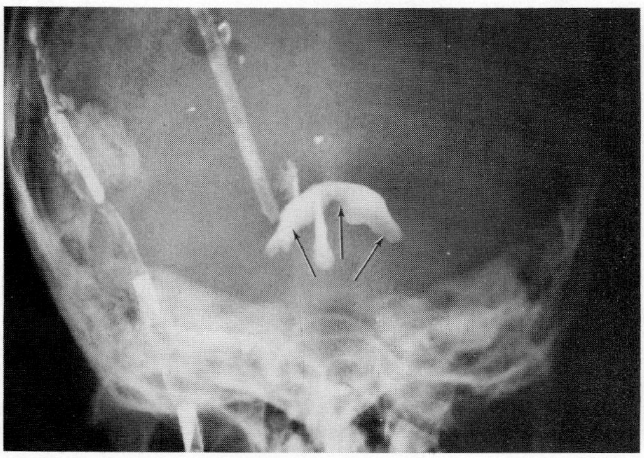

Figure 2–48e

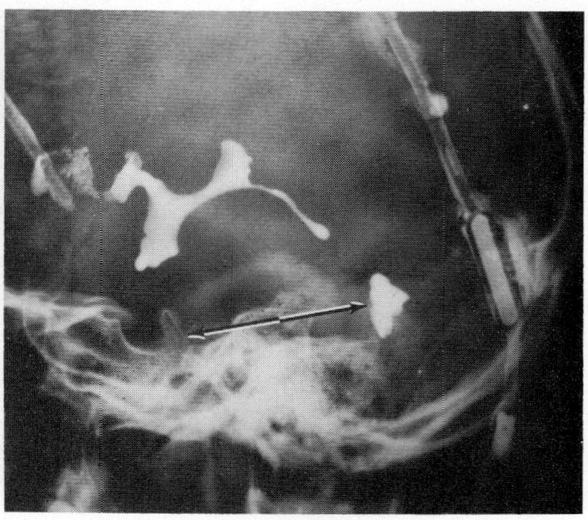

Figure 2–48f

g and h. At postmortem examination, a view of the base of the brain reveals diffuse enlargement of the left side of the pons and medulla (arrows on g). Cut sections through the pons show diffuse enlargement of the pons, more marked on the left side (arrows on h) and the hemorrhagic infarction of the central medulla (crossed arrow) that was the cause of this patient's demise.

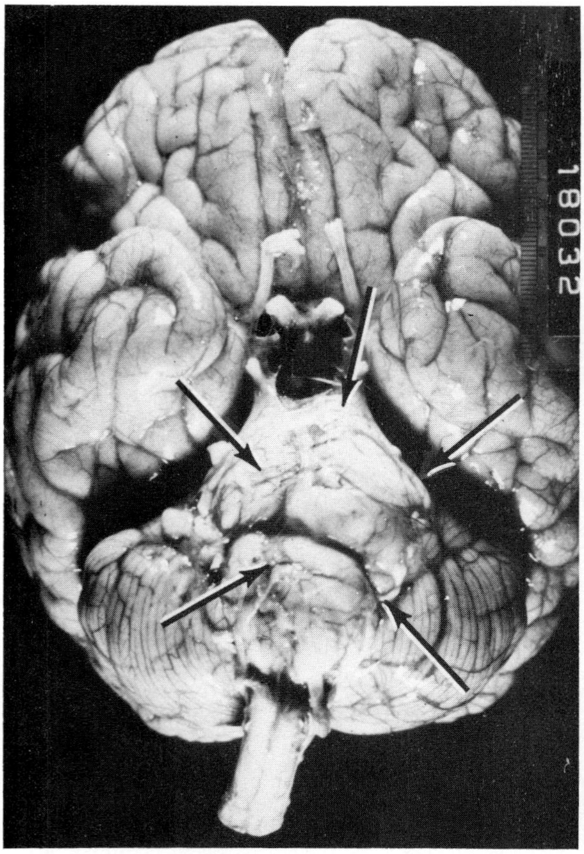

Figure 2–48g

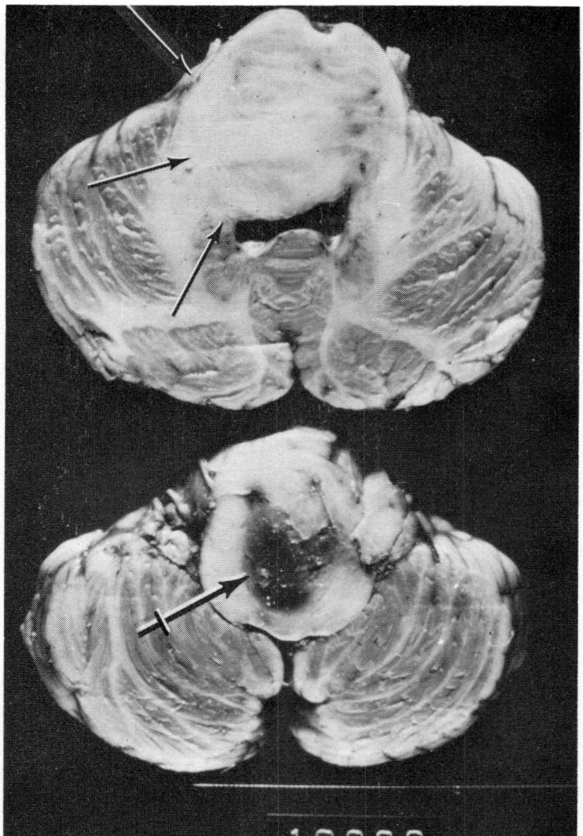

Figure 2–48h

MEDULLOBLASTOMA (Figure 2–49)

C. L. is a 21 year old man with a known medulloblastoma, who had had previous surgery and now entered with nausea, vomiting, and ataxia.

a and b. Posterior (a) and left lateral (b) radionuclide scans revealed a large area of increased activity in the left posterior fossa. A second small area of increased activity is noted in the left parietal area, possibly secondary to the shunt procedure.

c. The routine CT scan reveals the postsurgical changes in the posterior fossa; the fourth ventricle was never well seen.

d. After contrast infusion, there is marked enhancement of a large mass lesion in the left cerebellum. The area appears irregular in outline, and was felt to represent recurrent medulloblastoma (arrows).

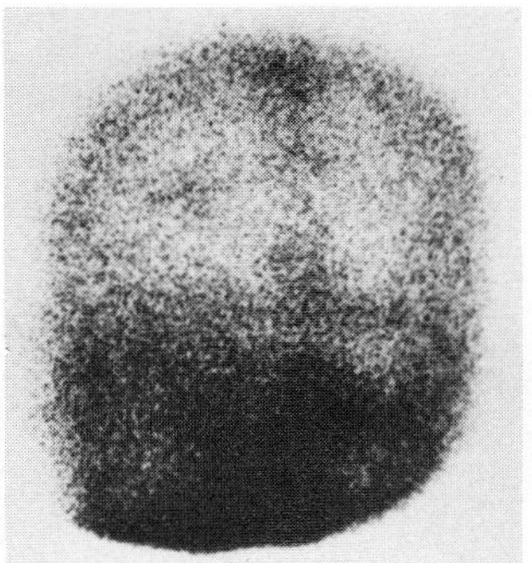

Figure 2–49a

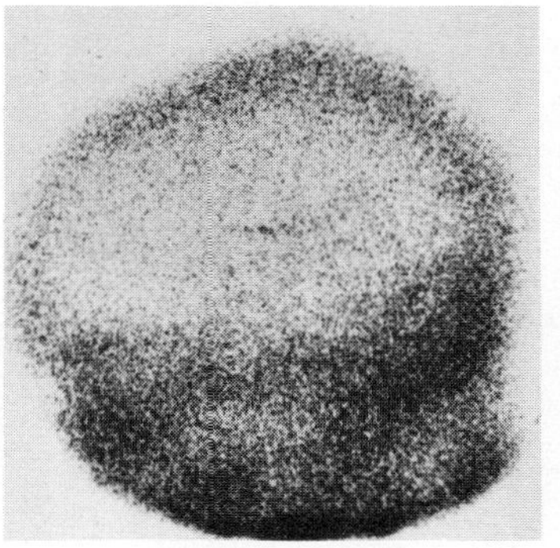

Figure 2–49b

1A

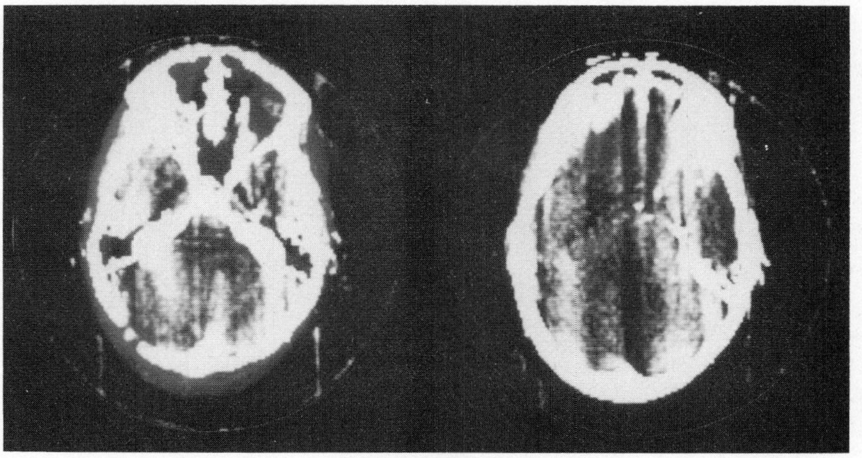

1B

Figure 2–49c

11B

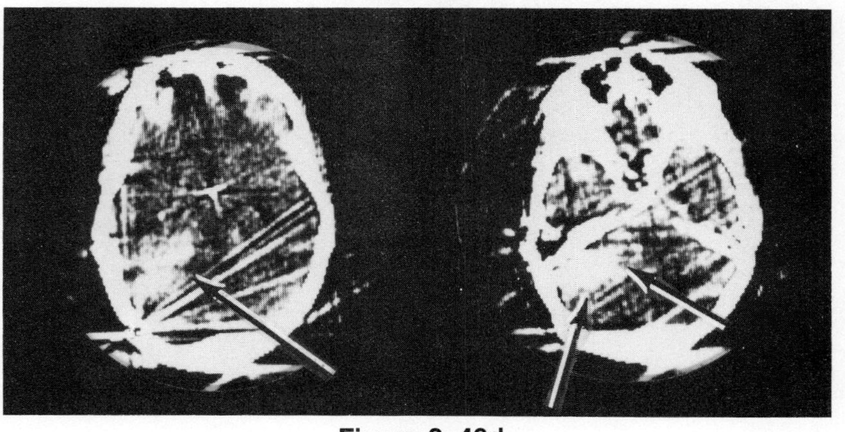

11A

Figure 2–49d

e and f. Left brachial arteriogram reveals the postsurgical changes and a large irregular area of stain corresponding to the abnormal area seen on the CT scan (see arrows). (The patient's condition deteriorated rapidly and he died shortly after these studies.)

g. Postmortem examination discloses that the entire left cerebellum appears to be replaced by the recurrent medulloblastoma (arrows). In addition, at the time of death the tumor had metastasized upward to involve the frontal lobes as well.

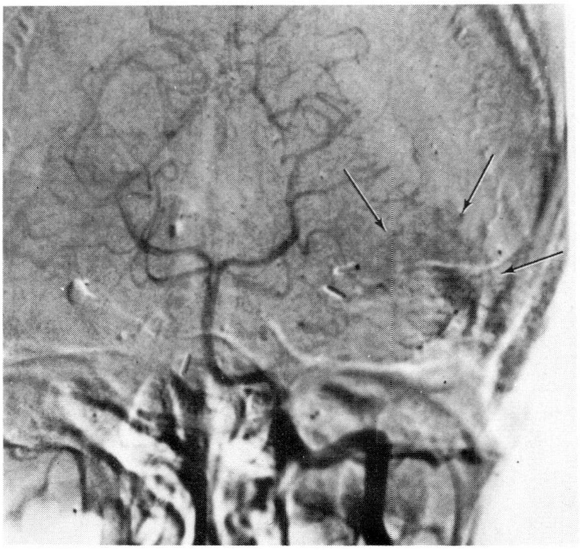

Figure 2–49e

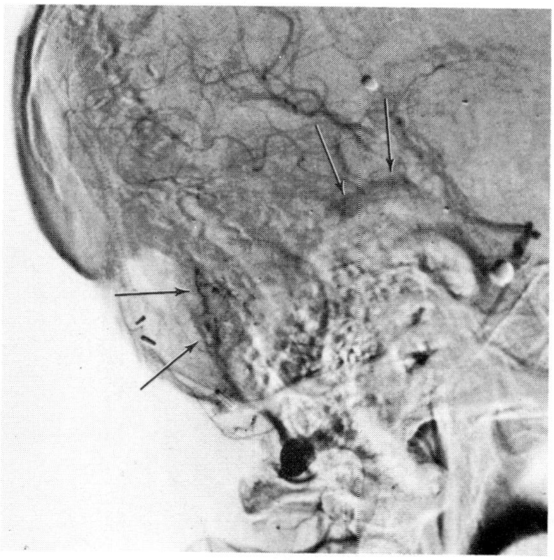

Figure 2–49f

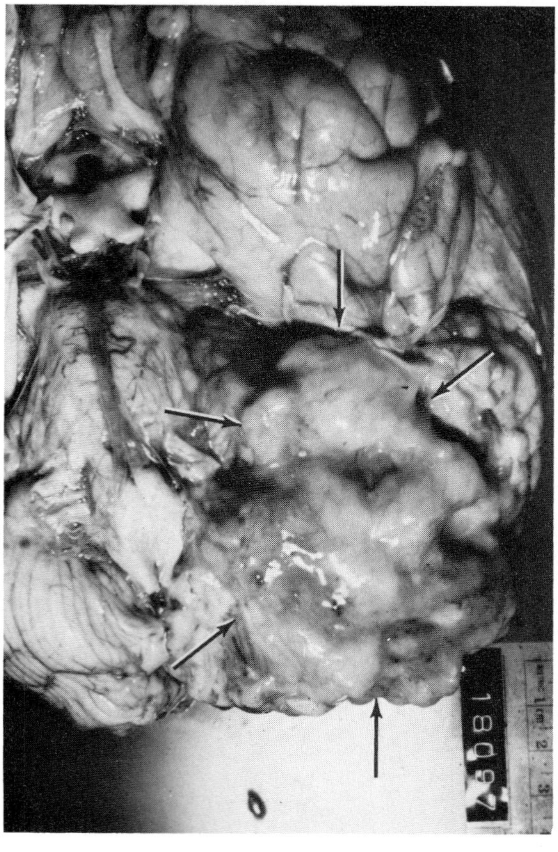

Figure 2–49g

CEREBELLAR ASTROCYTOMA (Figure 2–50)

R. E. is a 49 year old male who initially presented 2 years previously with left-sided hearing loss, nausea, vomiting, and ataxia.

a and b. Internal auditory canal tomograms reveal marked end of the left internal auditory canal (arrows). The right side appears normal.

c and d. Left lateral (c) and posterior views (d) obtained at the time of the original admission demonstrate an area of increased uptake of the radionuclide in the left cerebellum (arrows). Surgery revealed an astrocytoma that had eroded into the left internal auditory canal.

e. Radionuclide scan on the present admission shows the postsurgical changes in the posterior fossa on the left side, but no other abnormalities.

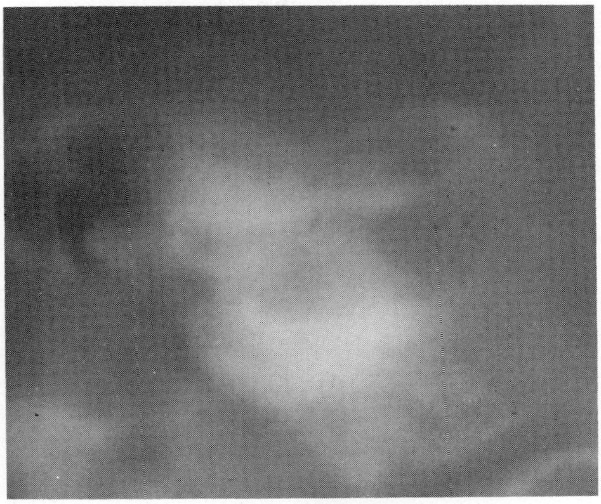

Figure 2–50a

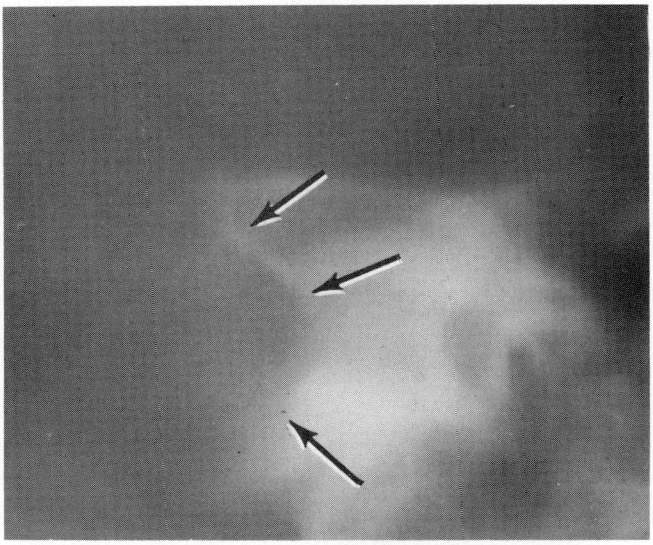

Figure 2–50b

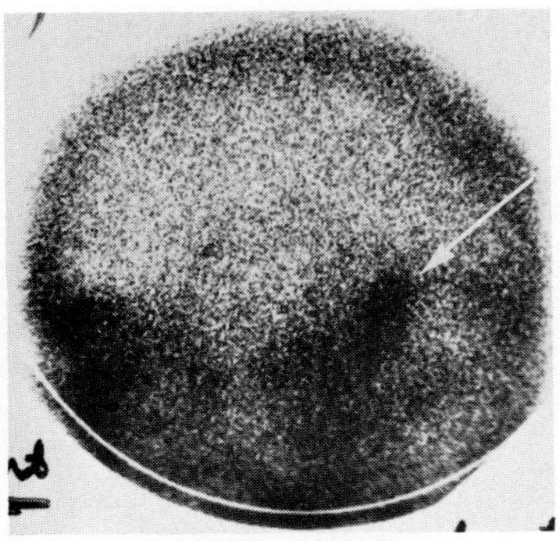

Figure 2–50c

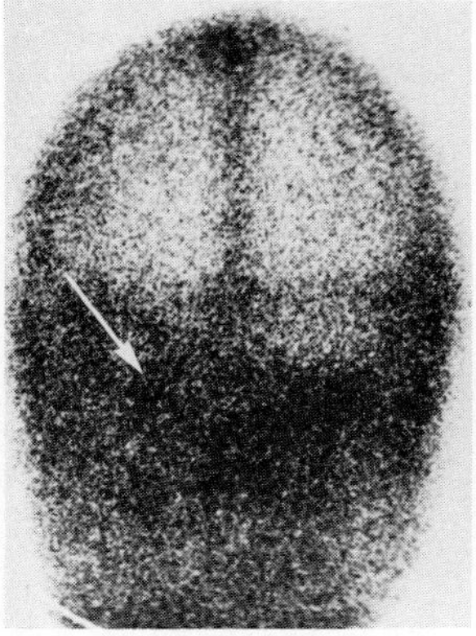

Figure 2–50d

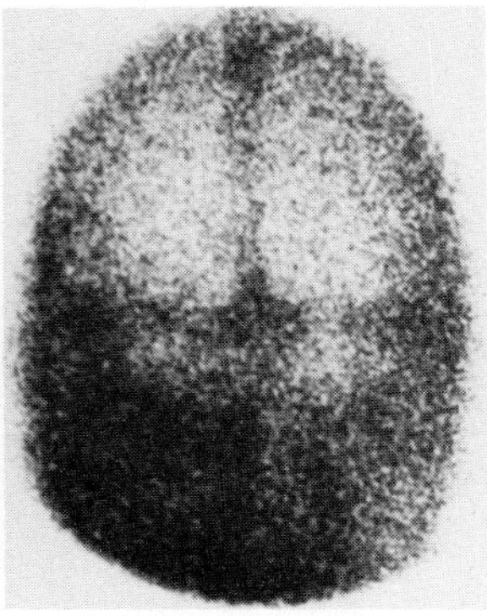

Figure 2–50e

f. The routine CT scan reveals a cystic area in the posterior fossa to the right of the midline adjacent to the right internal auditory canal (arrows). There was mild obstructive hydrocephalus.

g. Contrast enhancement reveals a thick rim of increased density around the previously noted cystic area. These findings are consistent with a diagnosis of cystic posterior fossa astrocytoma.

h. Right vertebral arteriogram demonstrates that the basilar artery is displaced to the left of the midline.

i. The lateral arterial phase reveals downward displacement of the posterior inferior cerebellar artery, close apposition of the basilar artery to the clivus, and a large avascular area in the right cerebellum (arrows).

Surgery revealed a cystic astrocytoma.

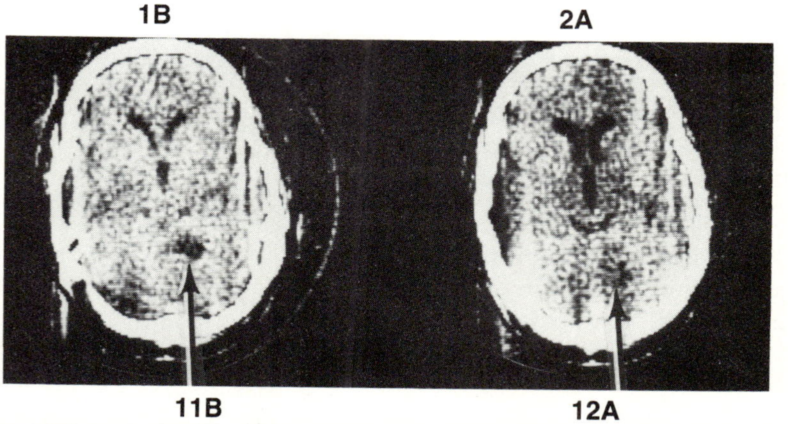

Figure 2–50f

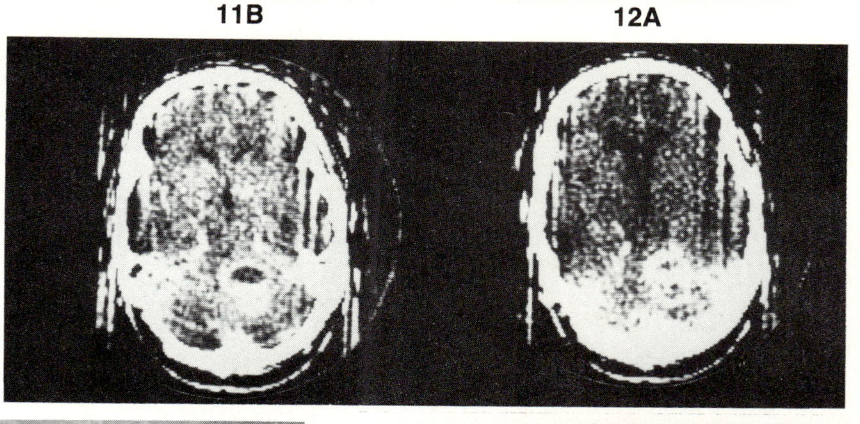

Figure 2–50g

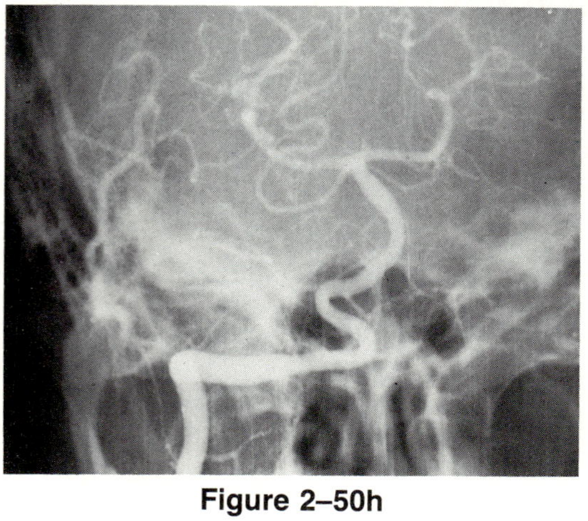

Figure 2–50h

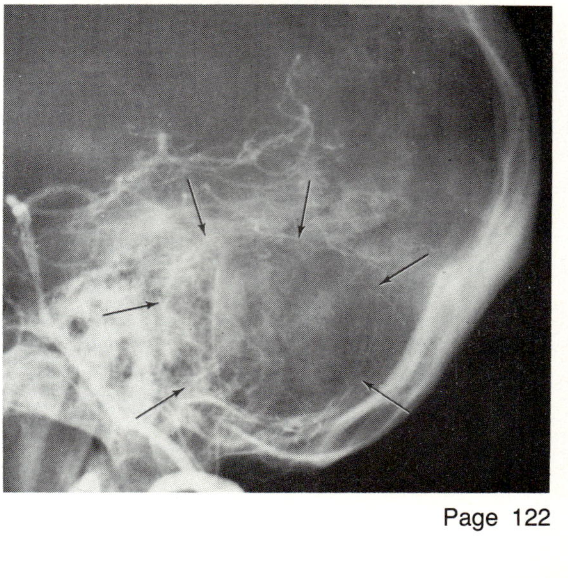

Figure 2–50i

CLIVUS MENINGIOMA (Figure 2–51)

This 76 year old female was transferred from a nursing home in a coma. There were no focal neurologic findings.

a and b. Two cuts from the postinfusion portion of the examination reveal a homogeneously enhancing mass (X) arising from the clivus. There is mild surrounding edema and the fourth ventricle is displaced posteriorly and flattened (arrow). The enlarged cerebellopontine angle cisterns (arrowhead) are consistent with an extra-axial mass.

c. The vertebral angiogram reveals that the basilar artery is displaced far posteriorly from the clivus (dotted line) around the large tumor arising from the clivus. This angiographic appearance is typical of an extra-axial mass. No blush could be identified.

Probable clivus meningioma, not surgically proved.

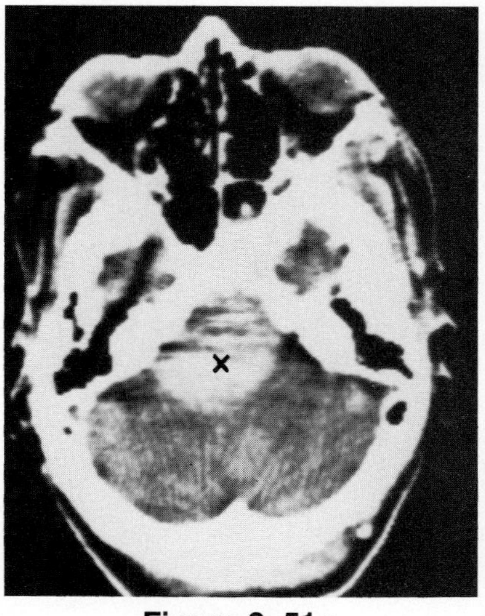

Figure 2–51a

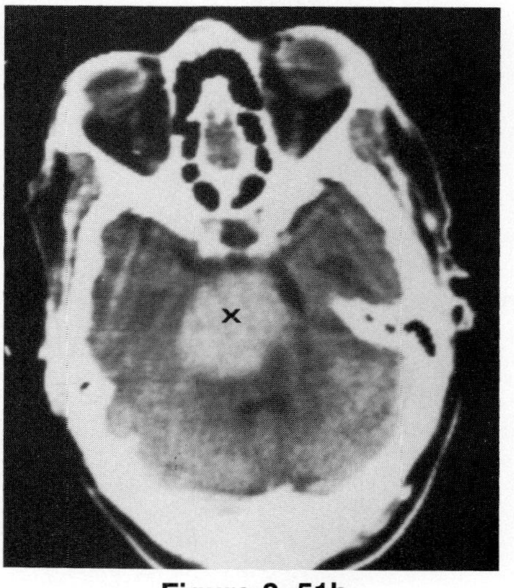

Figure 2–51b

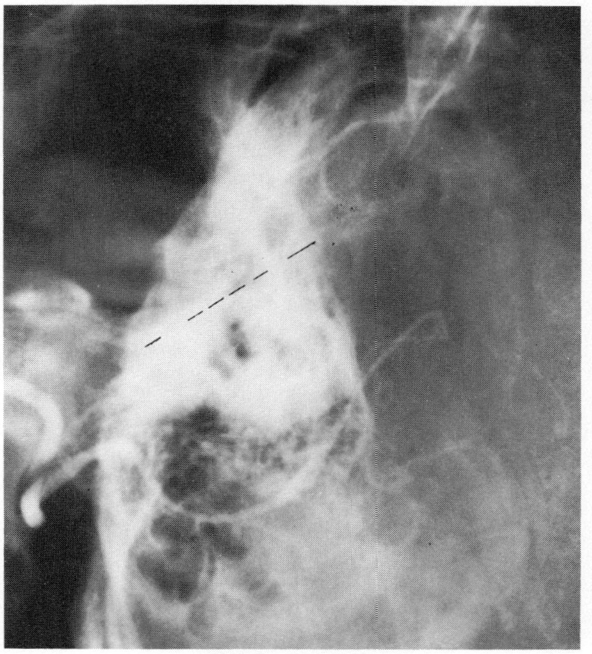

Figure 2–51c

CHAPTER 3

METASTASES

Patients with suspected brain metastases are examined by a routine scan followed by a scan with contrast enhancement. Because some of the smaller metastatic lesions have been undetectable prior to the infusion of contrast material, a scan with contrast enhancement is always done unless the patient has an allergy to the contrast material. Multiplicity of lesions is the classic presentation of metastases; however, there are a certain number of patients with metastases who have only one intracranial lesion. The patient's symptoms reflect the position of the metastatic lesion. The CT scan is more sensitive than the radionuclide scan for diagnosing metastatic lesions, especially for those lesions located in the midbrain and posterior fossa, particularly at the level of the pons.

The route and postinfusion studies are also useful for following response to treatment with radiotherapy or chemotherapy.

ADENOCARCINOMA, UNKNOWN PRIMARY (Figure 3–1)

E. C. is a 54 year old female who presented with left hemiparesis of gradual onset.

a. The routine scan demonstrates a calcified mass high in the right parietal parasagittal area (arrows on 3A and 3B). This mass is surrounded by marked edema, and there is shift of the midline to the left. Density, 46 to 64 u.

b. After infusion of contrast material, the mass is enhanced. The blush appears to be quite homogeneous. Density, 48 to 78 u. A

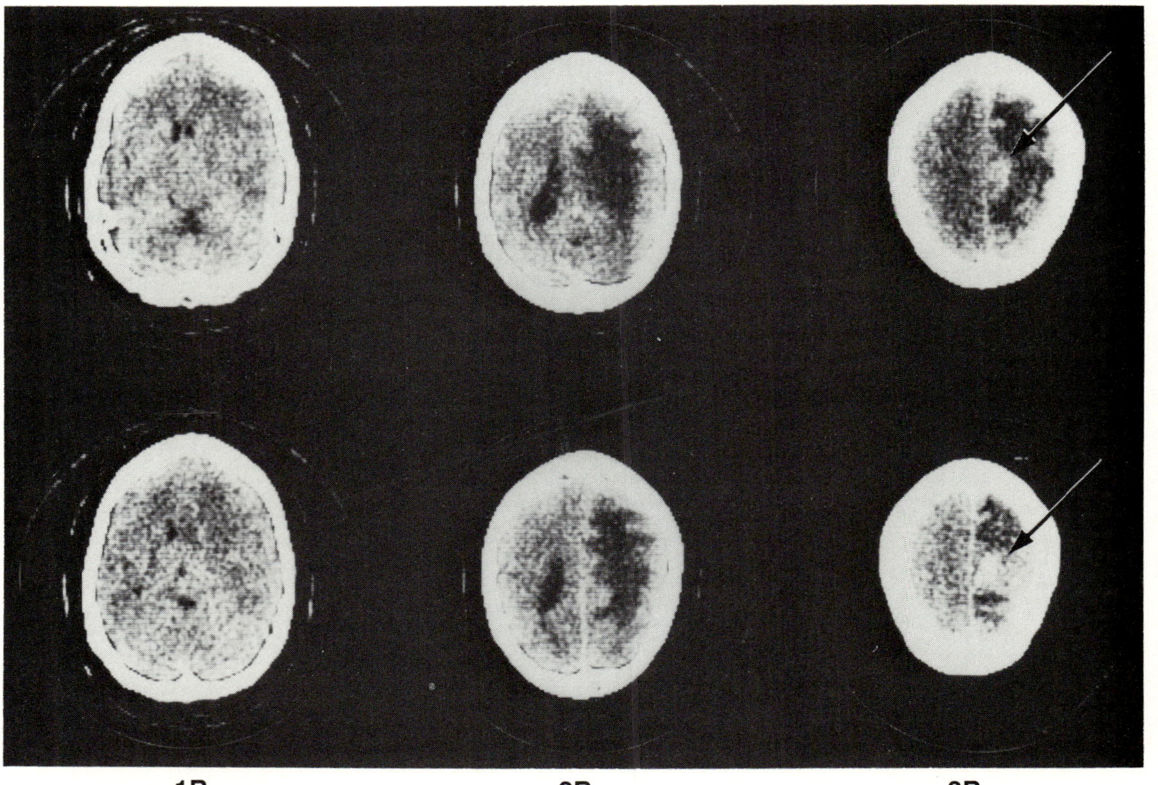

Figure 3–1a

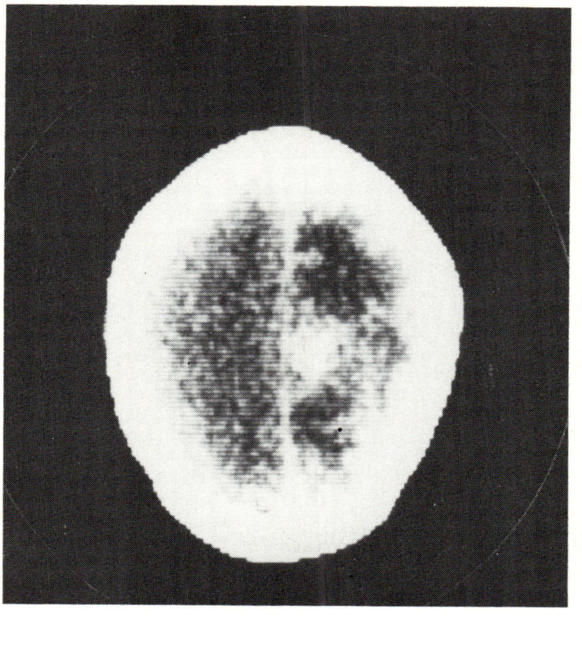

Figure 3–1b

parasagittal meningioma was thought to be the most likely diagnosis.

c. The early arterial phase of the right carotid arteriogram reveals forward displacement of the sylvian triangle (long arrow) and spreading of the vessels in the parietal area (short arrows).

d. A later arterial phase shows a moderate-sized branch of the middle meningeal artery coursing posteriorly (arrows).

e. On the anteroposterior arterial phase, a distal shift of the anterior cerebral artery is noted as it passes under the falx cerebri (arrow). There is downward displacement of the sylvian point (short arrow).

f. The venous phase reveals a well rounded tumor blush (arrows) high in the convexity region.

Although all the evidence seemed to support the diagnosis of a parasagittal meningioma, surgery revealed metastatic adenocarcinoma; the primary is unknown.

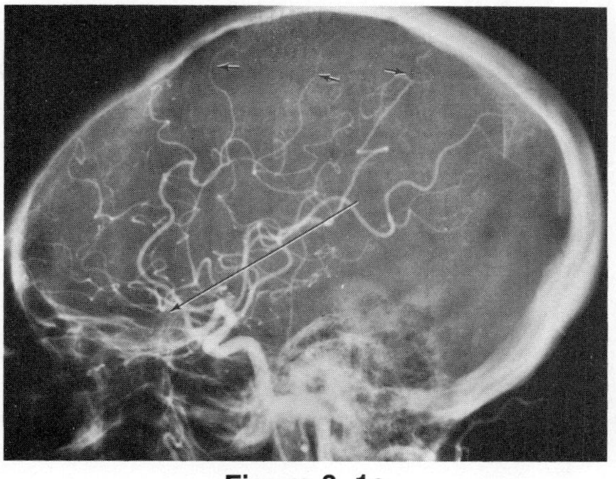

Figure 3–1c

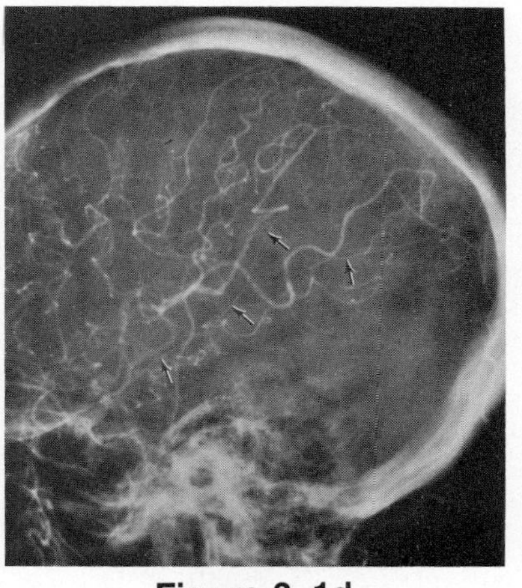

Figure 3–1d

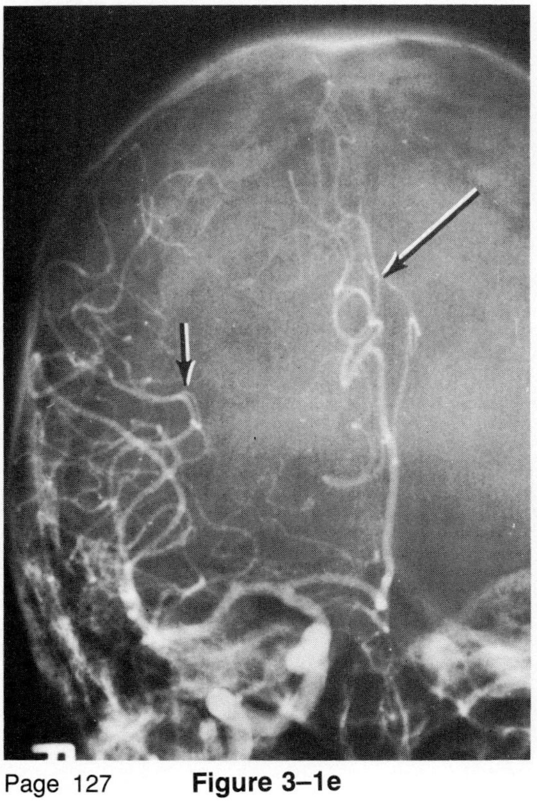

Figure 3–1e

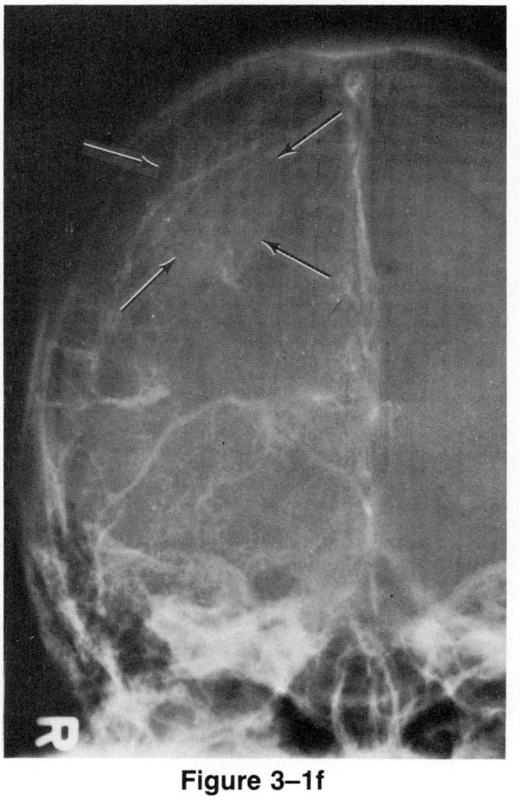

Figure 3–1f

METASTATIC LUNG CARCINOMA (Figure 3–2)

D. M. is a 57 year old woman who entered with a 2-week history of progressive right homonymous hemianopsia and increasingly bizarre behavior. The patient had a long history of psychiatric illness, but had otherwise been in good health. She had been a pack-a-day cigarette smoker for many years.

a. The initial chest x-ray reveals a small irregular mass lesion just beneath the medial end of the right clavicle (arrows). There appears to be some stranding toward the right hilar area.

b and c. Posterior (b) and left lateral (c) views of the radionuclide scan show an area of increased activity high in the left posterior parietal area.

d. The routine CT scan discloses a large lucent area deep in the left posterior parieto-occipital area. Density, 4 to 28 u. There is marked shift of the lateral ventricles from left to right.

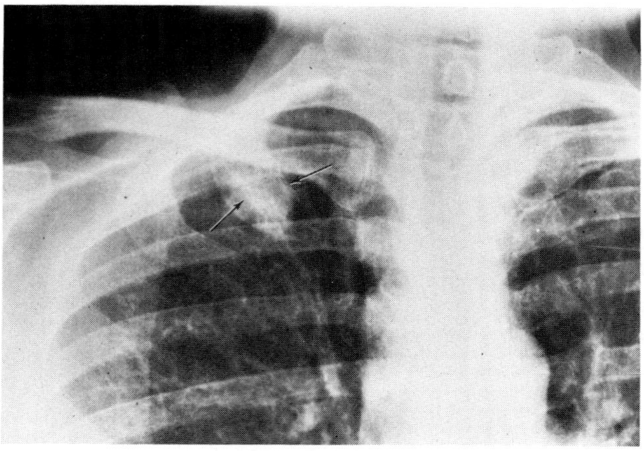

Figure 3–2a

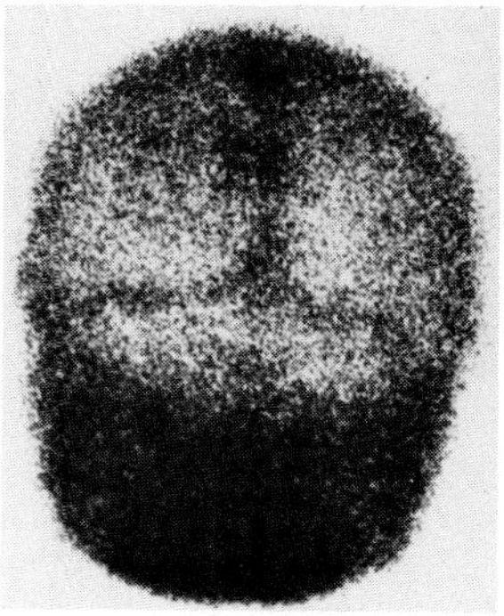

Figure 3–2b

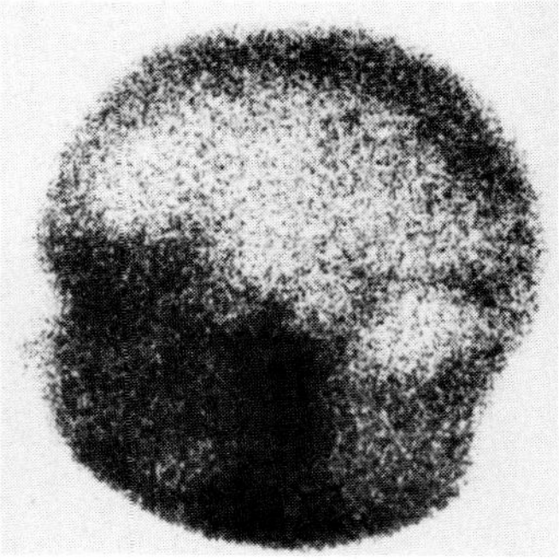

Figure 3–2c

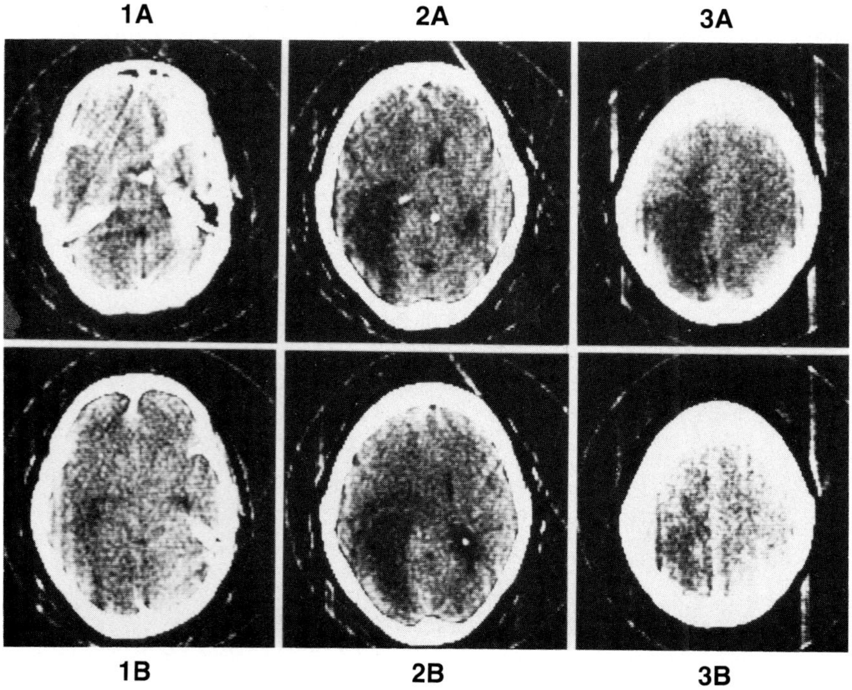

Figure 3–2d

e. Following the infusion of contrast material, a rim of enhancement is noted around this large lucent area. The cystic lesion has a bilobed appearance.

f. The anteroposterior arterial phase of the left carotid arteriogram shows a marked distal shift of the anterior cerebral artery under the falx cerebri (upper arrow), with downward displacement of the sylvian point (lower arrow).

g. The lateral arterial phase reveals marked forward displacement of the sylvian triangle (long arrow) and a large avascular area in the left posterior parieto-occipital region.

Surgery revealed a cystic lesion containing straw-colored fluid. The cyst wall was adenocarcinoma, consistent with a primary lung carcinoma.

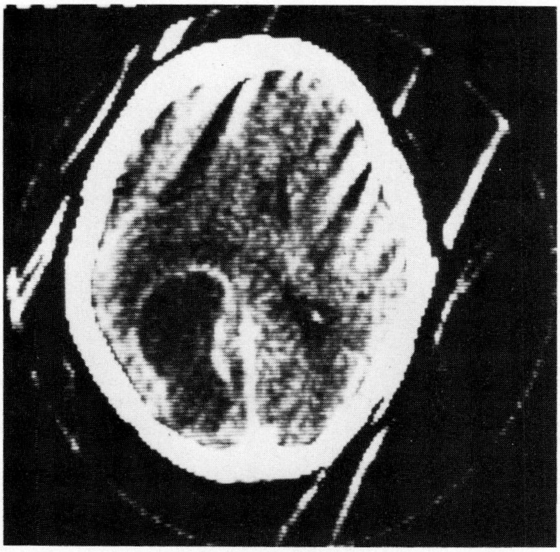

Figure 3–2e

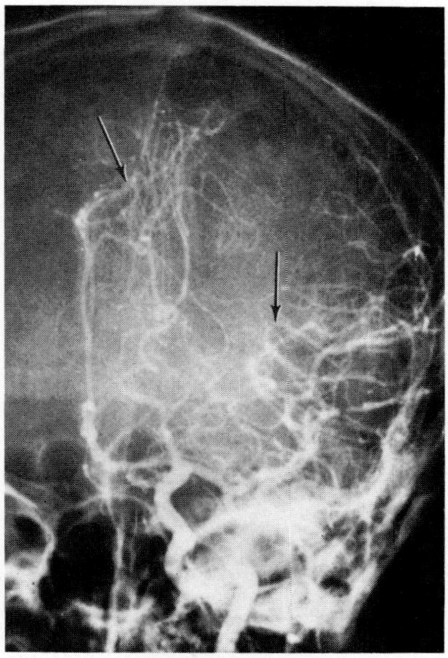

Figure 3–2f

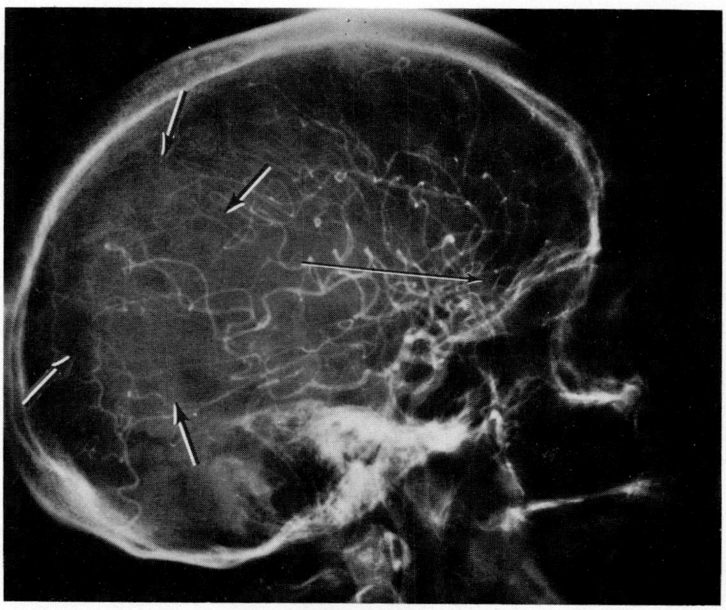

Figure 3–2g

METASTASES, LUNG PRIMARY (Figure 3–3)

H. S. is a 53 year old female who had sought treatment 3 years before admission for a "lump" on her scalp. Biopsy at that time revealed metastatic squamous cell carcinoma. A primary could not be found. At the present admission the patient complains of personality changes that have been progressive over several months. Chest x-ray now reveals a left hilar mass.

a and b. The left lateral (a) and anterior (b) views of the radionuclide scan show an area of increased uptake with a central lucency in the left frontal region adjacent to the midline.

c. The routine CT scan reveals a large lucent area in the left frontoparietal region. There appears to be a ring of increased density deep in this lucent area, best seen on cuts 2A and 2B (arrows). There is marked shift of the midline to the right side.

d. After contrast infusion, there is a dense ring of enhancement in the area of increased density that was noted on the initial scan, along with a large amount of surrounding edema.

e. The anteroposterior arterial phase of the left carotid arteriogram demonstrates a "round" shift of the anterior cerebral artery—a classic sign seen with a frontal lesion (arrows).

f. The lateral arterial phase reveals

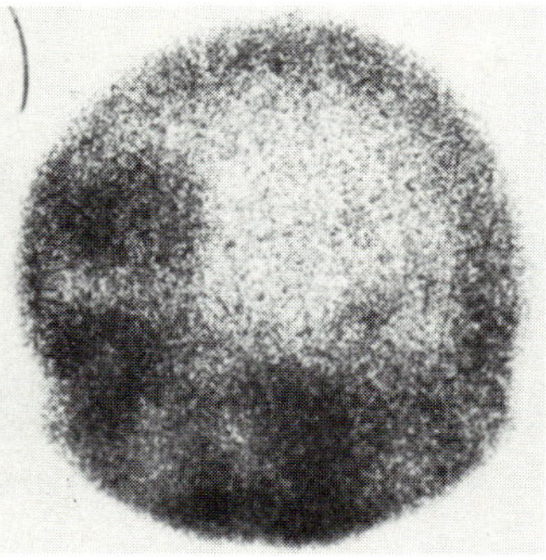

Figure 3–3a

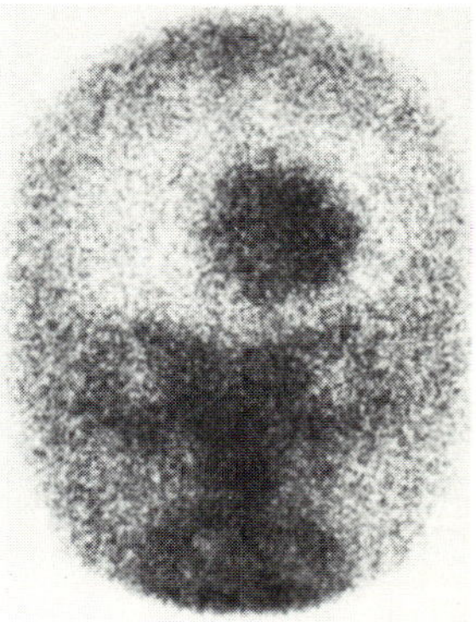

Figure 3–3b

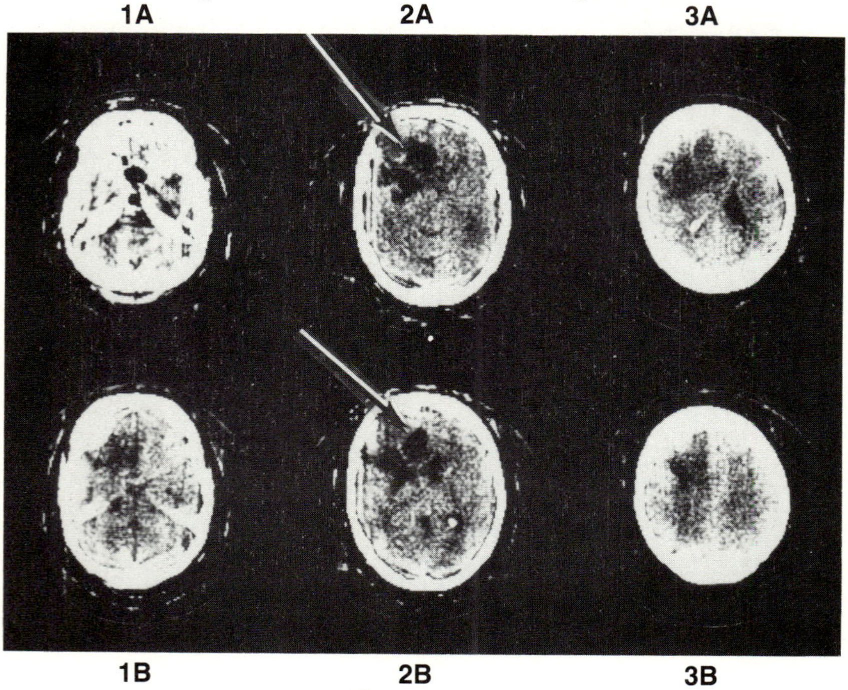

Figure 3–3c

11A 12A 13A

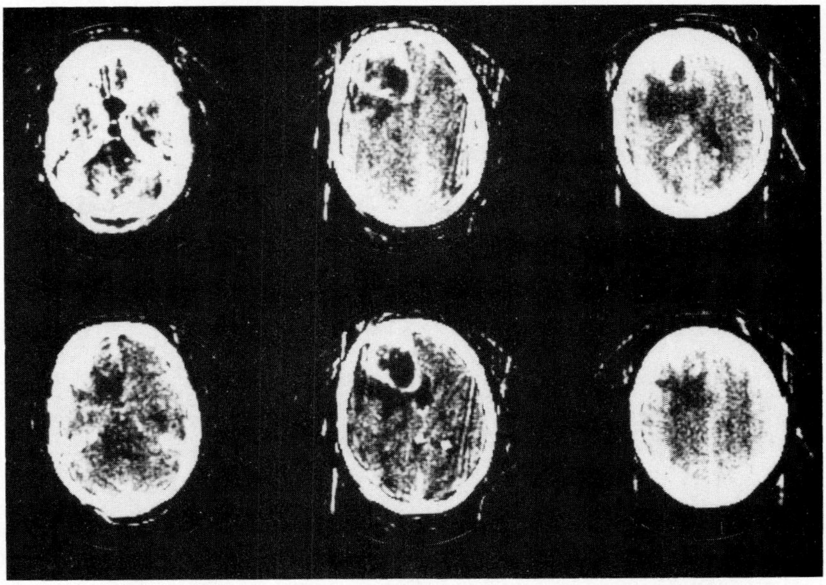

11B 12B 13B

Figure 3–3d

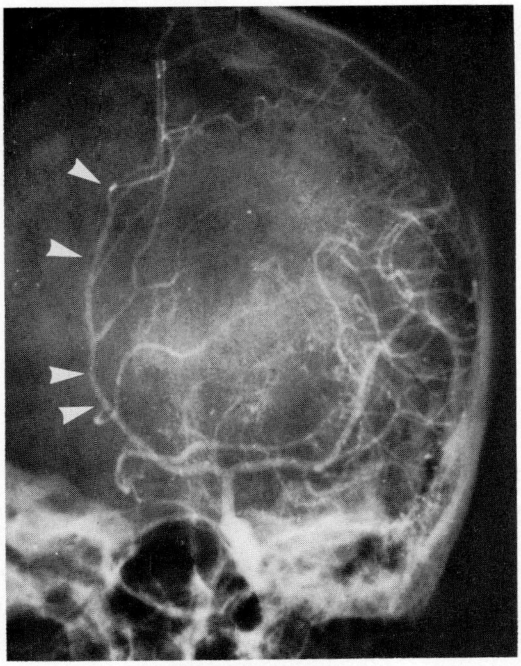

Figure 3–3e

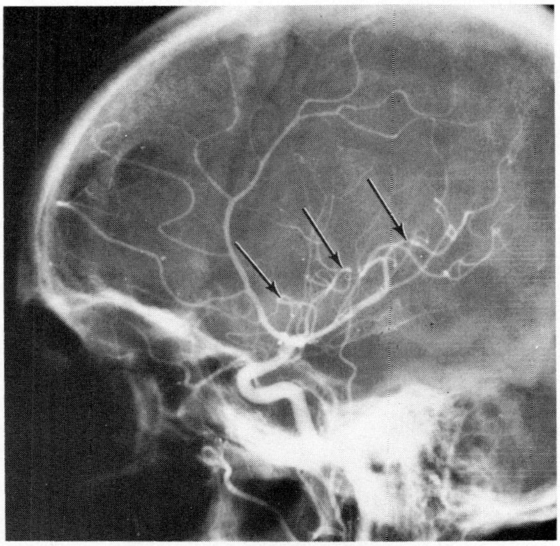

Figure 3–3f

stretching of all the frontal pole vessels and downward and posterior displacement of the sylvian triangle (arrows).

g. On the late arterial phase a large avascular area is seen in the left frontal region. There appears to be a faint vascular stain of the rim of the tumor.

Surgery revealed metastatic squamous cell carcinoma, compatible with a primary lung carcinoma.

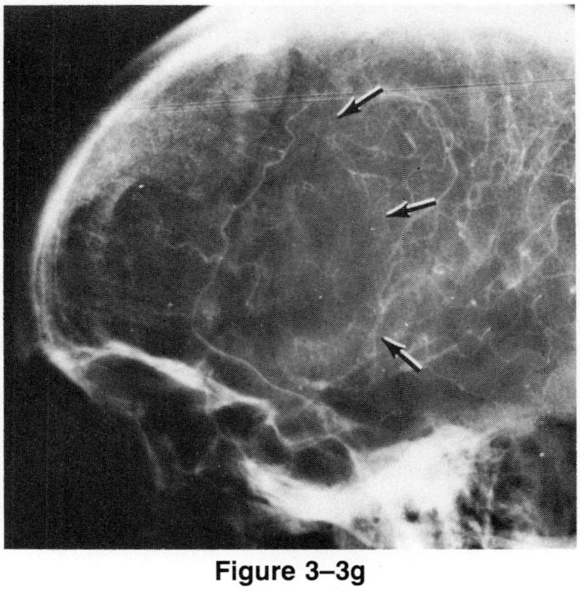

Figure 3–3g

METASTASES, LUNG PRIMARY (Figure 3–4)

E. J. is a 60 year old man with undifferentiated bronchogenic carcinoma of the right lower lobe of the lung and recent onset of headaches.

a. On the routine chest x-ray a large round mass lesion is noted in the right lower lung field.

b and c. The radionuclide scan is felt to be negative for intracranial metastases.

d. The routine CT scan reveals a cystic lesion in the left cerebellar hemisphere.

e. Contrast infusion discloses a thick ring of contrast enhancement about the previously noted cystic lesion. There is mild obstructive hydrocephalus.

Surgery revealed cystic metastases from the primary lung carcinoma.

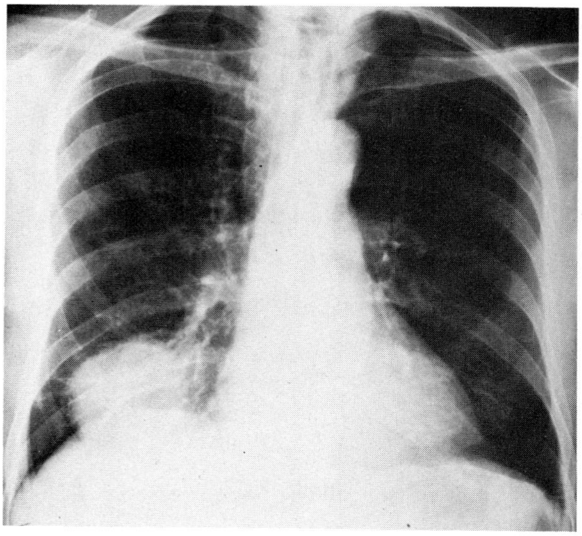

Figure 3–4a

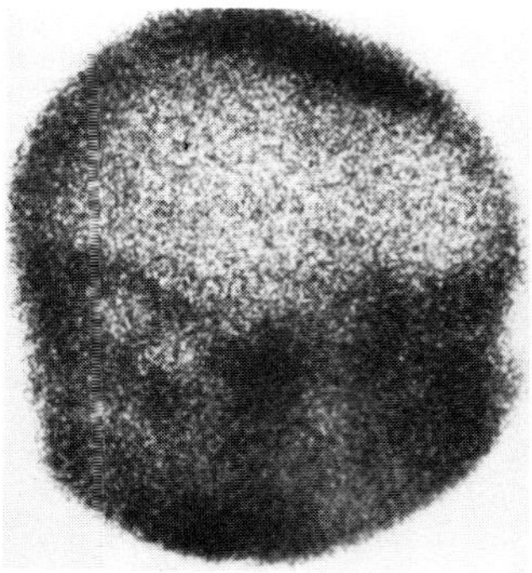

Figure 3–4b

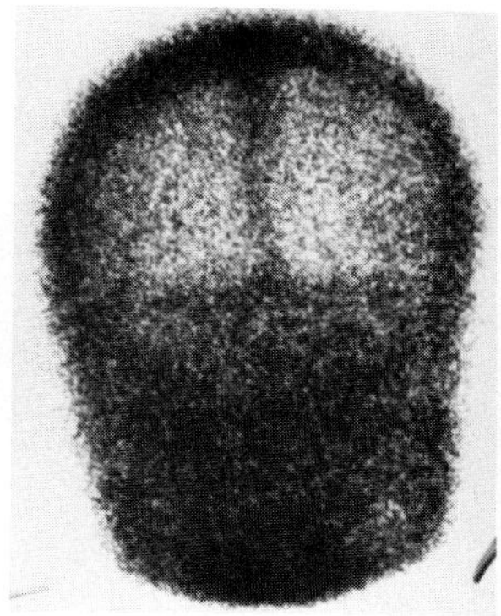

Figure 3–4c

1A

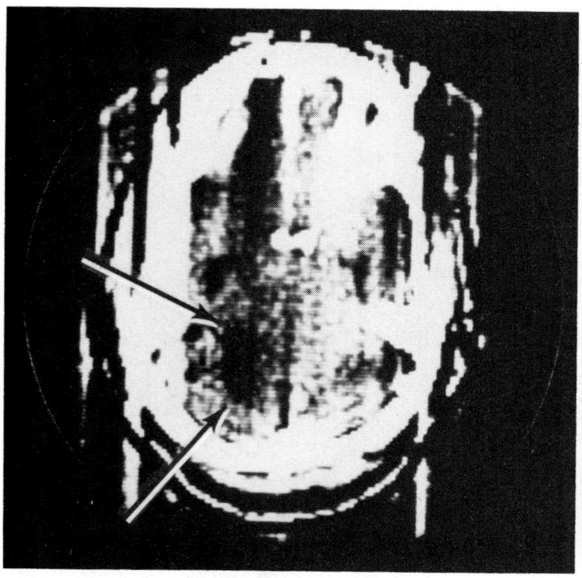

Figure 3–4d

11B

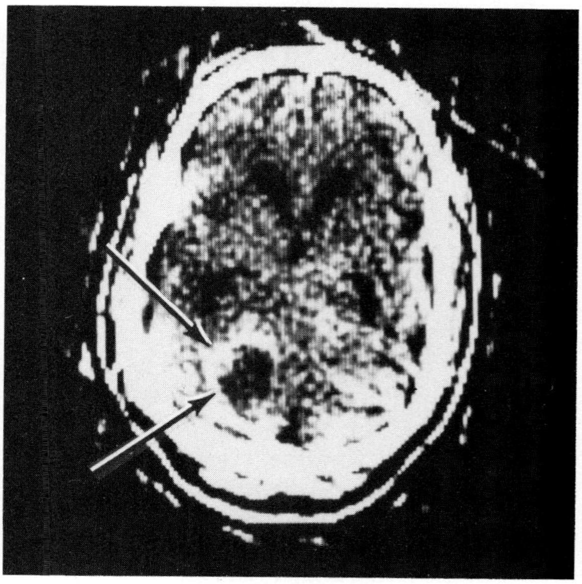

Figure 3–4e

METASTASES, LUNG PRIMARY (Figure 3–5)

N. N. is a 60 year old male with a known lung carcinoma and recent onset of a seizure disorder.

a. The routine chest x-ray reveals a large left hilar mass, with opacification and partial collapse of the left upper lobe. A faint air bronchogram is noted in the left upper lobe. The findings are compatible with a primary lung cancer.

b and c. The radionuclide scan appears within normal limits.

d. The routine CT scan (cut 1B) shows an area of linear increased density deep in the right temporal lobe region (arrow).

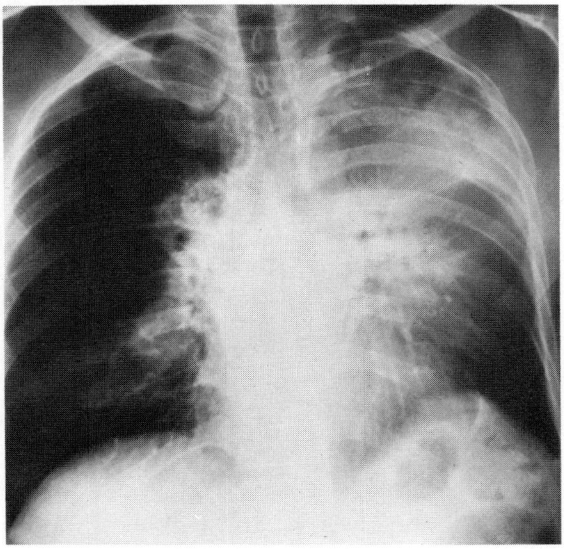

Figure 3–5a

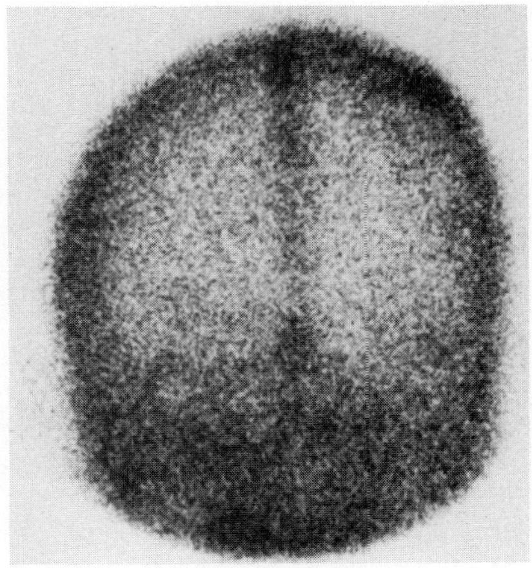

Figure 3–5b

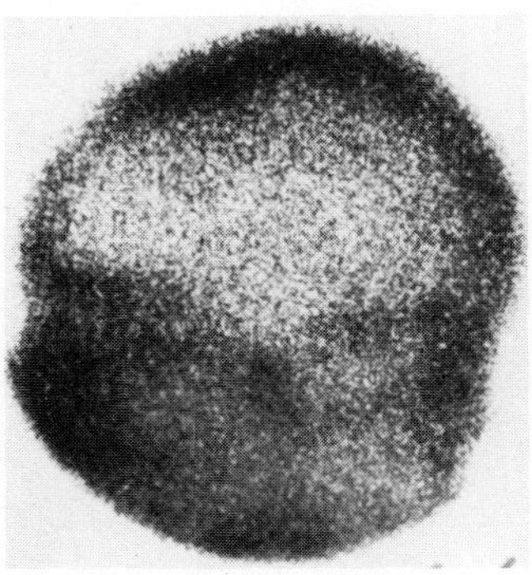

Figure 3–5c

1B

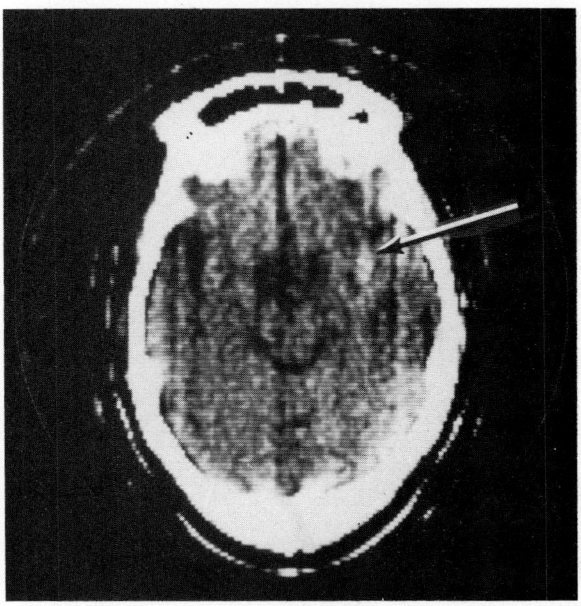

Figure 3–5d

e. After infusion of contrast material, there is marked enhancement of a mass lesion deep in the right temporal lobe–basal ganglia region.

f. Lateral view of the early arterial phase of the right brachial arteriogram discloses elevation of the sylvian triangle and supraclinoid portion of the internal carotid artery and its branches. An area of neovascularity can be seen just superior to the sella turcica on the lateral view (arrow).

11B

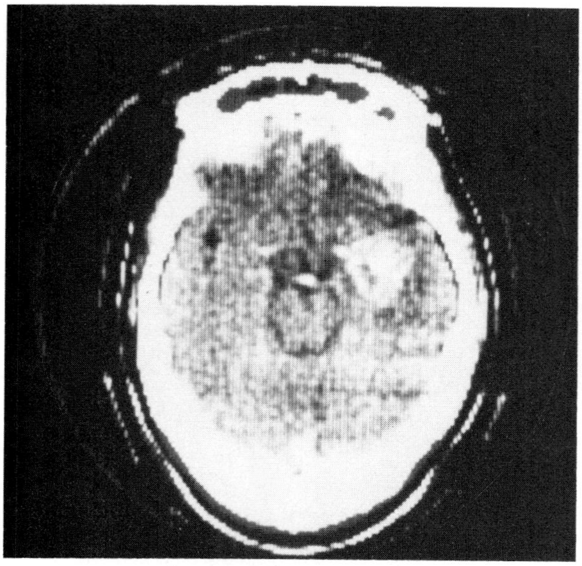

Figure 3–5e

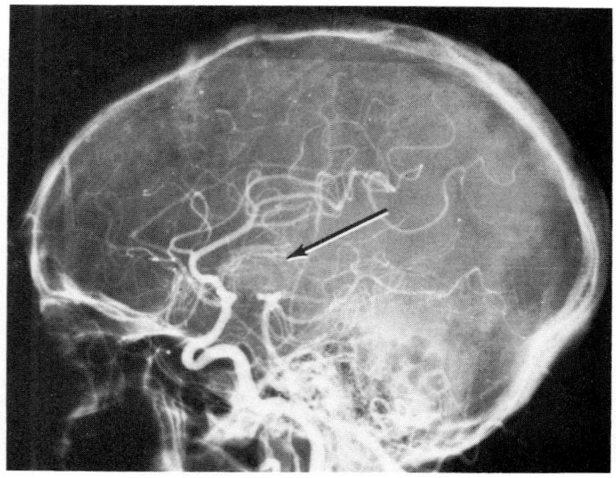

Figure 3–5f

g. The late arterial phase reveals several early draining veins (arrows).

h. The capillary phase shows better filling of the multiple early draining veins as they enter into the straight sinus (arrows).

i. The AP arterial phase is of poor quality, but the tumor blush can be faintly seen (arrows). This mass is thought to be a metastatic deposit from the patient's lung carcinoma.

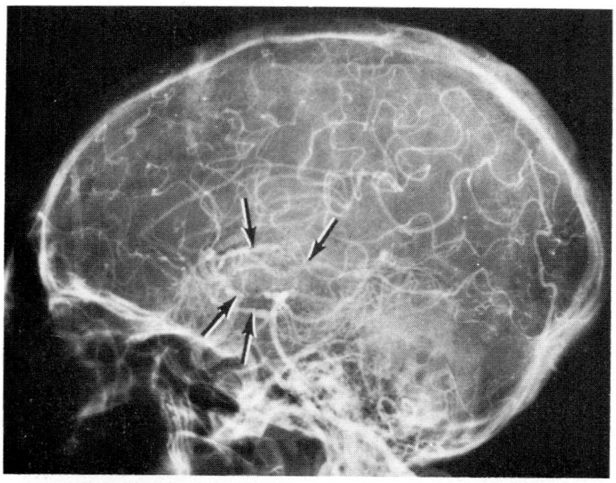

Figure 3–5g

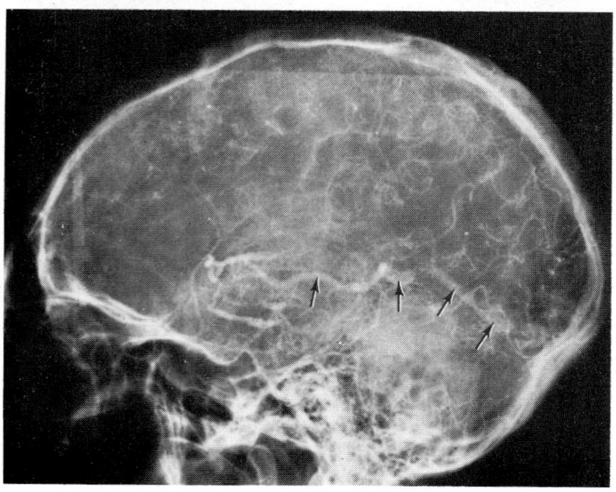

Figure 3–5h

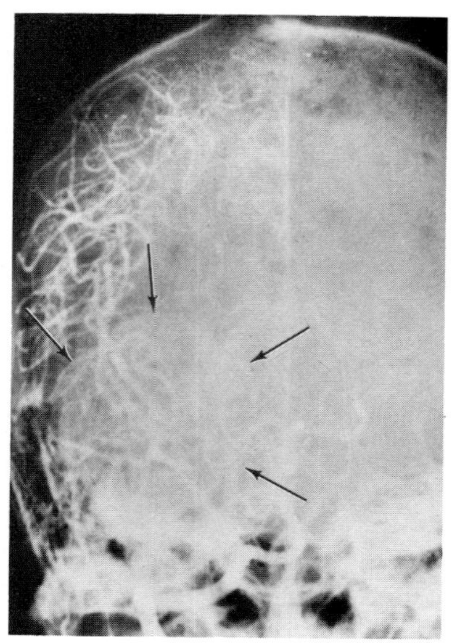

Figure 3–5i

METASTATIC MELANOMA (Figure 3–6)

M. M. is a 58 year old woman with a known malignant melanoma. She complains now of headaches.

a and b. The routine radionuclide scan appears within normal limits.

c. The routine CT scan (cuts 1A and 1B) reveals an area of lucency in the left posterior temporal lobe region. Density, 20 to 40 u (arrow). After the infusion of contrast material (cuts 11A and 11B), a small round metastasis in the center of the previously noted lucent area is enhanced. Density, 70 to 100 u. No other lesions noted.

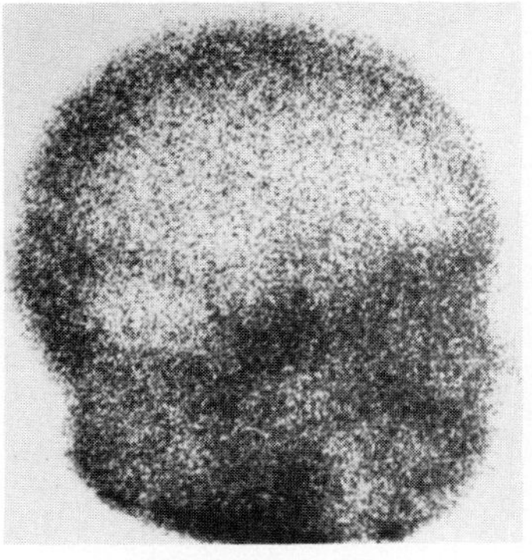

Figure 3–6a

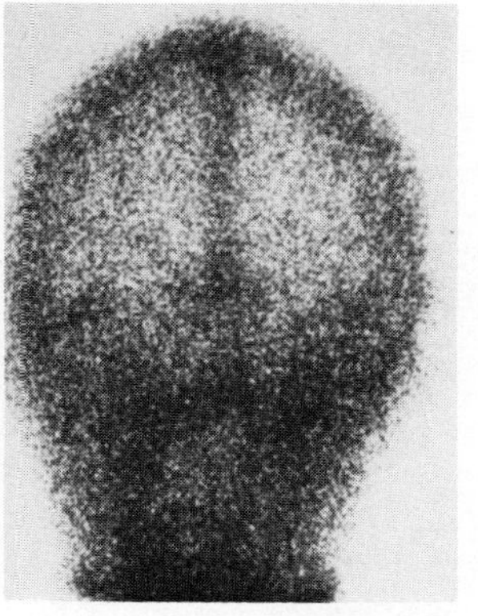

Figure 3–6b

1A 11A

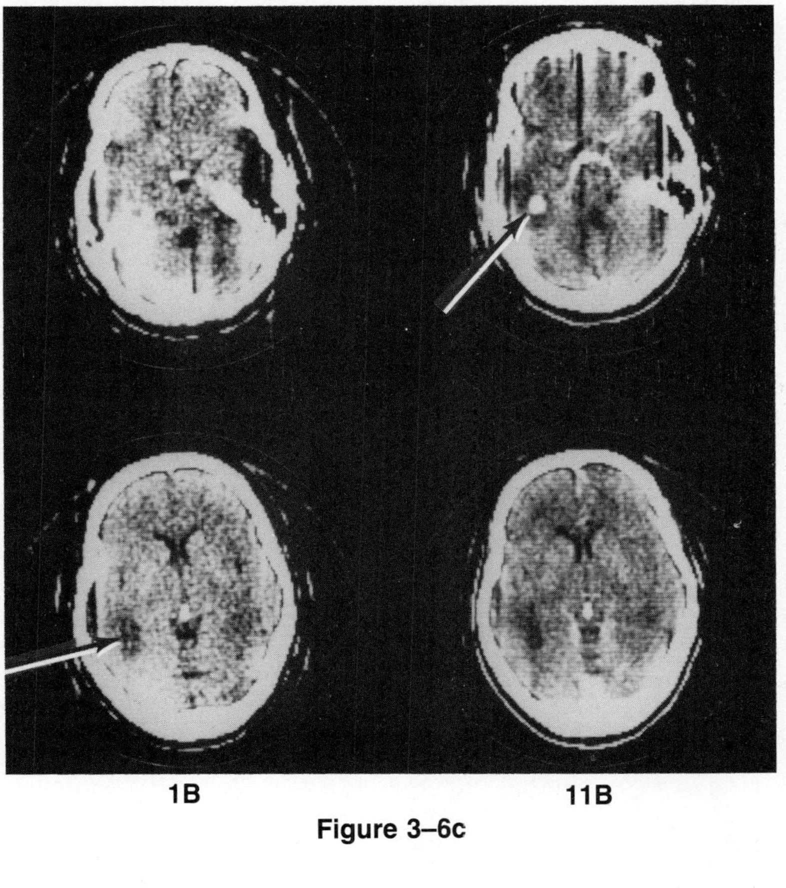

1B 11B

Figure 3–6c

d. Lateral arterial phase of the left carotid arteriogram shows elevation of the branches of the middle cerebral artery group (arrows) by an avascular posterior temporal lobe mass. The arteriogram was performed several weeks after the initial CT scan.

e and f. Anteroposterior arterial and venous phases reveal a distal shift of the anterior cerebral artery under the falx cerebri and an even greater shift of the internal cerebral vein (arrows). The sylvian point is displaced medially on the arterial phase (horizontal arrow on e).

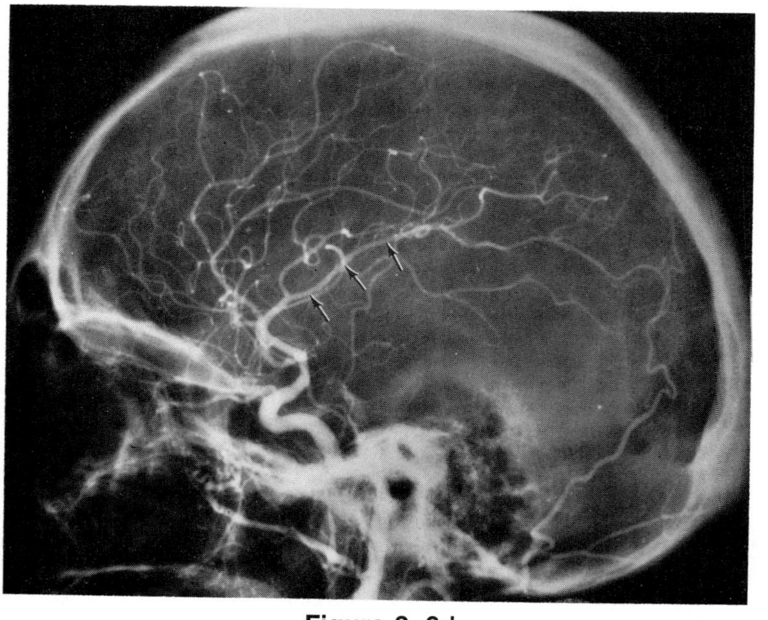

Figure 3–6d

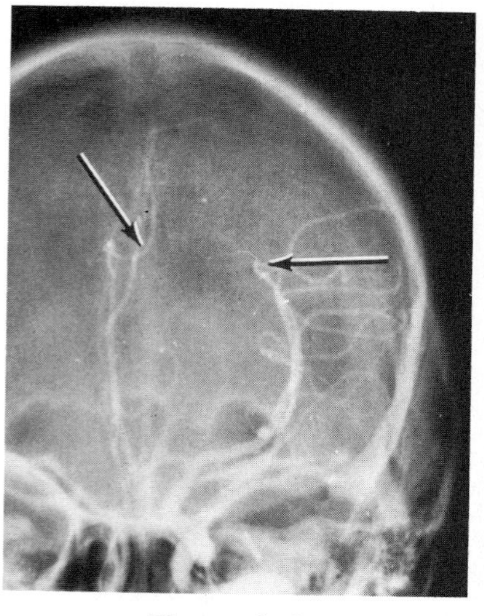

Figure 3–6e

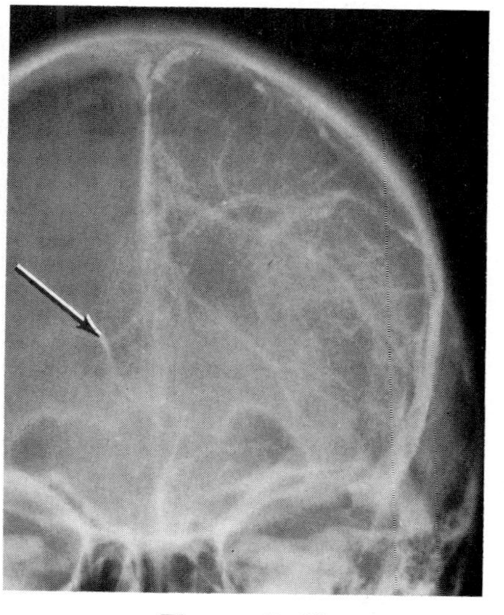

Figure 3–6f

g to j. Several months later, the radionuclide scan discloses multiple intracranial metastases.

k. A follow-up CT scan with contrast material also reveals multiple intracranial metastases.

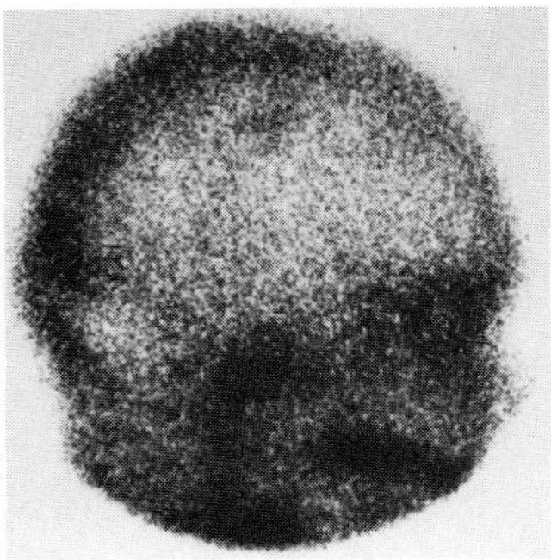

Figure 3–6g

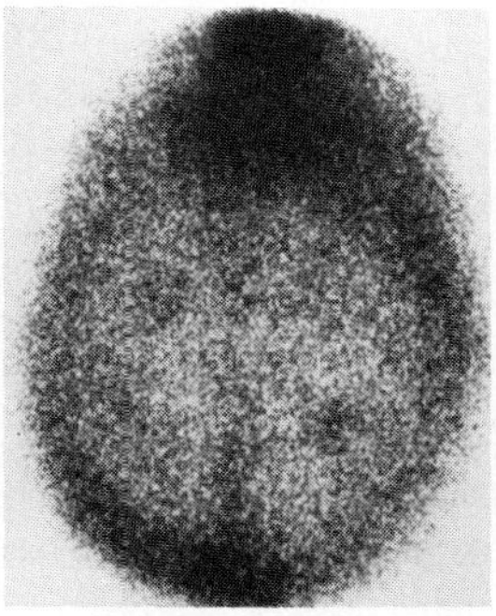

Figure 3–6h

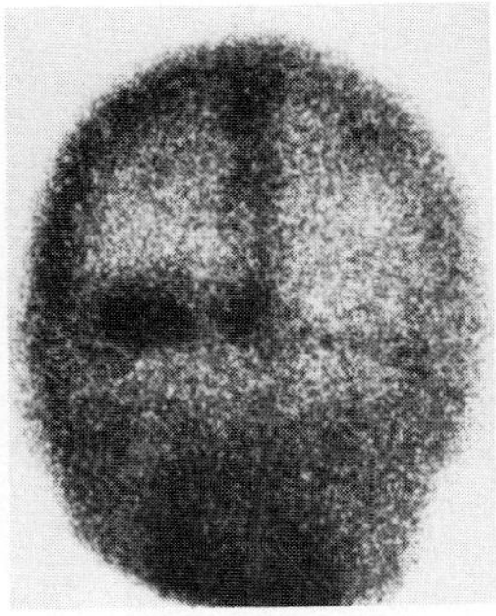

Figure 3–6i

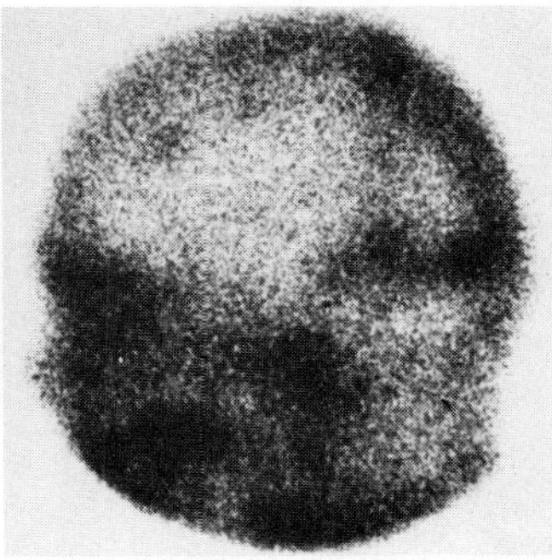

Figure 3–6j

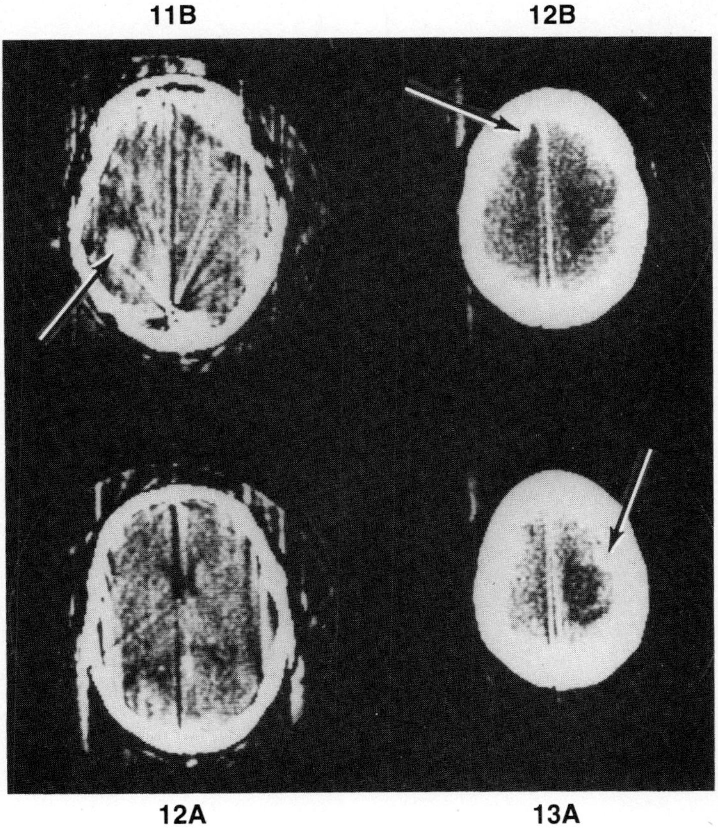

Figure 3–6k

METASTATIC LUNG CARCINOMA (Figure 3–7)

This 35 year old male had had an adenocarcinoma of the lung removed 6 months prior to admission. He now presents with a dense right hemiparesis.

a. The preinfusion scan demonstrates a very large cystic mass higher than cerebrospinal fluid density, which reflects the high protein content. There is a dense ring of peripheral tissue and a nodule of tumor in the wall of the cyst (N). There is marked shift of the lateral ventricles to the contralateral side.

b. The postinfusion portion of the examination reveals that there is dense enhancement of the ring of tissue and of the tumor module (N).

Surgery confirmed a solitary metastatic lesion with a cyst containing straw-colored fluid. A primary brain tumor could have this appearance but is unlikely to have such a smooth rim of enhancement or such a dense rim on the preinfusion portion of the study. The history of previous lung tumor makes the diagnosis of metastatic disease most likely.

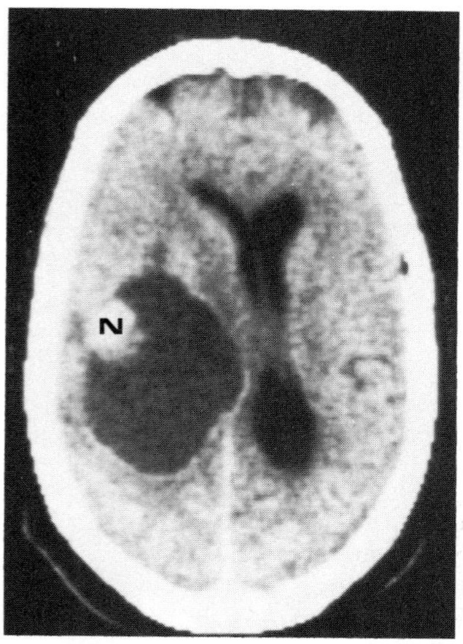

Figure 3–7a

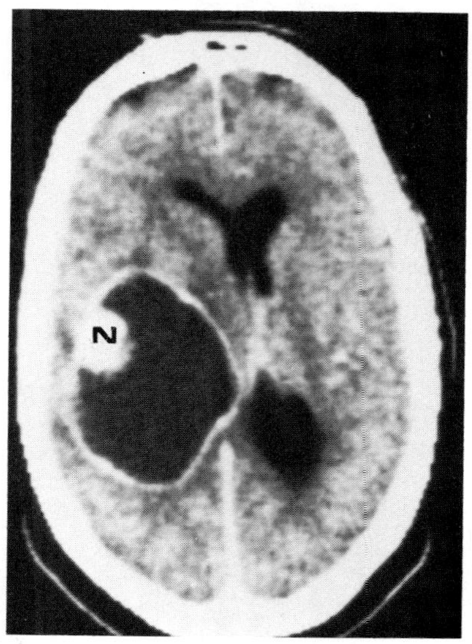

Figure 3–7b

METASTATIC BREAST TUMOR (Figure 3–8)

This 47 year old female presented with a history of changing mental status. She had had a mastectomy approximately 4 years prior to admission.

a and b. The preinfusion portion of the study appears normal.

c and d. The postinfusion portion of the examination reveals very subtle enhancement of several small round lesions (arrows).

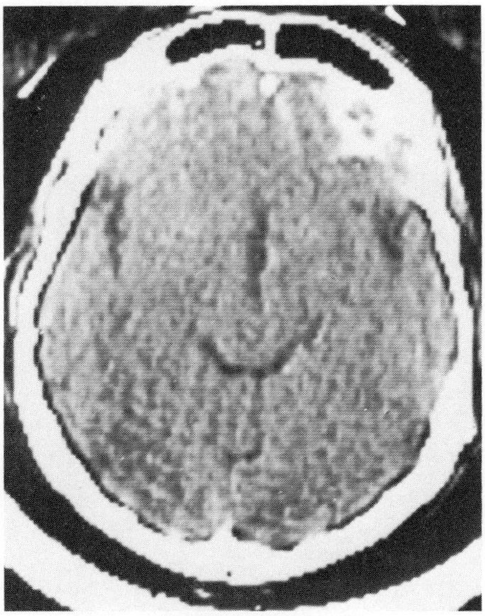

Figure 3–8a

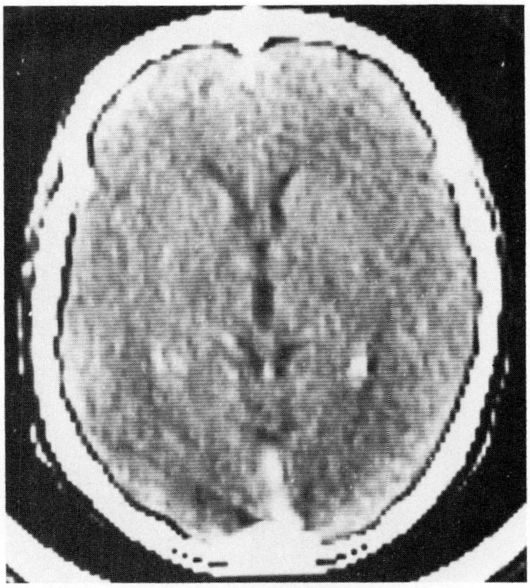

Figure 3–8b

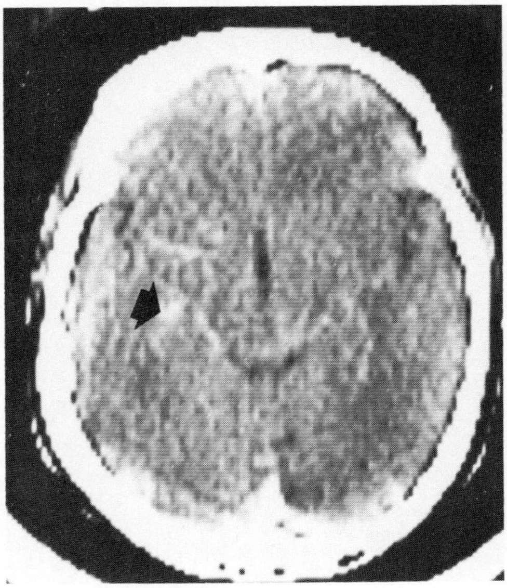

Figure 3–8c

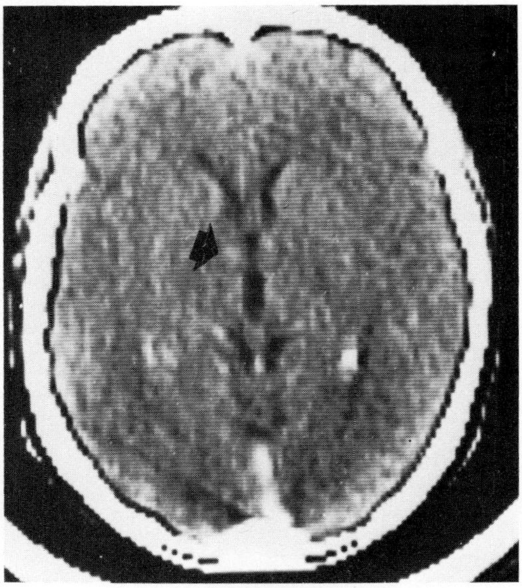

Figure 3–8d

e and f. Following the injection of twice the normal amount of contrast material (600 ml of 30 per cent contrast material) and a delay of ½ hour, the scan was repeated and revealed a myriad of enhancing metastatic deposits, now readily visible. We have found this technique to be helpful in patients in whom metastases are strongly suspected but the routine studies are normal.

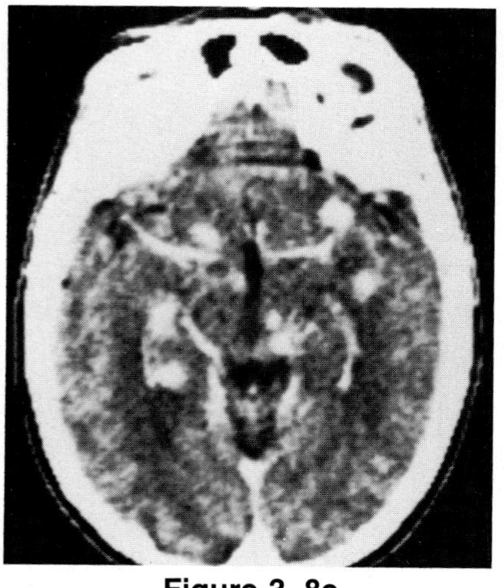

Figure 3–8e

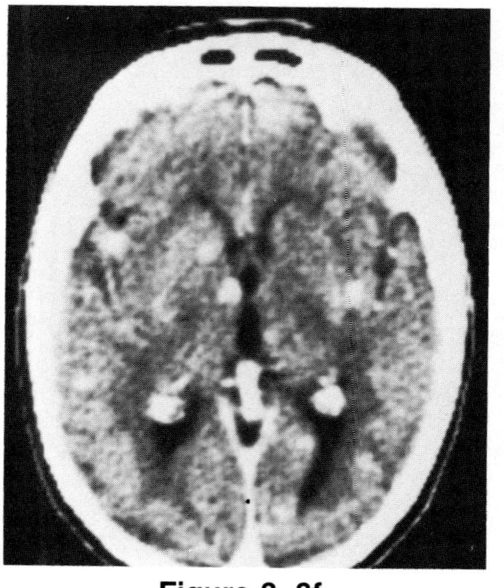

Figure 3–8f

MULTIPLE METASTASES, LUNG PRIMARY (Figure 3–9)

This 54 year old male presented with ataxia and headache. The chest x-ray revealed a right upper lobe mass.

a to d. Multiple postinfusion cuts reveal innumerable metastatic lesions in both the infratentorial and supratentorial distribution. Note that the lesions are round and enhance homogeneously—this is a rather typical finding with metastatic lesions. Some of the lesions appear to have necrotic centers, also common with metastases.

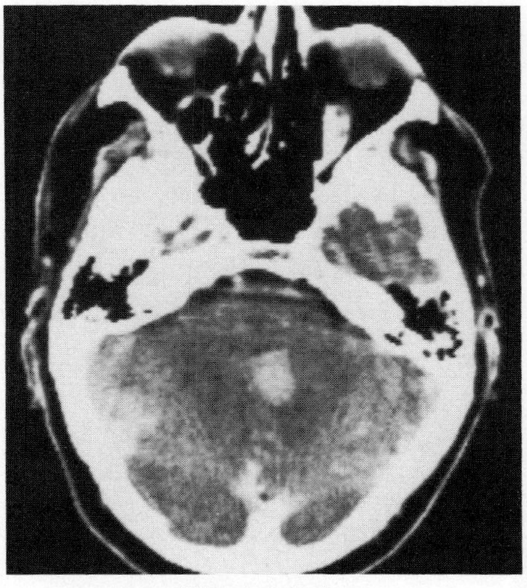

Figure 3–9a

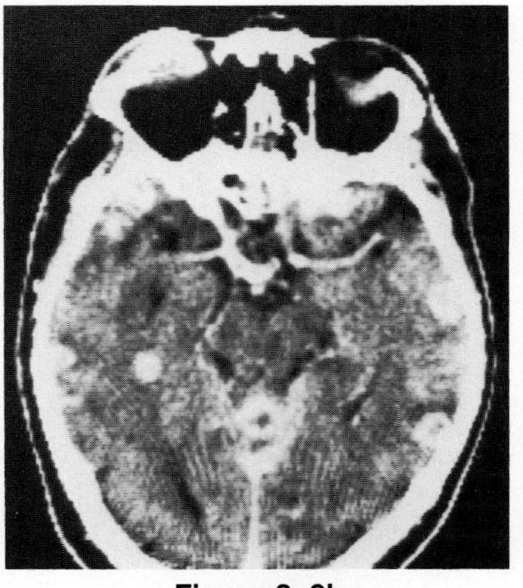

Figure 3–9b

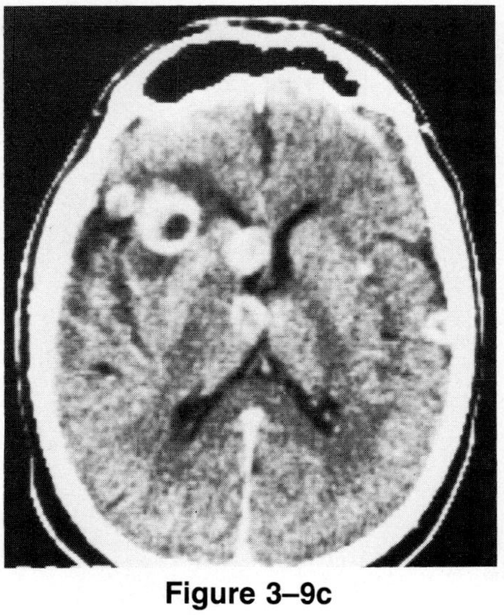

Figure 3–9c

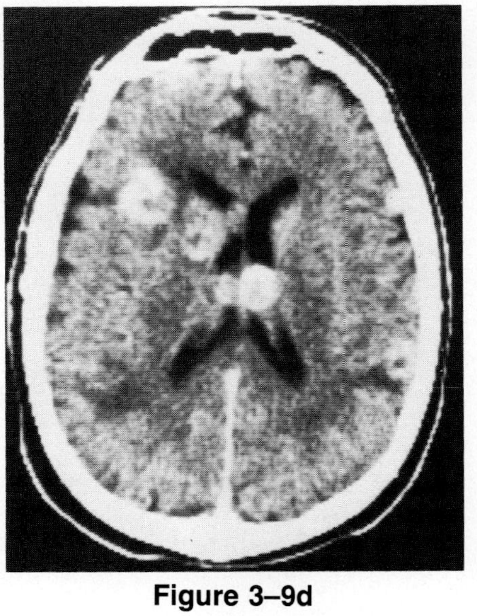

Figure 3–9d

MULTIPLE METASTASES, LUNG PRIMARY (Figure 3–10)

This 67 year old male had had a squamous cell carcinoma of the lung removed approximately 1½ years prior to admission. He presents now with nausea, vomiting, and left-sided weakness.

a. The preinfusion scan appears within normal limits except for moderate enlargement of the lateral ventricles seen on the higher cuts.

b to d. The postinfusion portion of the study reveals multiple metastatic lesions. There are a large number of metastatic deposits in the cerebellum and multiple smaller metastatic deposits in the supratentorial distribution. The metastases in the posterior fossa have resulted in the obstructive hydrocephalus. The supratentorial metastases were "balancing" and therefore there is no shift of the midline structures. Note that in general metastatic squamous cell carcinoma tends to be of low density on the preinfusion scan, while metastatic adenocarcinoma *tends* to be of higher than normal brain density on the preinfusion scan (see Fig. 3–11).

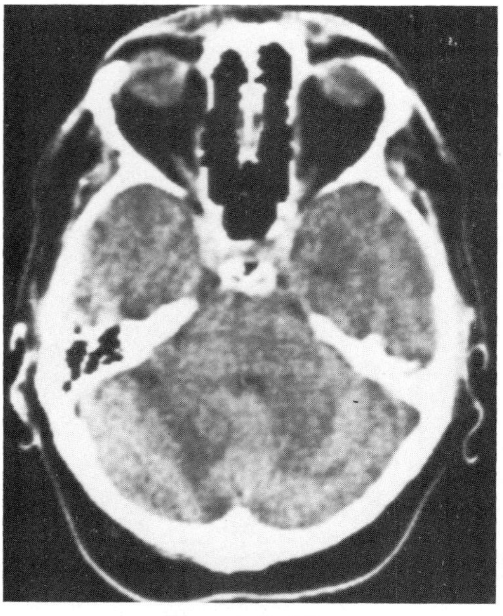

Figure 3–10a

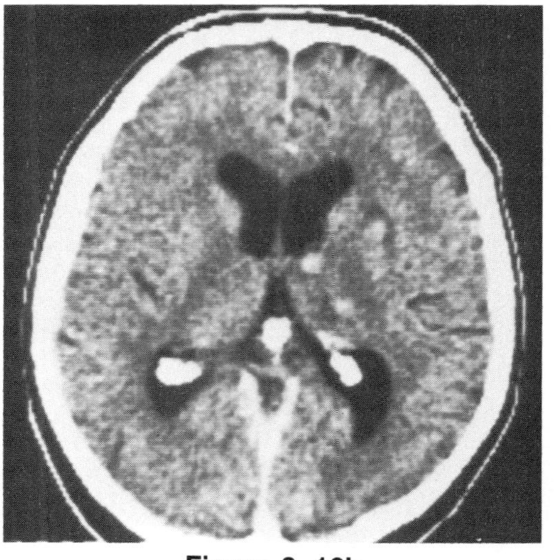

Figure 3–10b

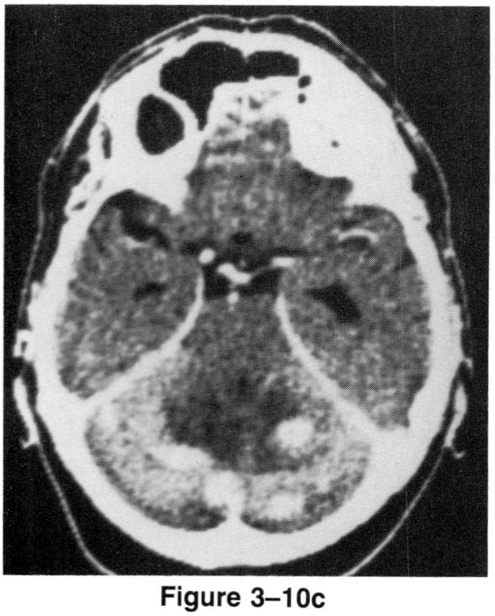

Figure 3–10c

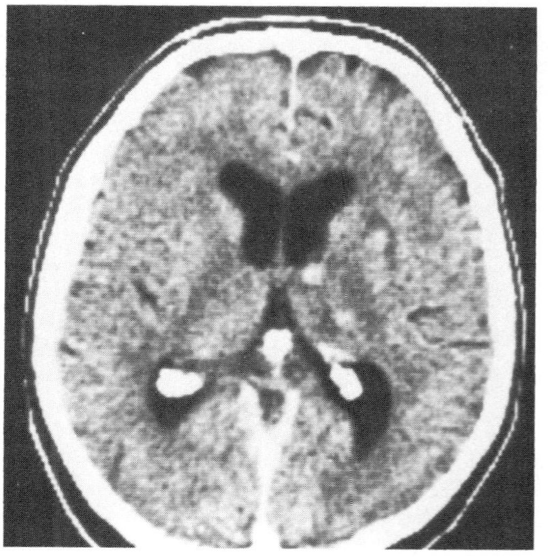

Figure 3–10d

MULTIPLE METASTASES, BREAST PRIMARY (Figure 3–11)

This 59 year old female presented with confusion and ataxia.

a and b. The preinfusion scan reveals subtle rounded areas of higher than normal brain density (arrows).

c to f. The postinfusion scan reveals multiple, rounded, enhancing lesions.

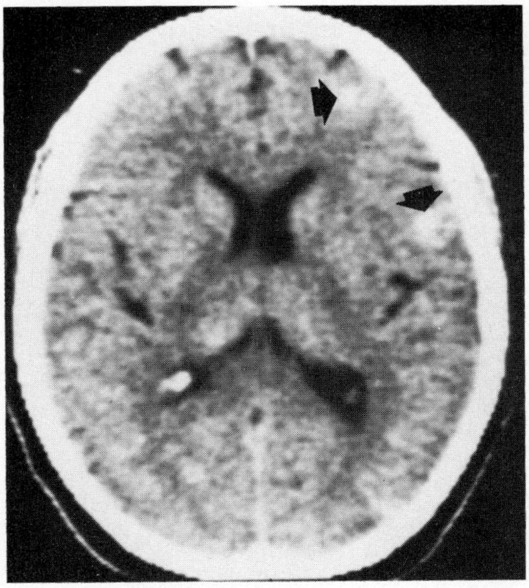

Figure 3–11a

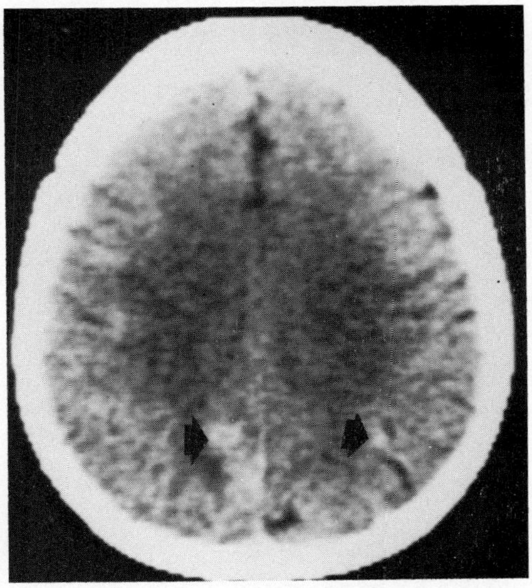

Figure 3–11b

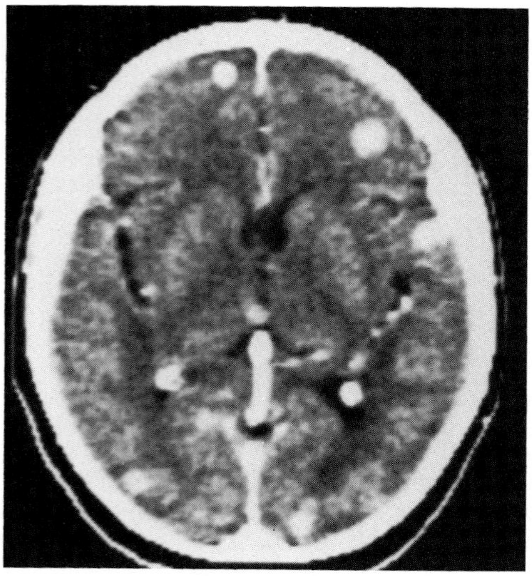

Figure 3–11c

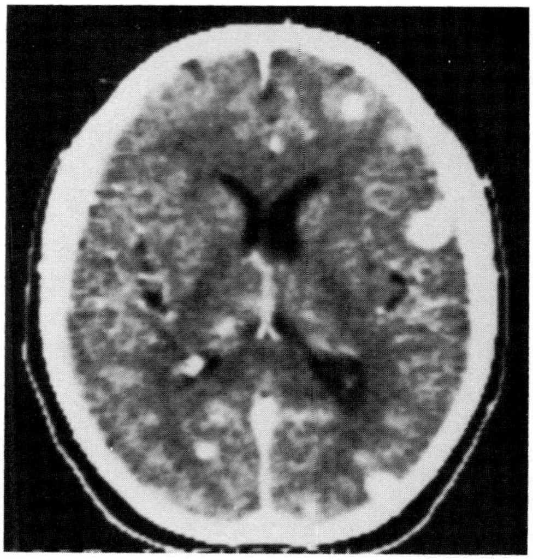

Figure 3–11d

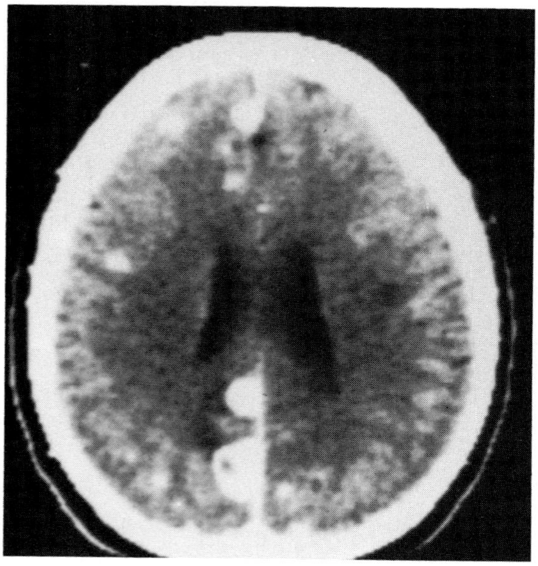

Figure 3–11e

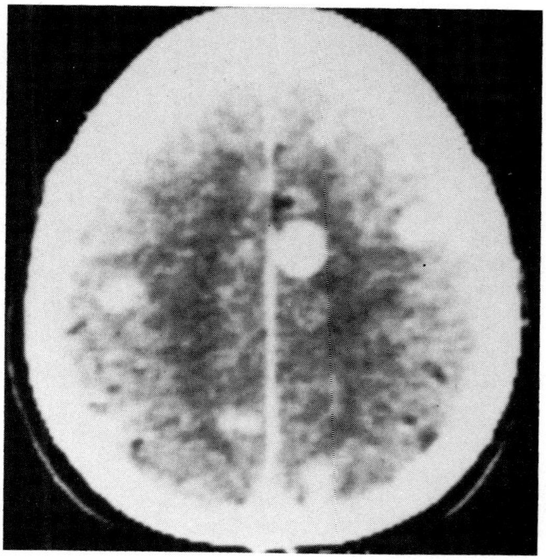

Figure 3–11f

EXTRACRANIAL METASTASIS WITH INTRACRANIAL EXTENSION (Figure 3–12)

B. D. is a 61 year old female with recent onset of progressive right exophthalmos. Physical examination revealed a palpable mass in the right lacrimal gland region. Routine skull films revealed destruction of the zygomatic process of the frontal bone and of the roof of the right orbit.

a to c. The radionuclide scan reveals a large area of increased uptake in the right orbit and the right frontal lobe. This is best seen (a) on the anterior view, (b) on the "orbital" view (arrows), and (c) on the vertex view.

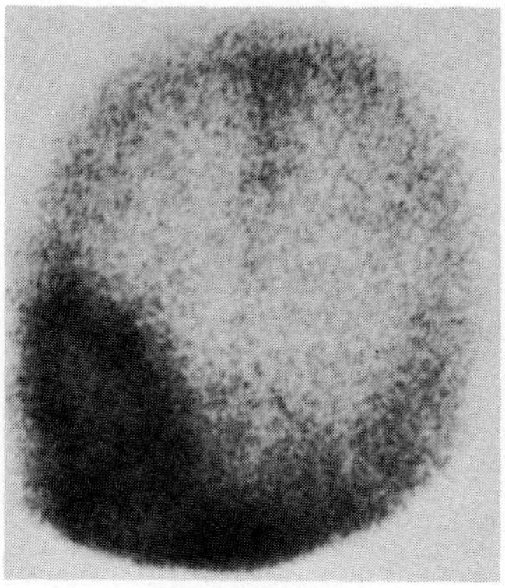

Figure 3–12a

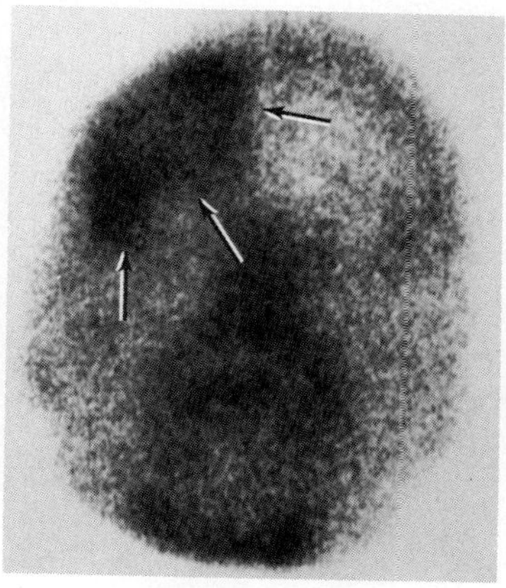

Figure 3–12b

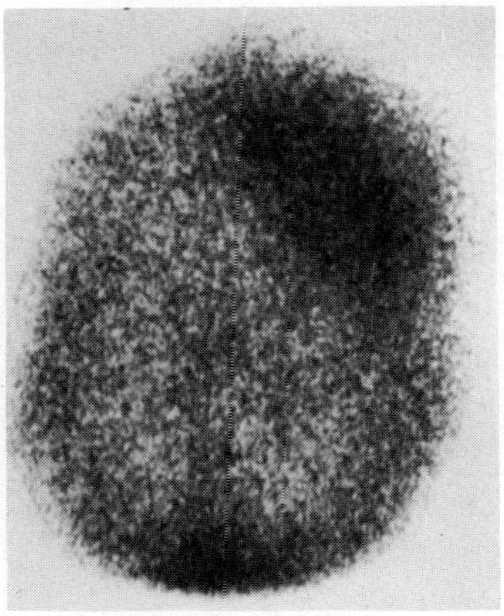

Figure 3–12c

d. In the routine CT scan, cuts 1A and 1B disclose a mass lesion behind the right orbit that extends into the temporal fossa (arrows) and is also noted to extend into the right frontal lobe of the brain. Exophthalmos is present on the right side. Contrast infusion provides enhancement of the mass and permits identification of the intracranial extension with its surrounding edema. There is shift of the lateral ventricles to the left.

A splenic flexure carcinoma was detected, and although a lytic metastasis from colon carcinoma does not seem likely, no other primary could be found. It was elected to treat this lesion with radiotherapy.

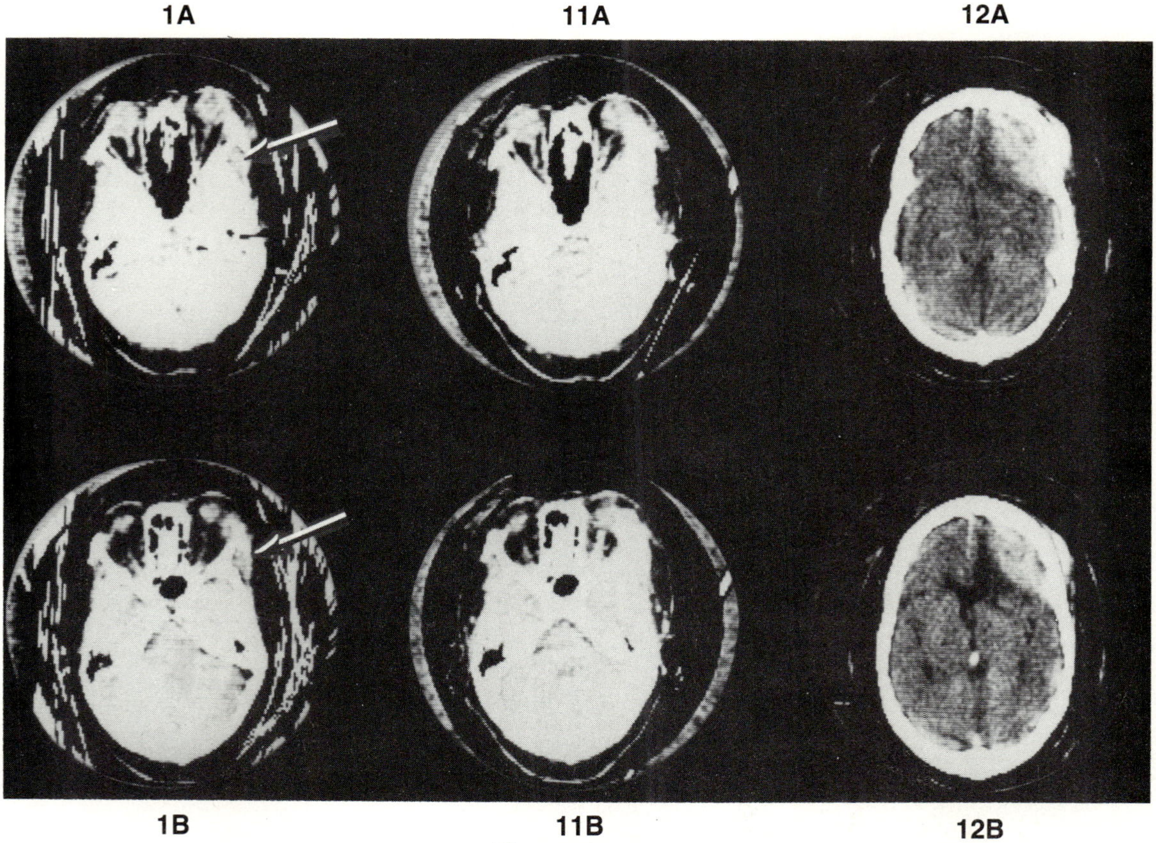

Figure 3–12d

RECURRENT SQUAMOUS CELL CARCINOMA OF THE FACE WITHOUT INTRACRANIAL EXTENSION (Figure 3–13)

A. M. is an 86 year old male with recurrent squamous cell carcinoma of the nose and face. The computed tomogram was obtained to determine whether there was intracranial extension of the tumor.

a. The routine CT scan reveals a bulky tumor mass involving the left maxillary and ethmoid sinuses (arrows), as well as the soft tissues of the face. No evidence of intracranial extension is noted on the preinfusion scan. Density, 34 to 46 u.

1A 2A

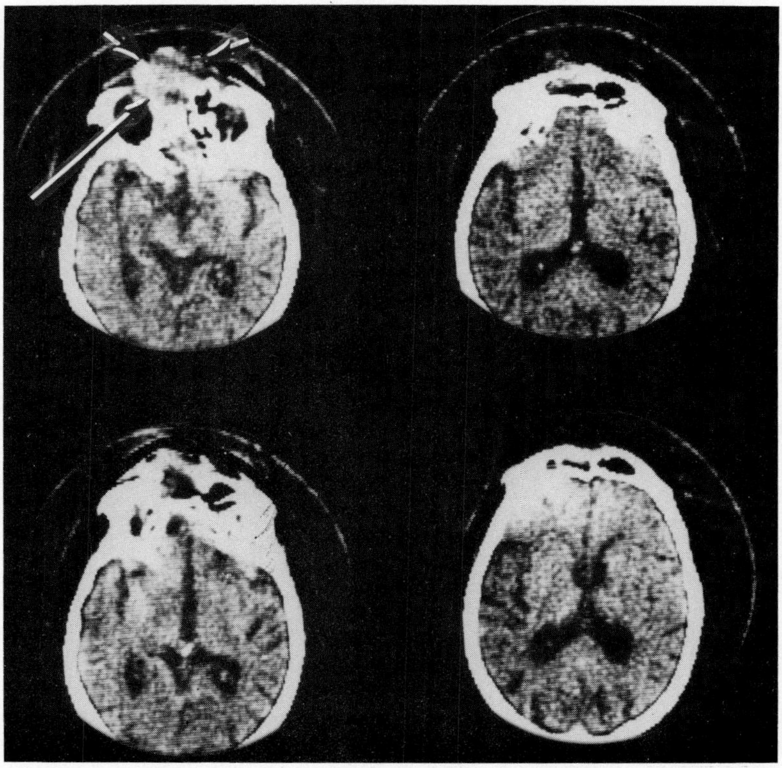

1B 2B

Figure 3–13a

b. After contrast enhancement there is a marked increase in the density of the mass, to 46 to 62 u. The tumor appears to cross the midline and probably involves the right ethmoid sinus as well. There is no evidence of intracranial extension. Moderate atrophy is also noted.

12A

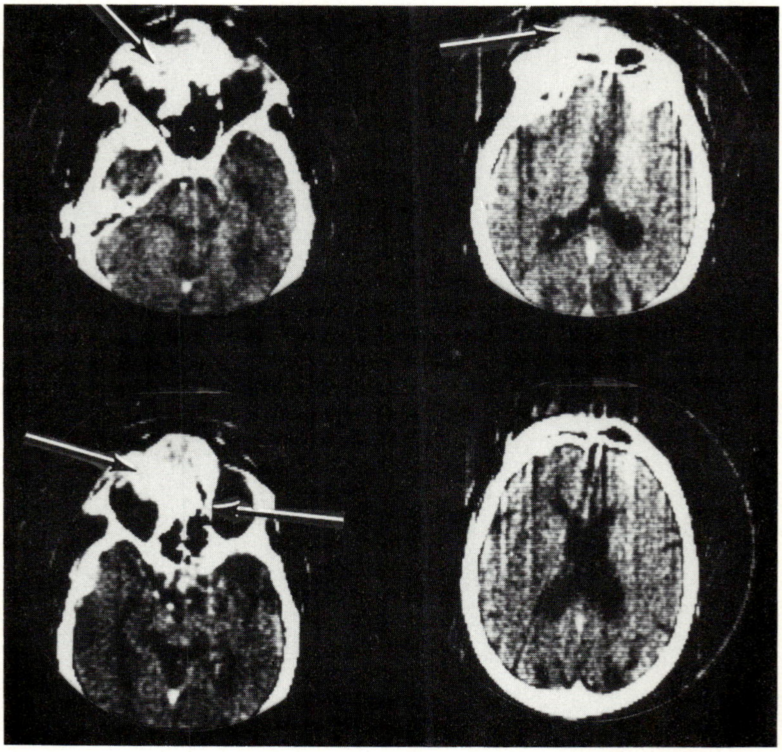

11B 12B

Figure 3–13b

BRAIN ABSCESS (Figure 3–14)

G. S. is a 54 year old male with lymphocytic leukemia. The radionuclide scan of the liver showed a space-occupying lesion. Two weeks ago, during the course of chemotherapy, the patient began having headaches, and, more recently, syncopal episodes.

a and b. The posterior (a) and left lateral (b) views of the radionuclide scan reveal an area of increased activity in the left occipital lobe just above the transverse sinus. There is a suggestion of central lucency.

c. The routine CT scan shows a large area of lucency in the left occipital lobe. There is shift of the midline to the right and anterior displacement of the choroid

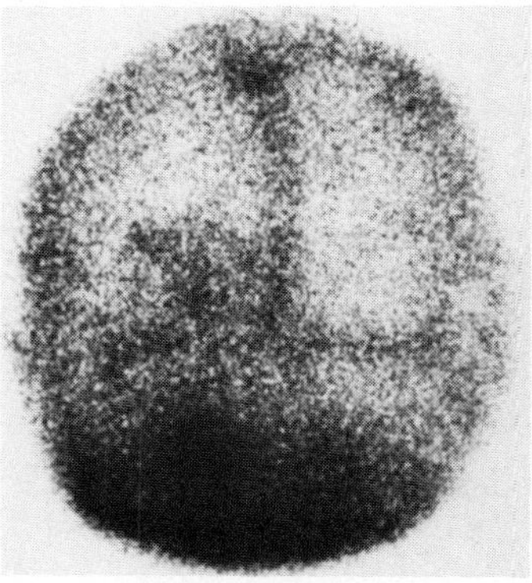

Figure 3–14a

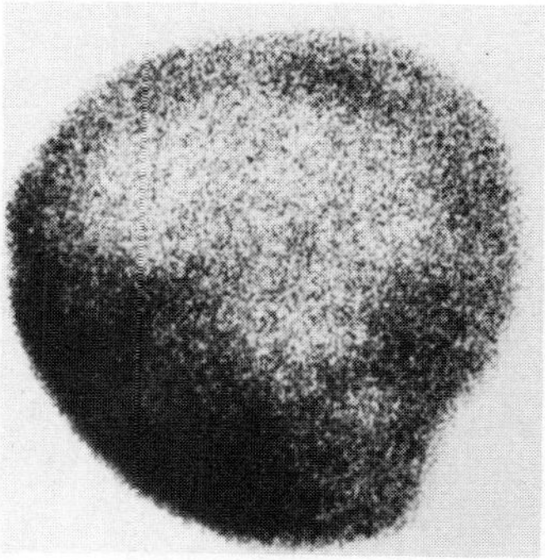

Figure 3–14b

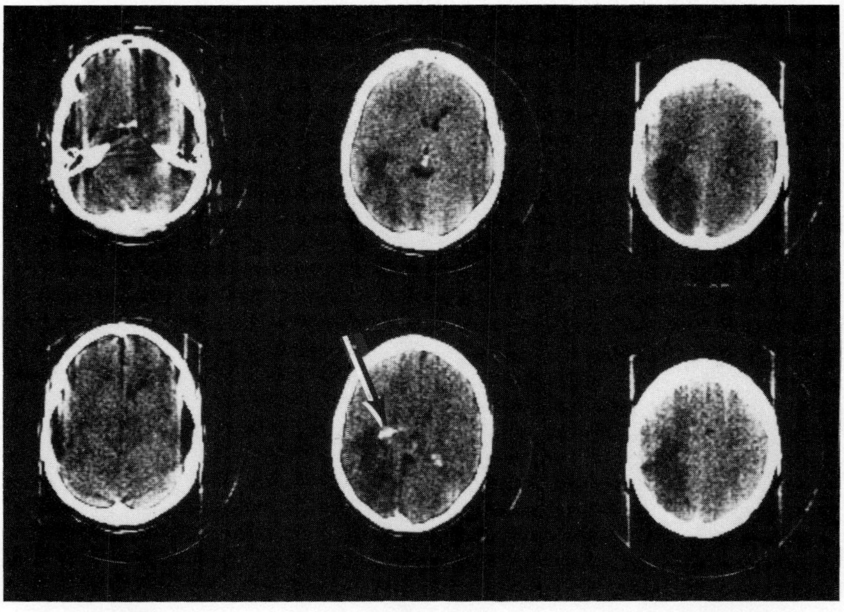

Figure 3–14c

plexus calcification of the left lateral ventricle (arrow on cut 2B).

d. After contrast infusion, there appears to be a multiloculated lesion in the left occipital pole with surrounding edema.

e. The lateral arterial phase of the left carotid arteriogram displays forward and upward displacement of the sylvian triangle.

f. The capillary phase reveals a large avascular area in the left posterior parietal and occipital poles. A vascular capsule could not be identified.

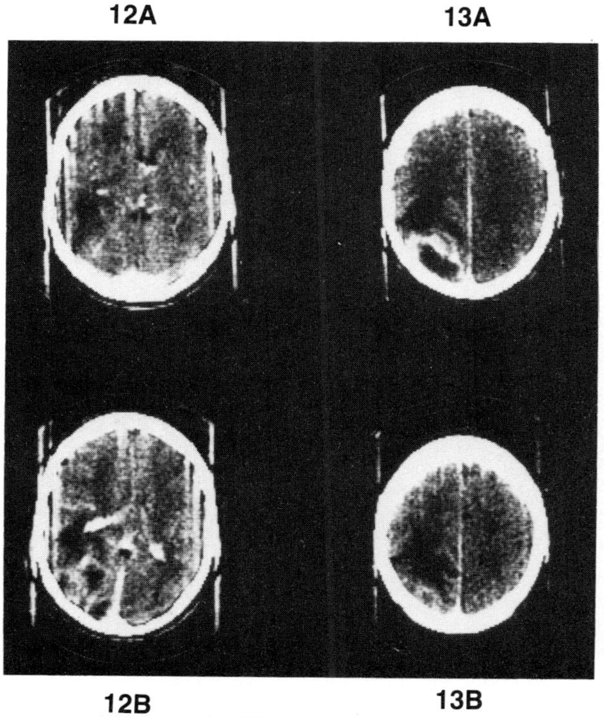

Figure 3–14d

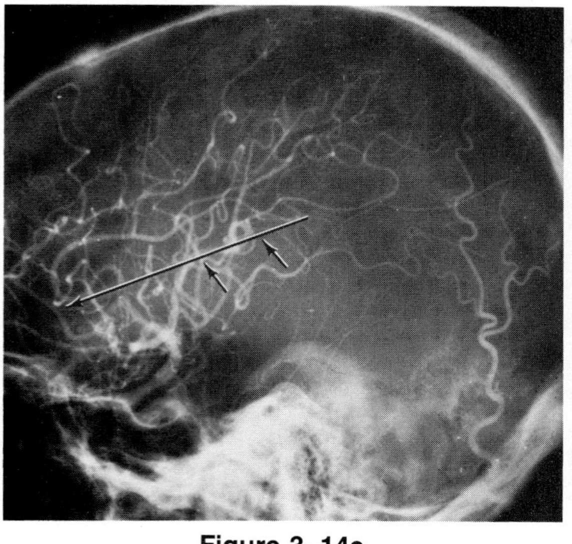

Figure 3–14e

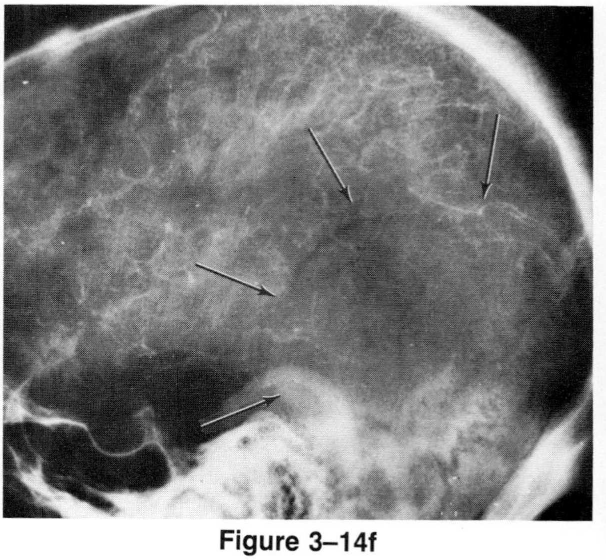

Figure 3–14f

g. There is a distal shift of the anterior cerebral artery under the falx cerebri (arrow).

h. There is greater shift of the internal cerebral vein than of the anterior cerebral artery (arrow). This is a typical finding with posteriorly placed lesions.

Surgery revealed a left occipital lobe abscess.

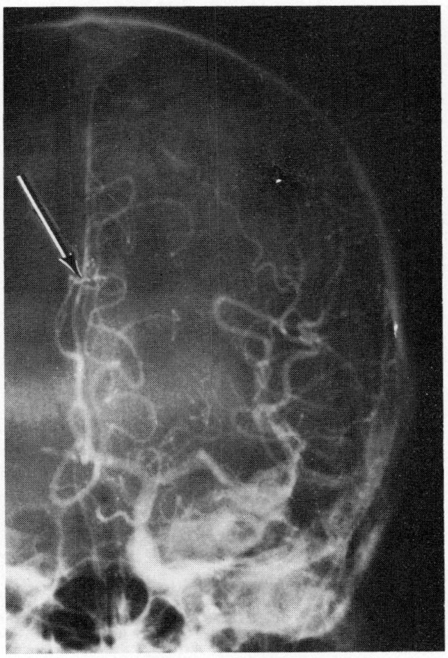

Figure 3–14g

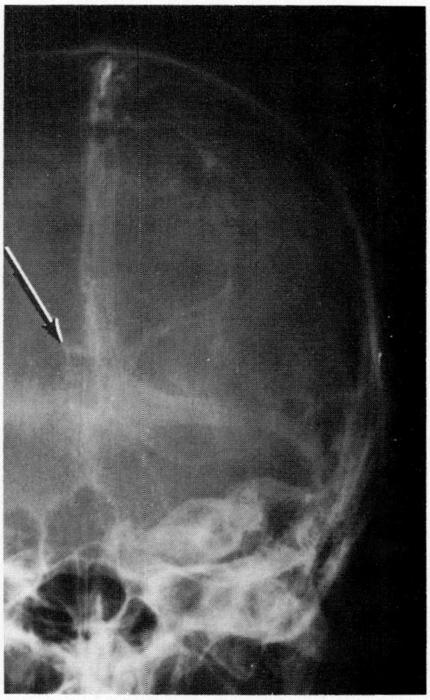

Figure 3–14h

CHAPTER 4

VASCULAR DISEASES

Infarcts

Areas of infarction usually appear as areas of lucency on the preinfusion scan. The age of the infarct cannot usually be determined by the scan appearance. These areas of lucency have a variety of patterns, depending upon the area of the brain that is involved with the infarct. They can vary in size from very small to rather large areas that occupy an entire major vessel distribution. These large areas of infarction are seen most often in the distribution of the middle cerebral artery, but occasionally the anterior cerebral distribution is involved. More rarely the entire distribution of the internal carotid artery may be involved, i.e., the entire hemisphere may be lucent. Most often, in the case of infarcts there will be no evidence of shift of the midline structures. However, with an acute infarct there may occasionally be a small amount of mass effect or even a rather dramatic mass effect with marked shift of the third and lateral ventricles. In these cases an infusion scan is helpful to distinguish between an area of infarction with mass effect and a tumor.

The postinfusion scan may reveal one of several changes: (1) there may be no change in the infarct; (2) the area of infarction may become less apparent; or (3) uncommonly, if the initial scan is negative, the area of infarction may become apparent only after the infusion of contrast material—presumably this is because the normal brain takes up the contrast material whereas the area of infarction does not. The implication of this last statement is that if the patient's clinical appearance suggests an infarct and the initial scan is negative, then an infusion of contrast material may be in order for complete evaluation. Since the postinfusion scan may reveal no change—especially early after the acute insult—infusion study may be academic once an area of intracerebral hemorrhage has been ruled out. (4) On the postinfusion scan, there will occasionally be a marked uptake of the contrast material in the area of infarction because of "luxury perfusion." In these cases the preinfusion scan may show an area of infarction or may even have a normal appearance. The arteriogram may or may not show an area of vascular occlusion with collateral flow; on the other hand, the "luxury perfusion" may be visible on the computed tomogram even without evidence of major vascular occlusion on the arteriogram. (5) Hemorrhagic infarcts are also seen.

Another pattern of vascular enhancement on the postinfusion scans is dense "finger-like" projections of enhancement extending into the brain from the outer convexity with intervening areas of lucency.

Not all infarcts are apparent at the time of the acute insult; approximately 50 to 60 per cent of infarcts will be detectable by computed tomography after the first 7 days.

INFARCT SECONDARY TO SICKLE CELL DISEASE (Figure 4–1)

P. T., a 25 year old female with known sickle cell anemia, presented at this time with mild weakness of the right arm that rapidly progressed to a dense right hemiparesis. In spite of preventive measures, the patient's clinical course progressively and relentlessly deteriorated until death on the day after admission.

a. The routine CT scan reveals a large, somewhat irregular area of lucency in the left frontoparietal region. There is no evidence of shift of the ventricles, and the density of the area measured from 16 to 30 u. The infarct is visible from cuts 1A to 3A. This is a typical appearance of an area of infarction. In this young patient the infarct is secondary to the patient's underlying sickle cell anemia.

1A 2A 3A

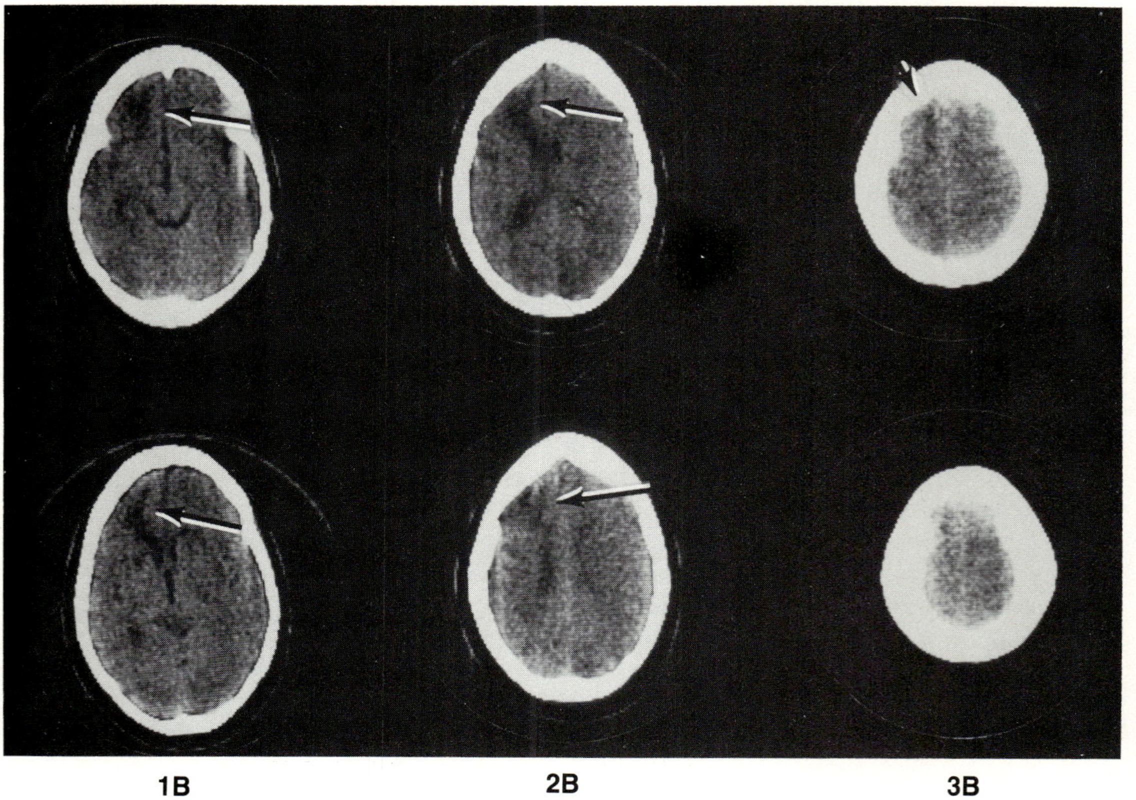

1B 2B 3B

Figure 4–1a

b and c. At the time of postmortem examination, it is apparent that the area of infarct corresponds well to that seen on the CT scan. There is loss of brain substance in this area, as well as diffuse softening of the brain in the area of the left frontal lobe (arrows).

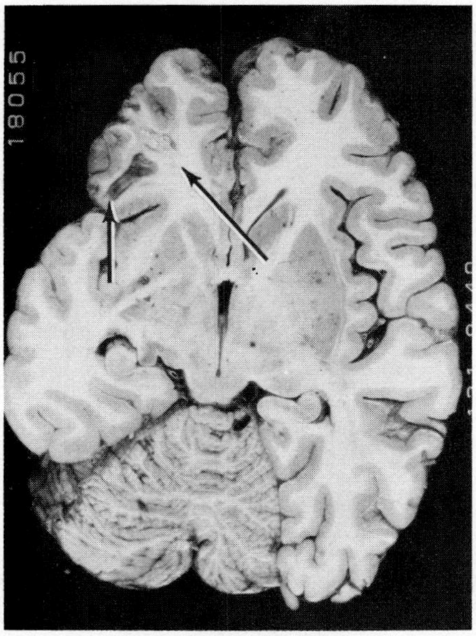

Figure 4–1b

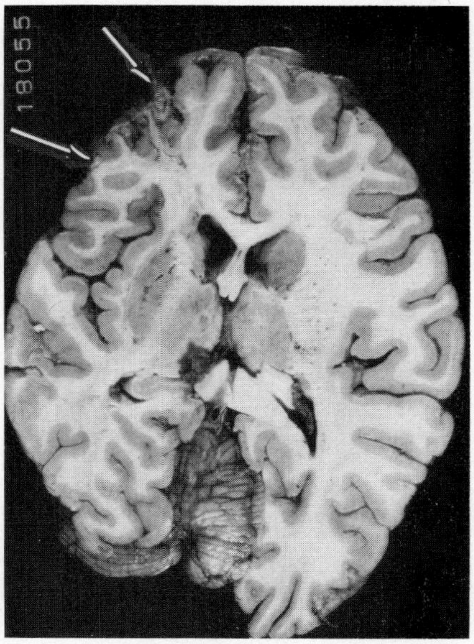

Figure 4–1c

OLD CEREBRAL INFARCT (Figure 4–2)

H. F., an elderly gentleman, gave a history of an old "stroke" many years prior to this study. He never recovered use of his left side.

The routine scan reveals a large area of lucency on the right side that corresponds to the distribution of the right middle cerebral artery. This entire area measured in the density range of cerebrospinal fluid, and this is apparently an area of infarction in the right middle cerebral artery distribution that has progressed to an area of porencephaly.

1A 2A 3A

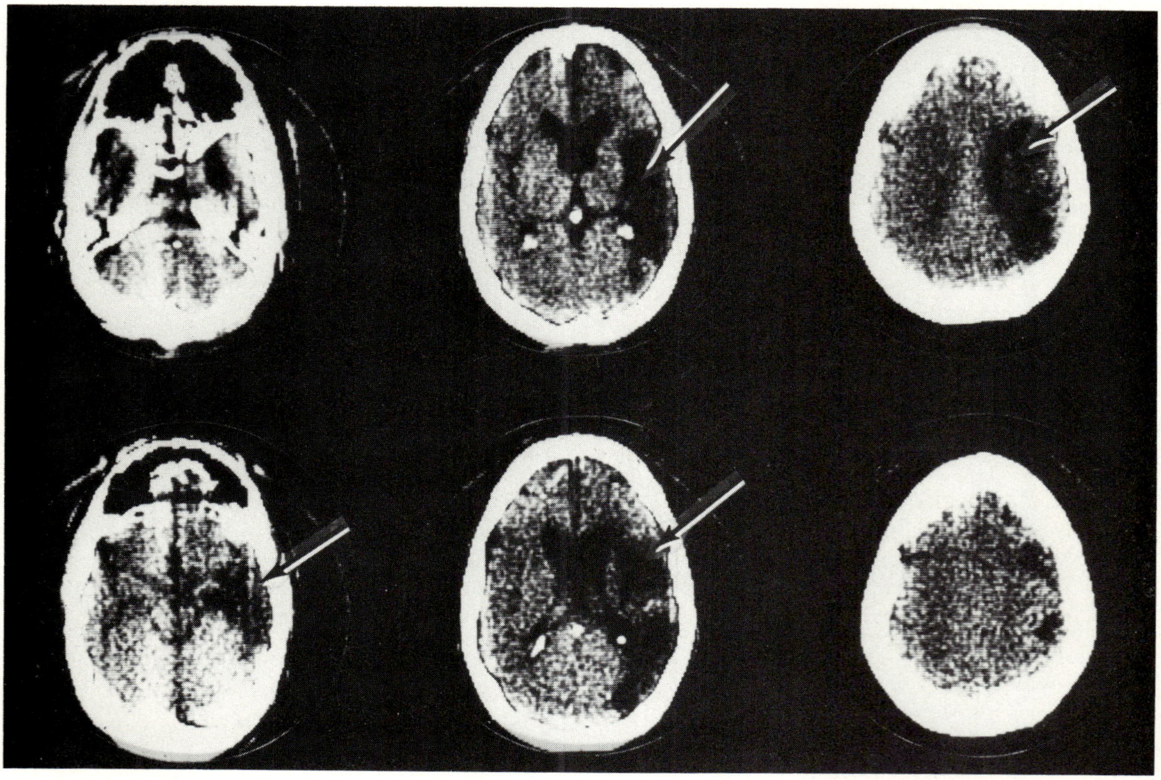

1B 2B 3B

Figure 4–2

LARGE INFARCT WITH MASS EFFECT (Figure 4–3)

E. W. is a 47 year old female with a gradual onset of a left hemiparesis and deepening coma.

The routine CT scan reveals a very large lucent area on the right that measured from 16 to 36 u. There is marked shift from right to left. This represents a very large infarct in the distribution of the right internal carotid artery associated with marked mass effect. This was biopsy proved.

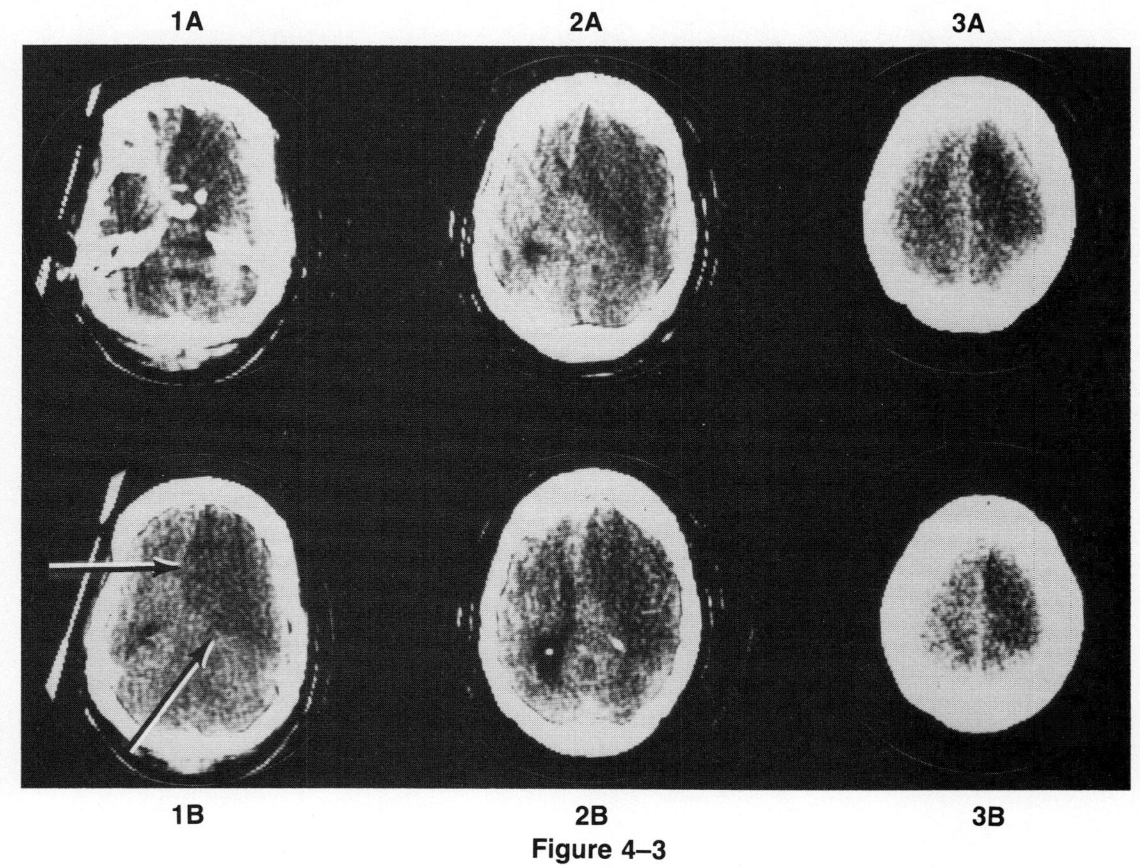

Figure 4–3

MULTIPLE SMALL INFARCTS (Figure 4–4)

This patient had multiple small areas of infarction which varied in density from 0 to 32 u. The possibility of multiple small emboli should be raised in this case.

1A 2A 3A

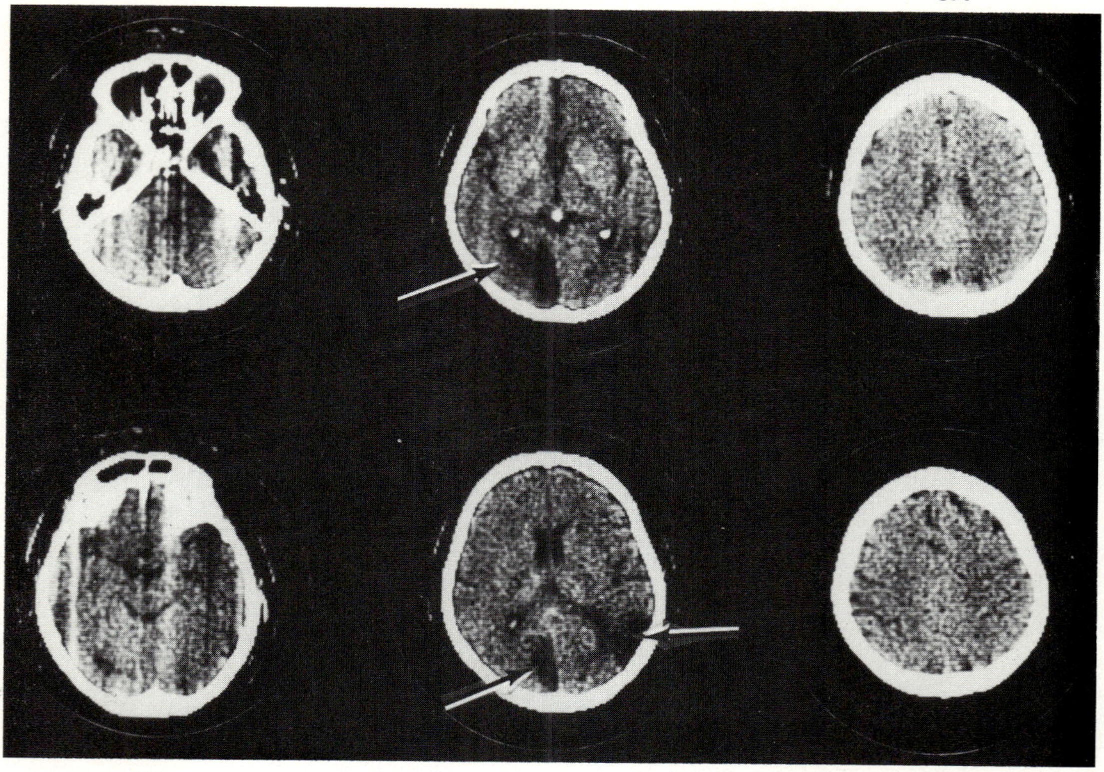

1B 2B 3B

Figure 4–4

ACUTE INFARCT (Figure 4–5)

This 67 year old male presented with the history of sudden onset of a left hemiparesis.

a and b. The preinfusion portion of the examination reveals an area of lucency in the right middle cerebral artery distribution (arrows).

c and d. After the infusion of contrast material, the area of lucency is less apparent (arrows). At times the postinfusion scan may appear entirely normal. Therefore, if only a postinfusion scan is performed, the acute infarct may be overlooked.

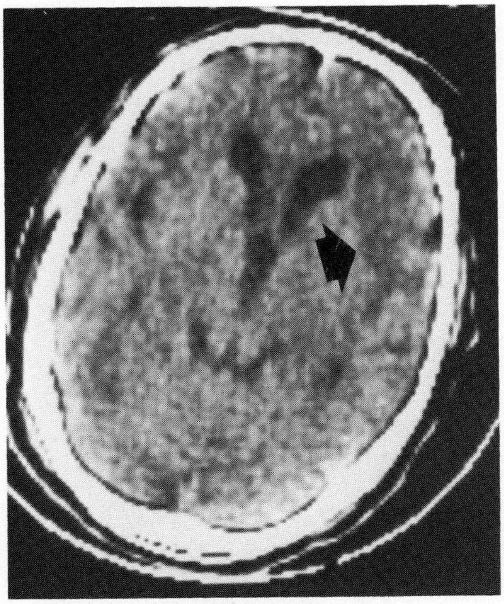

Figure 4–5a

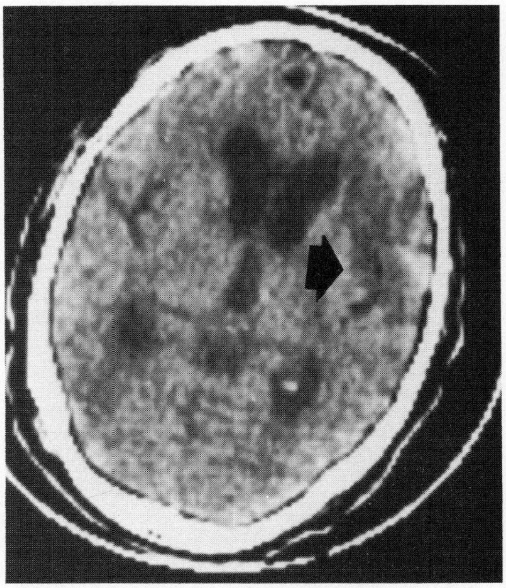

Figure 4–5b

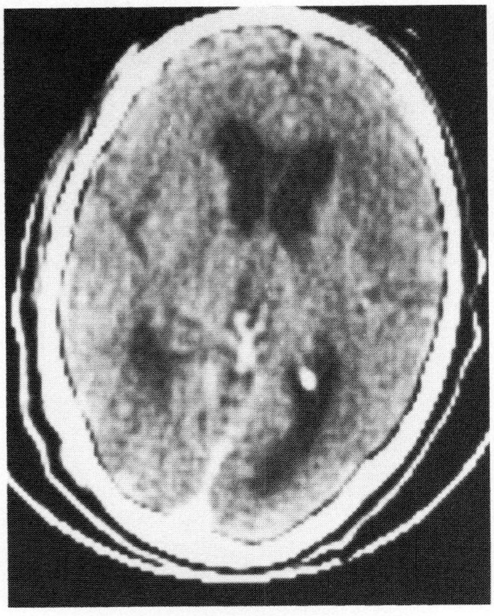

Figure 4–5c

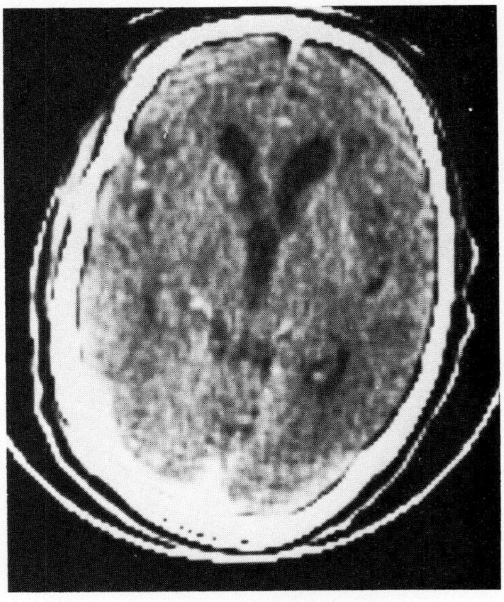

Figure 4–5d

CALCIFIED INFARCT (Figure 4–6)

This 73 year old male presented for routine study with a history of a cerebrovascular accident 10 years previously.

a and b. The CT scan reveals an area of lucency in the left anterior and middle cerebral artery distribution consistent with an area of infarction. The infarct is old and it is associated with enlargement of the ipsilateral ventricle. In addition, there is an area of calcification in the middle of the area of infarction, which is believed to be dystrophic calcification secondary to the infarct. This appearance is rare but not unseen.

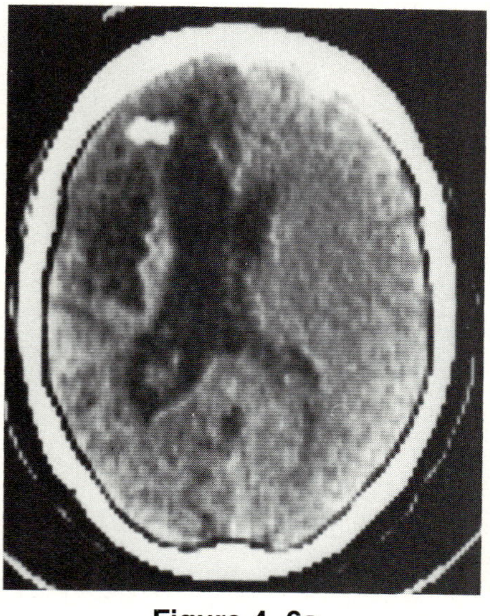

Figure 4–6a

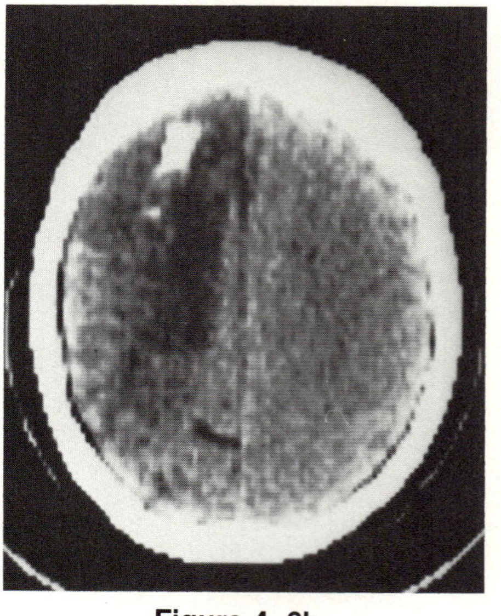

Figure 4–6b

CEREBRAL INFARCT (Figure 4–7)

G. M. is an elderly gentleman who presented with transient episodes of aphasia and right-sided weakness. The aphasia cleared, but the right-sided weakness remained.

a. The routine CT scan reveals an area of lucency in the distribution of the left middle cerebral artery without evidence of shift. The findings are consistent with a left middle cerebral infarct.

b. On the percutaneous left carotid arteriogram, a complete occlusion of the left internal carotid artery is seen at the level of the bifurcation (arrow).

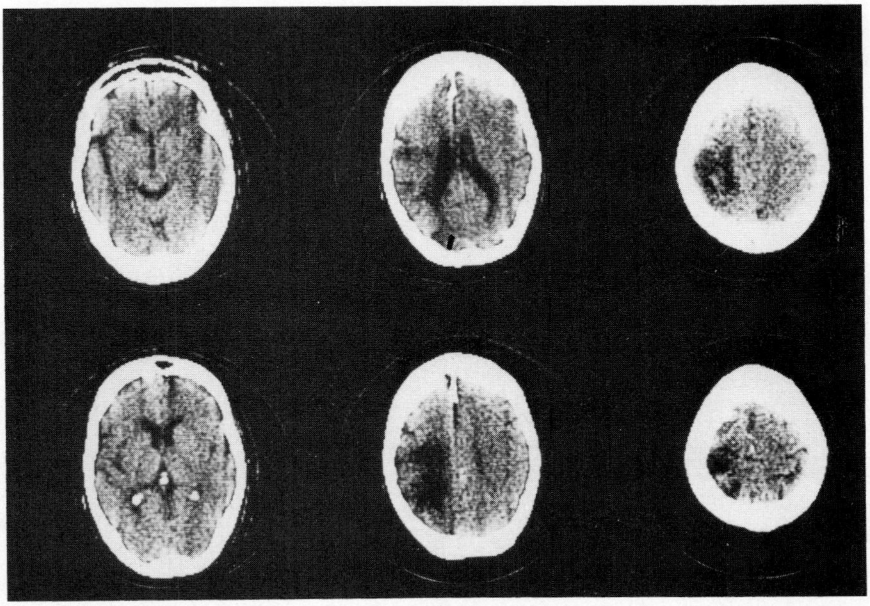

Figure 4–7a

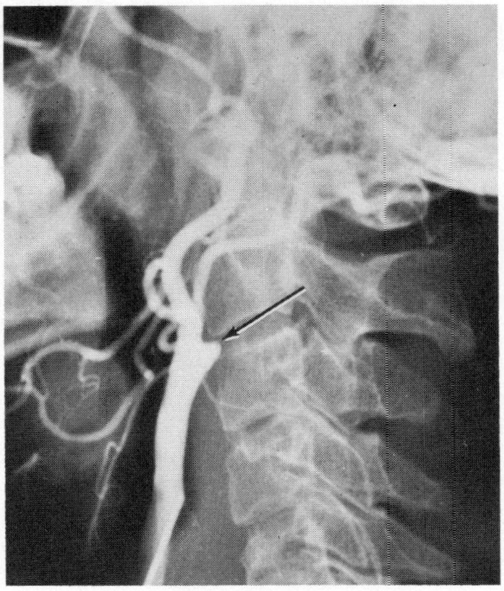

Figure 4–7b

c and d. The right brachial arteriogram reveals crossover to fill the entire left side as well. A small aneurysm is also noted in the cavernous portion of the internal carotid artery on the right side (arrow). The bifurcation on the right side did not have a significant stenosis.

The infarct in this case is presumably ischemic, possibly at the time of occlusion of the left internal carotid artery.

When working a patient up for carotid bifurcation disease in the neck, it is safest to begin with the right brachial arteriogram. Both a neck-chest and an intracranial series should be performed in a biplane projection. One should always be alert to the possibility of intracranial vascular stenosis, as well as the occasional unsuspected brain tumor. By evaluating the presence or absence of crossover filling from the right side, one can get some idea of the patency of the left carotid circulation. Following right brachial arteriography, percutaneous puncture of the left carotid artery is then performed with biplane study of the carotid bifurcation and the intracranial circulation.

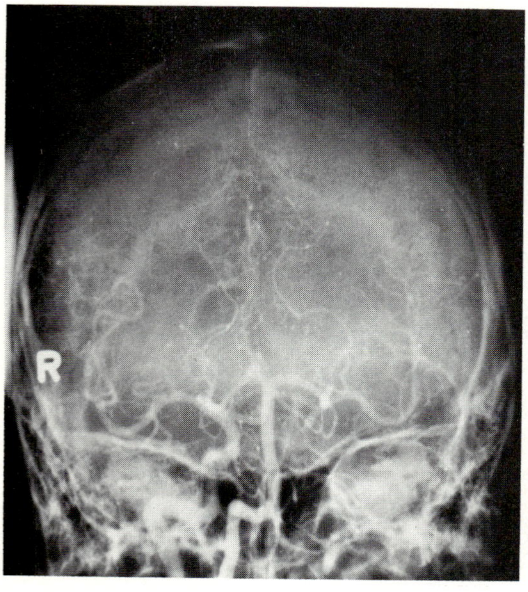

Figure 4–7c

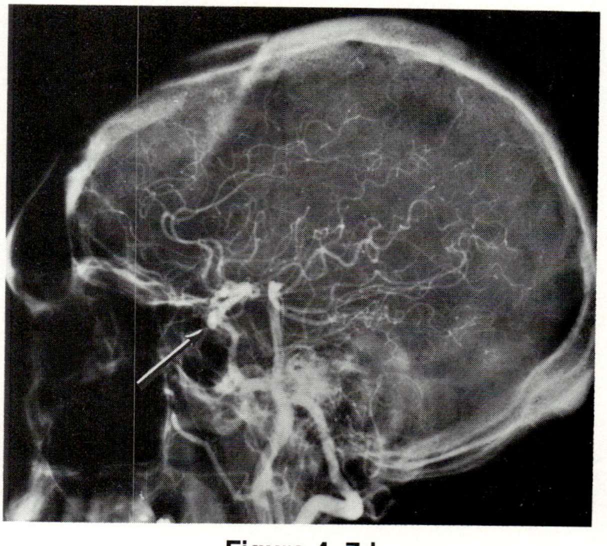

Figure 4–7d

INFARCT WITH LUXURY PERFUSION (Figure 4–8)

S. K., a 52 year old male, presented initially with a right retinal stroke. Later in his hospitalization he developed confusion of sudden onset and a left hemiparesis. He had a right carotid bruit.

a. Radionuclide scan: The vertex view reveals some increase in uptake deep in the right hemisphere.

b and c. The lateral views appear within normal limits.

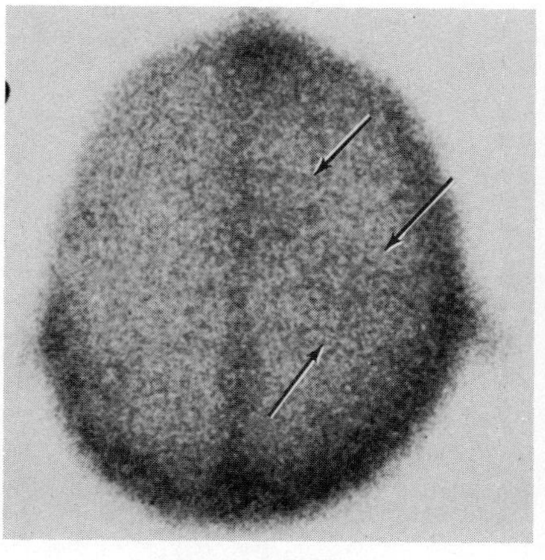

Figure 4–8a

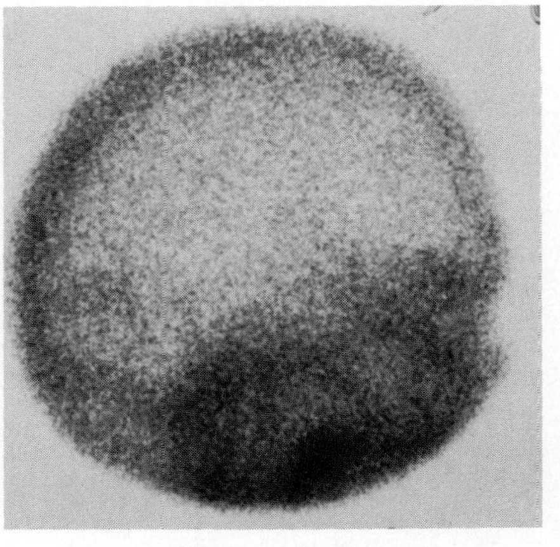

Figure 4–8b

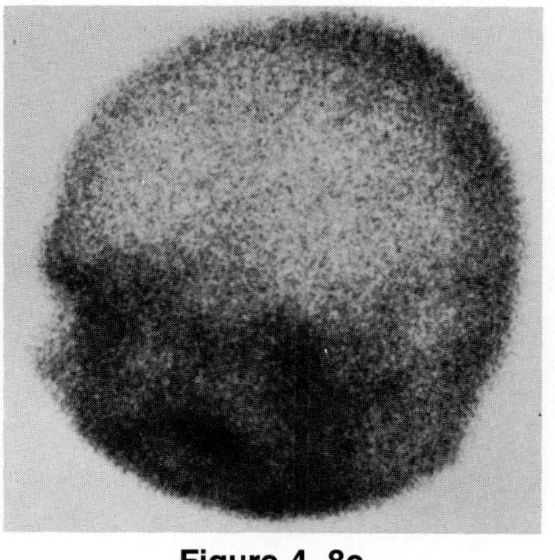

Figure 4–8c

d. The routine CT scan also appears within normal limits. The area of infarction visualized post infusion measured 24 to 44 u on the initial scan—well within normal limits.

e. Post infusion a large area of marked enhancement is noted in the distribution of the right middle cerebral artery. This represents the "luxury perfusion" appearance that can be seen occasionally on the arteriograms as well as on the CT scans.

2A

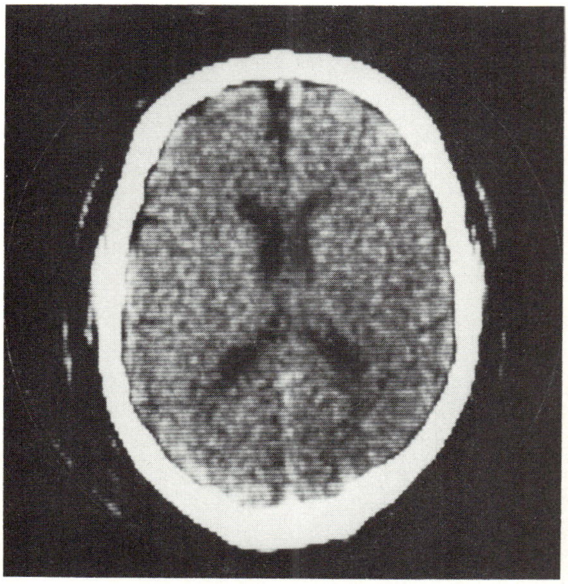

Figure 4–8d

11A 12A 13A

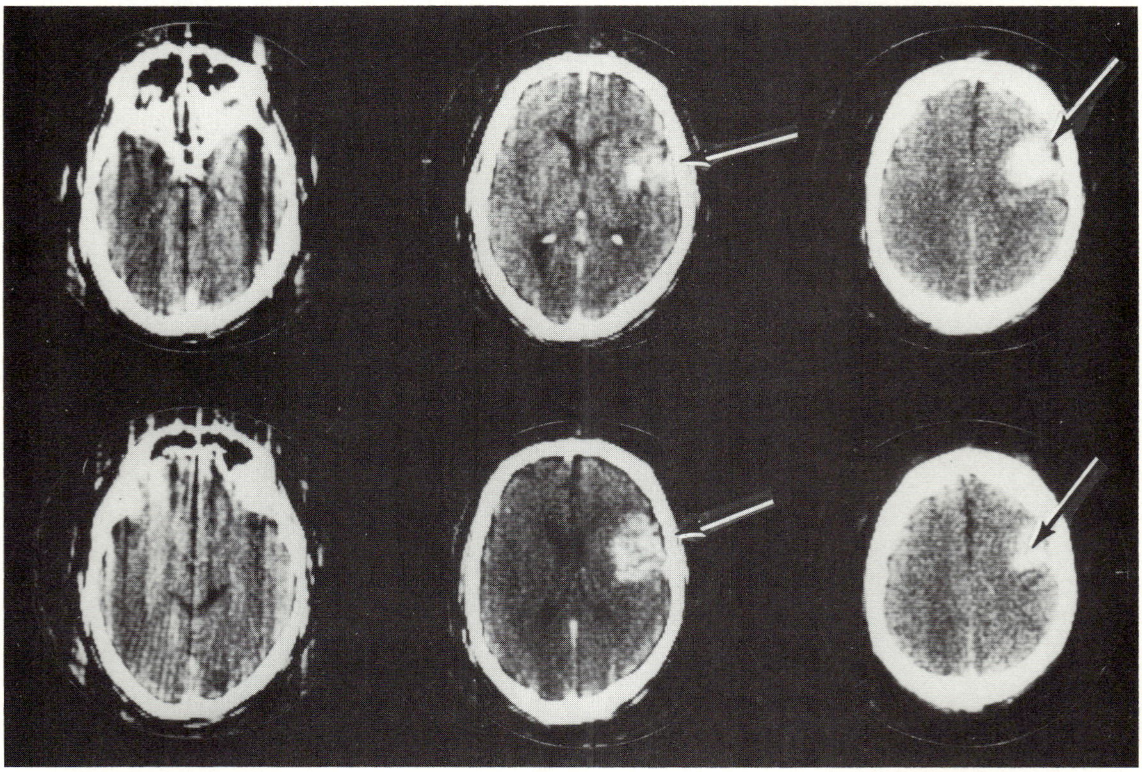

11B 12B 13B

Figure 4–8e

INFARCT WITH LUXURY PERFUSION (Figure 4–9)

C. H. is a 54 year old male who presented with a sudden onset of confusion and right hemiparesis.

a and b. The left lateral (a) and posterior (b) views of the radionuclide scan reveal an area of increased uptake in the left middle cerebral artery distribution. The findings are consistent with an area of infarction.

c. The routine CT scan shows mild atrophy but no evidence of infarction. Density in the area of infarction was 16 to 34 u.

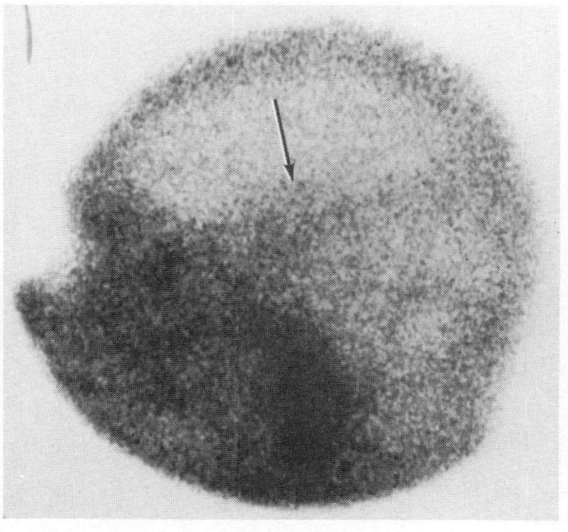

Figure 4–9a

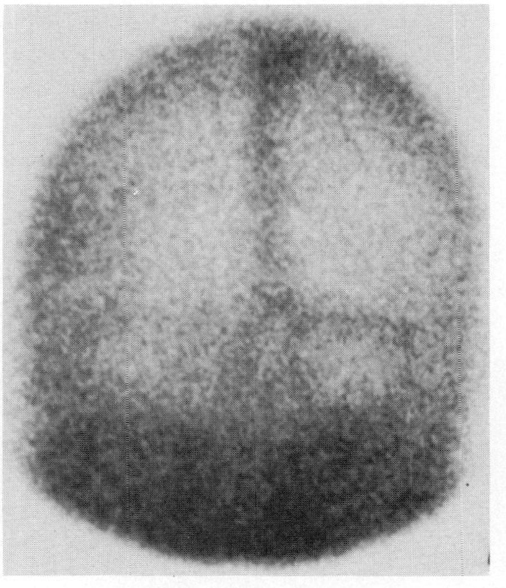

Figure 4–9b

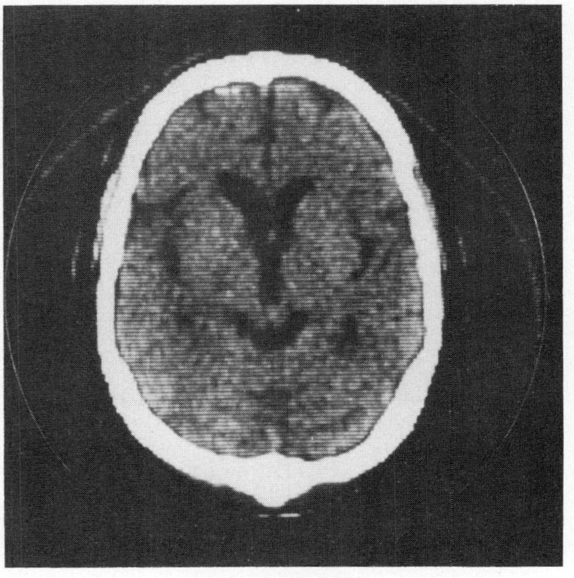

Figure 4–9c

d. However, after infusion there is a large irregular area of enhancement that is apparent on all the postinfusion views. Density, 54 to 84 u (arrows). The value of the infusion study in this patient is questionable. The history was that of an infarction, and the nuclide scan substantiated that diagnosis. Once the routine CT scan has ruled out an area of hemorrhage or the presence of a tumor, further demonstration of the area of infarction becomes academic. Of course, performing an infusion study on all such patients will increase the accuracy of diagnosis and decrease the number of false negative scans.

11A 12A 13A

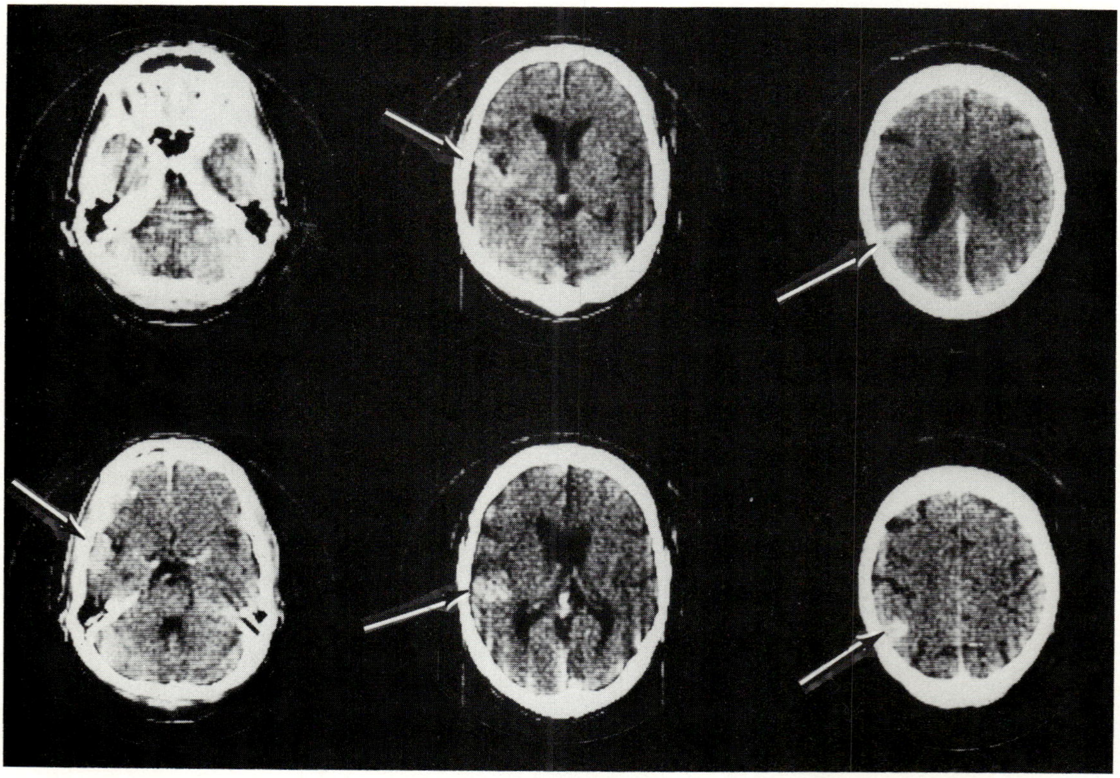

11B 12B 13B

Figure 4–9d

INFARCT WITH LUXURY PERFUSION (Figure 4–10)

S. B. is a 55 year old female who entered the hospital with a 15-year history of uncontrolled hypertension and acute onset of left arm weakness.

a and b. The anterior (a) and right lateral (b) views of the radionuclide scan reveal a flame-shaped region of increased uptake in the anterior portion of the right middle cerebral artery distribution. The angiogram phase (not shown) demonstrates decreased perfusion on the right on the initial views, with increased perfusion on the right side on the delayed views. These are classic findings for a right middle cerebral artery infarct.

c. On the routine CT scan, a mottled area of increased and decreased density is seen in the middle cerebral artery distribution on the right side. There is no mass effect noted. Density, 24 to 50 u.

d. Post infusion there is marked enhancement in this area, with the density increasing to 36 to 96 u. This is luxury perfusion.

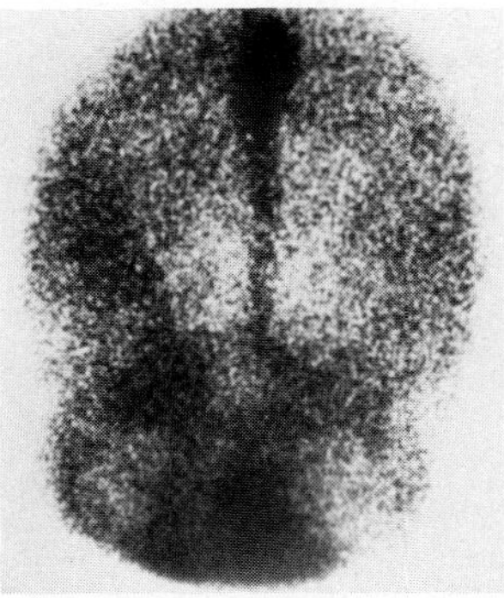

Figure 4–10a

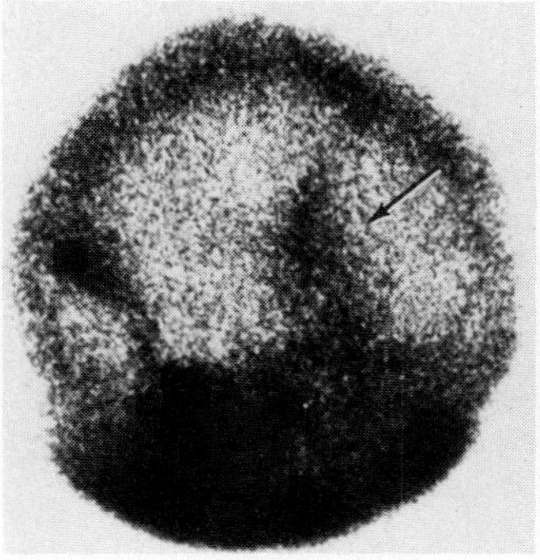

Figure 4–10b

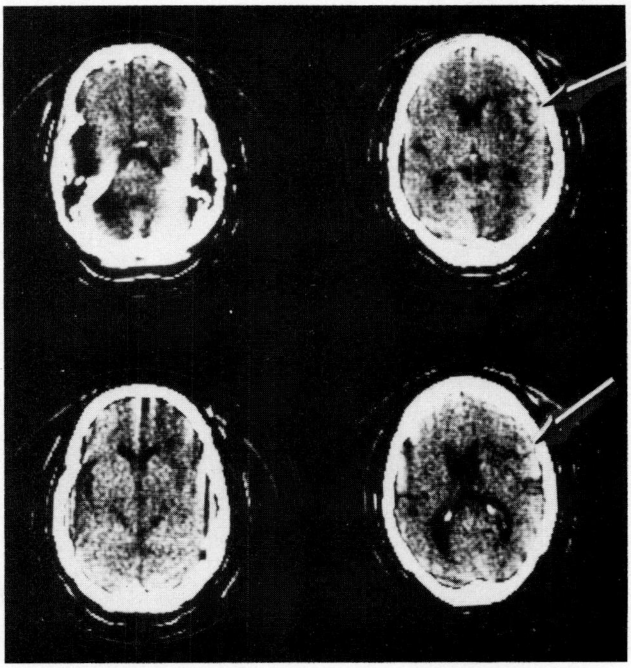

Figure 4–10c

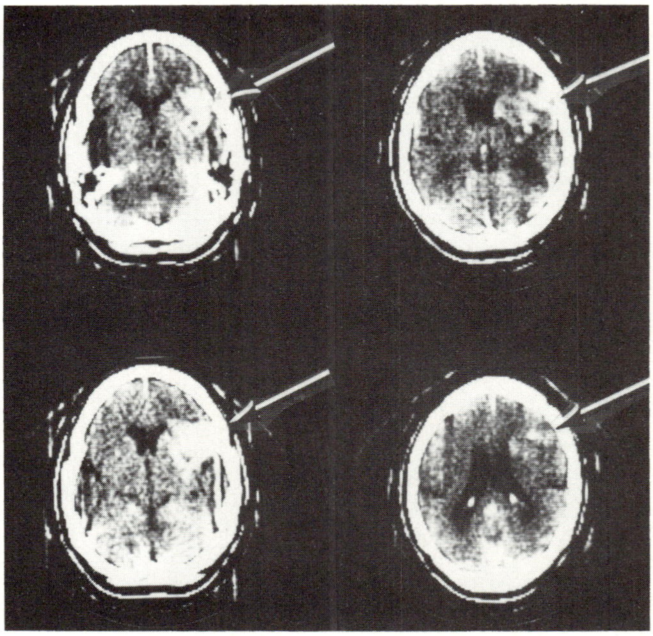

Figure 4–10d

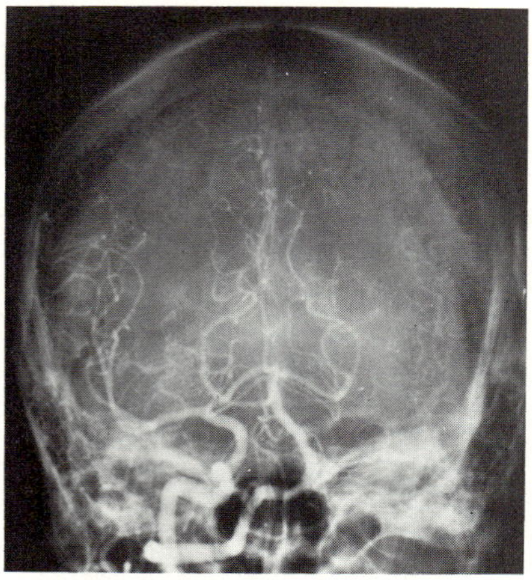

Figure 4–10e

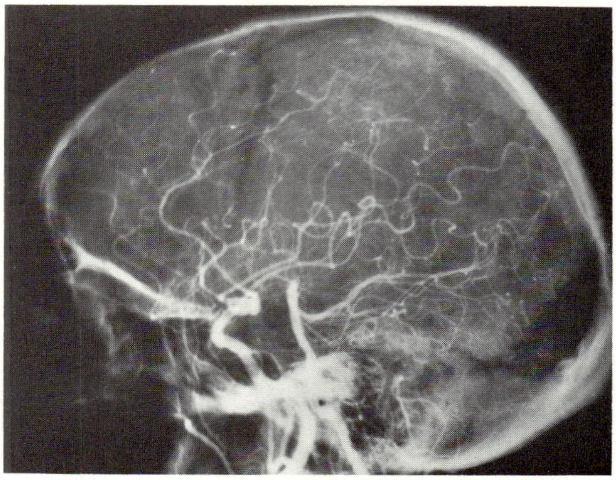

Figure 4–10f

e to g. The right brachial arteriogram shows no evidence of vascular occlusion. The AP view reveals no evidence of shift. The arterial phase on the lateral view (f) demonstrates no abnormalities. On the venous phase there is a faint blush consistent with luxury perfusion in the infarcted area (arrows), and this is the arteriographic reflection of the findings noted on the postinfusion CT scan.

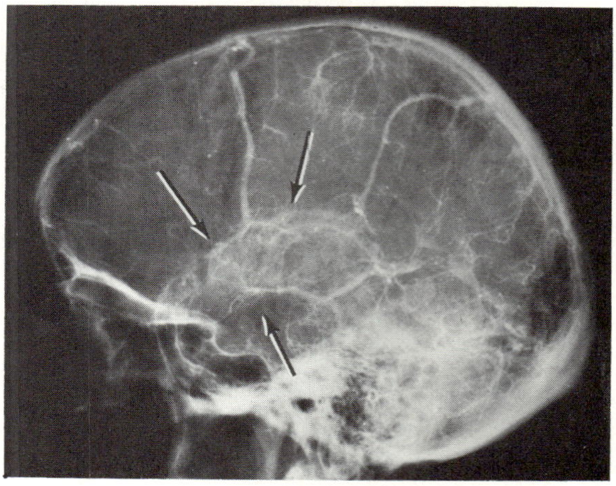

Figure 4–10g

INFARCT WITH LUXURY PERFUSION (Figure 4–11)

This 62 year old female is 10 days "post-CVA."

a. The preinfusion scan appears within normal limits. The lateral ventricles are top-normal in size.

b. Post infusion there is enhancement and "luxury perfusion" in the left middle cerebral artery distribution; density, 48 to 100 u.

2A 2B

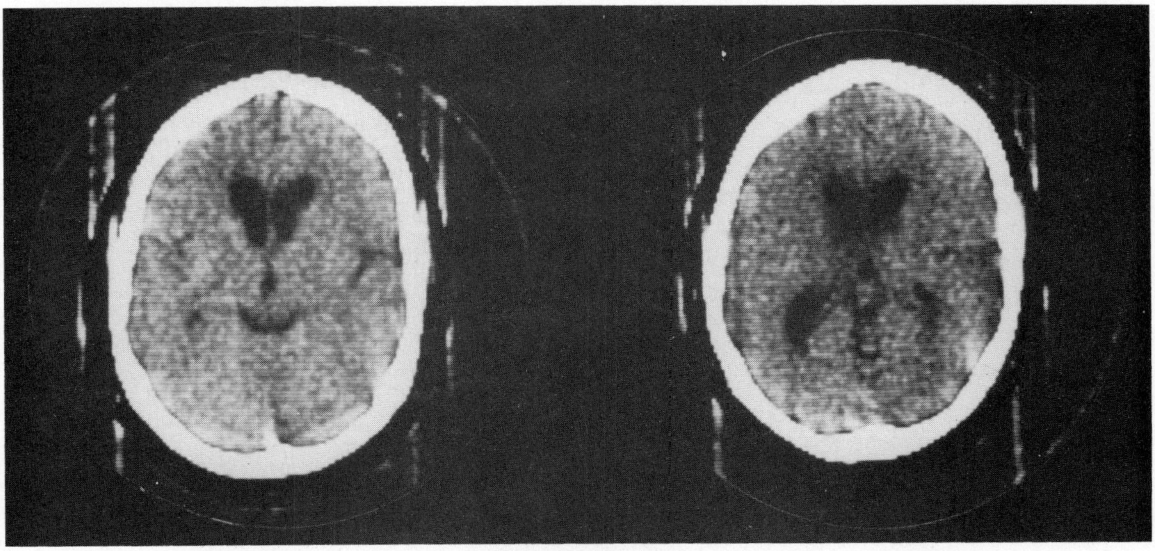

Figure 4–11a

11A 12A 13A

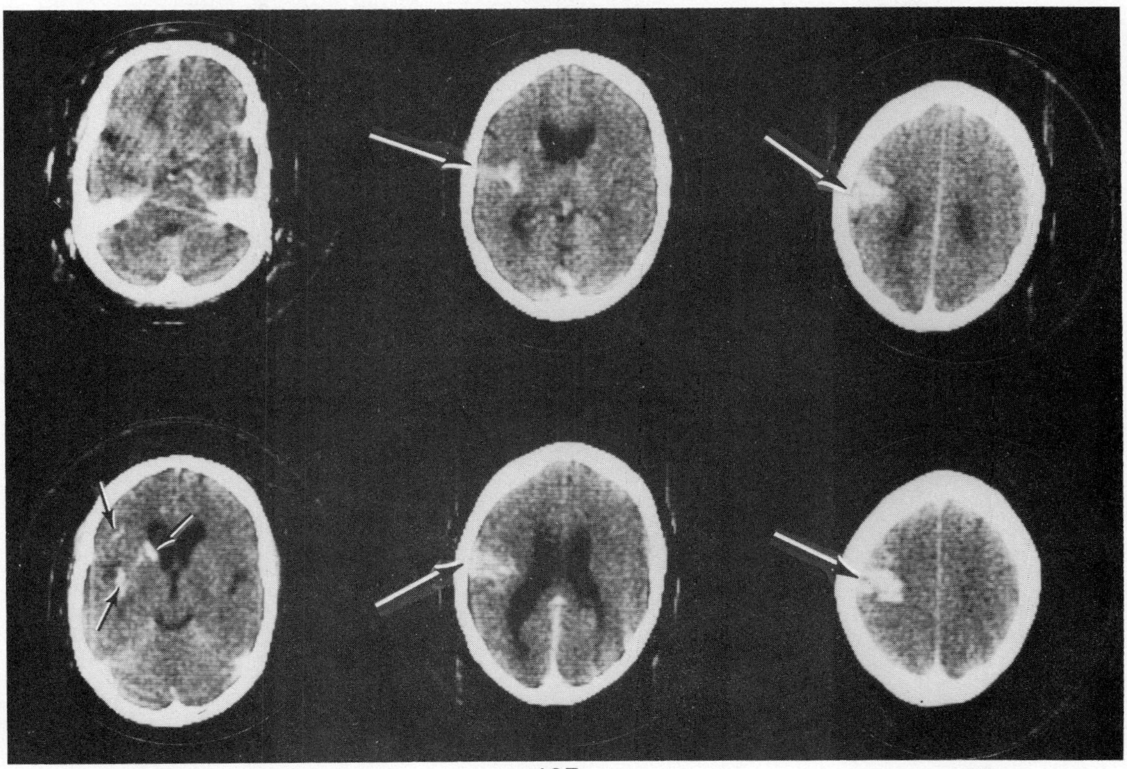

11B 12B 13B

Figure 4–11b

INFARCT WITH MASS EFFECT (Figure 4–12)

S. S. is a 66 year old female who developed incoherent speech and right-sided weakness 3 days prior to this scan.

The routine CT scan reveals an irregular area of decreased density in the left basal ganglia region which measured from 16 to 30 u (arrows). Some mass effect is noted with this area of infarction, with slight compression of the frontal horn of the left lateral ventricle, and the slight shift of the third ventricle. Incidentally, there is enlargement of the prepontine and cerebellopontine angle cisterns (arrows on 1A), raising the possibility of pontocerebellar atrophy or degeneration.

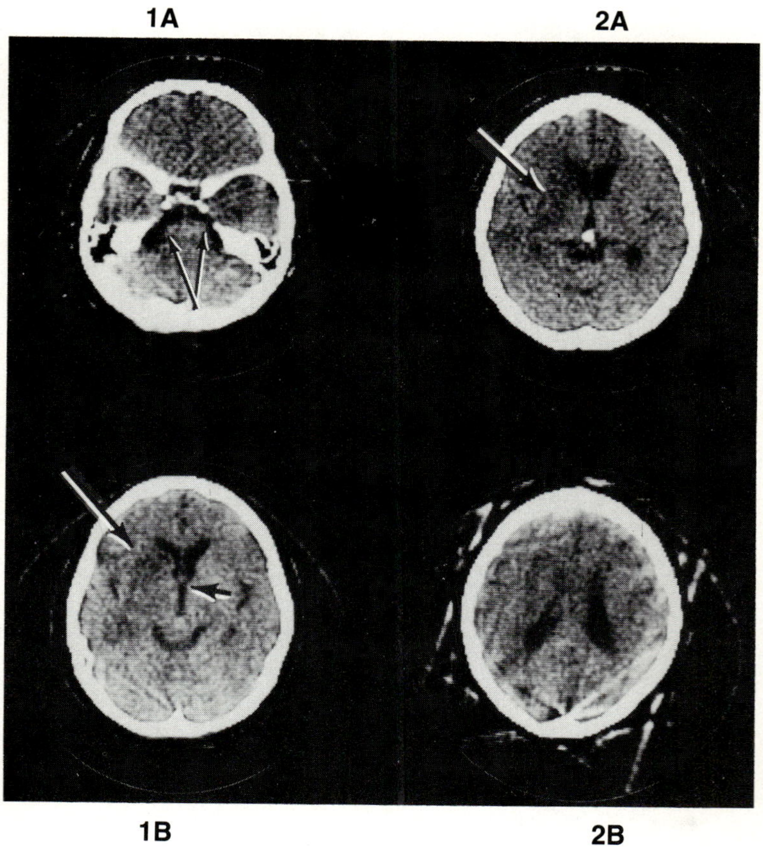

Figure 4–12

INFARCT AND SMALL ASYMPTOMATIC MENINGIOMA (Figure 4–13)

L. W. is a 52 year old female who presented with a right hemiparesis of acute onset.

a. The routine CT scan shows a large low density area in the distribution of the left middle cerebral artery. There is no evidence of mass effect.

b. The postinfusion scan reveals no real change in the area of infarction; however, a small round area of enhancement is noted adjacent to the straight sinus on the right side (long arrow).

c. Postmortem examination of the brain discloses the large area of softening in the left hemisphere (arrows), correlating perfectly with what is present on the CT scan.

d. In addition, a small asymptomatic meningioma is attached to the falx cerebri just at the level of its attachment with the tentorium. This photograph of the embedded sectioned specimen reveals both the meningioma and its meningeal attachment. The meningioma measured 13 mm in its longest dimension.

2B

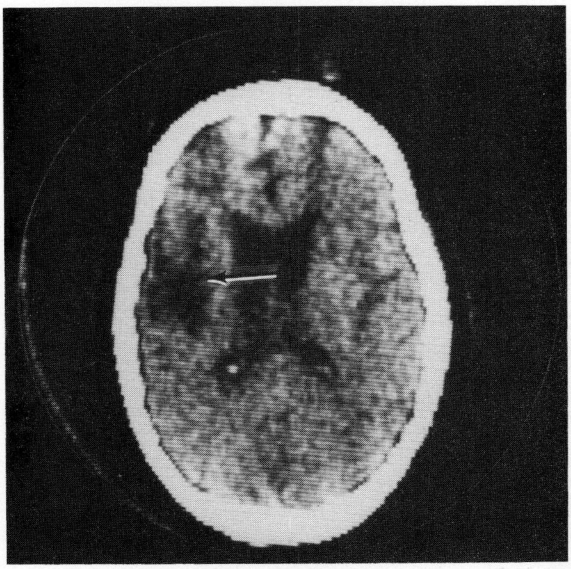

Figure 4–13a

12B

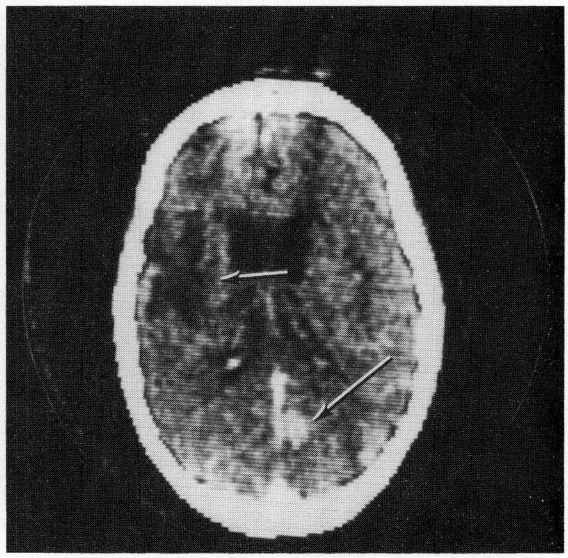

Figure 4–13b

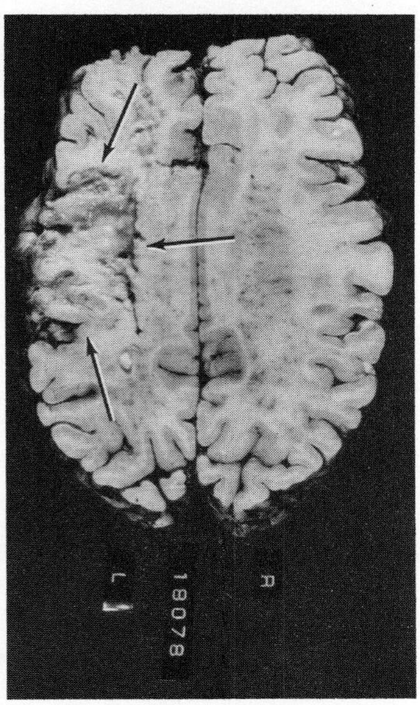

Figure 4–13c

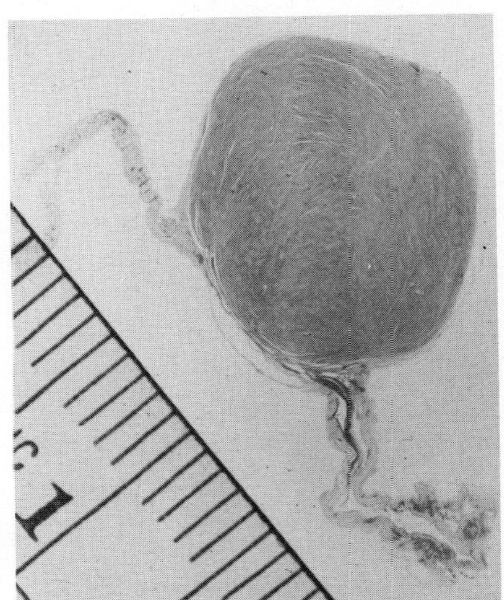

Figure 4–13d

Spontaneous Intracerebral Hematomas

Intracerebral hematomas are diagnosed beautifully by the method of CT scanning. The high density of clotted blood makes the area of abnormality readily apparent on the scan. These intracerebral hematomas can range in size from a very small lesion to one of spectacularly large size. The small hematomas with a wide symptom complex are those that occur in the pons and brain stem. In the past, these pontine and brain stem hemorrhages have been suspected but never proved. The radionuclide scan is normal acutely, and these hematomas begin to resorb very early after they occur. The areas of clotted blood may at times be surrounded by an area of edema even in the acute stage; certainly they develop an area of surrounding lucency after resorption begins.

Hypertensive basal ganglia hematomas are readily diagnosed. The clinical history of acute onset of a contralateral hemiparalysis and decreased level of consciousness is the initial clue to the diagnosis. On the CT scan the areas of spontaneous hemorrhage are often quite large and generally occur in the region of the basal ganglia. The classic angiographic appearance with contralateral shift of the anterior cerebral artery and an even greater shift of the internal cerebral vein is often seen. The lenticulostriate arteries may be displaced either medially or laterally, depending upon the position of the hemorrhage, and these changes can be readily correlated with the CT findings. The usual density of clotted blood is approximately 56 to 90 u, but may extend over a larger density range. There is essentially no change in the appearance of these areas of hemorrhage after the infusion of contrast material. We have occasionally seen cases of spontaneous intracerebral hematomas even in the absence of hypertensive disease; in these cases an occult arteriovenous malformation should be suspected.

BRAIN STEM HEMORRHAGE (Figure 4–14)

L. R. is a 38 year old female hypertensive who presented with nausea, dizziness, nystagmus, and vomiting of acute onset.

The radionuclide scan is within normal limits. The routine CT scan reveals a small area of increased density in the posterior fossa just to the left of the fourth ventricle. This area measured 44 to 68 u (arrow). There is also a small amount of edema noted anterior to this. No deformity of the fourth ventricle appears and no other abnormalities are noted. This represents a small brain stem and/or cerebellar hemorrhage.

This type of abnormality has been suspected for some time but could not be proved premortem prior to CT scanning. The range of size of posterior fossa hemorrhages is of course quite variable. A large hemorrhage is fatal very early, whereas a small area of hemorrhage presents acutely and resolves over a period of time.

This case illustrates an important concept—that of the "partial volume phenomenon." The density of the area of hemorrhage in this case was from 44 to 68 u. This density is lower than we would anticipate for clotted blood. Because the routine scan cuts are 8 mm thick, a small area of increased density may extend only partially into the scan slice thickness and thus will not fill up the 8 mm thickness. If this is the case, the computed density will also include the adjacent normal brain (or another structure) and thus lower the average density in the small column of tissue, ultimately lowering the anticipated density value of the lesion. The reverse is true for a relatively low density mass. This "partial volume phenomenon" can be seen with any combination of densities, and should be borne in mind when a density measurement is made on a relatively small abnormal area.

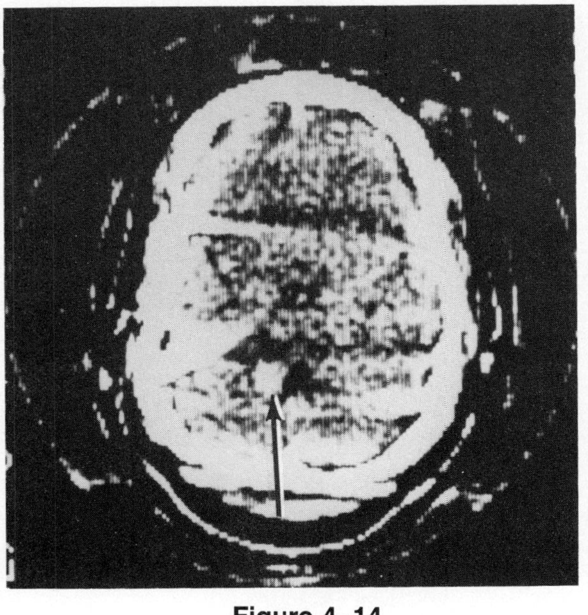

Figure 4–14

MASSIVE BRAIN STEM HEMORRHAGE (Figure 4–15)

E. F., an elderly woman, presented to the emergency room with bilateral flaccid paralysis and coma of sudden onset. No further history was available.

a. The computed tomogram reveals a very large high density lesion in the pons and medulla, extending off laterally. The density measured from 56 to 88 u. This represents a very large brain stem hemorrhage.

b. Cut 2A shows the upward extent of the hemorrhage. Clotted blood is present in the third ventricle (crossed arrow), extending upward in the cerebral peduncles (arrows). There is moderate acute obstructive hydrocephalus.

This patient was being sustained on a respirator at the time of this study; however, there is no chance of recovery from a devastating injury such as this massive hemorrhage into such a critical area.

1A

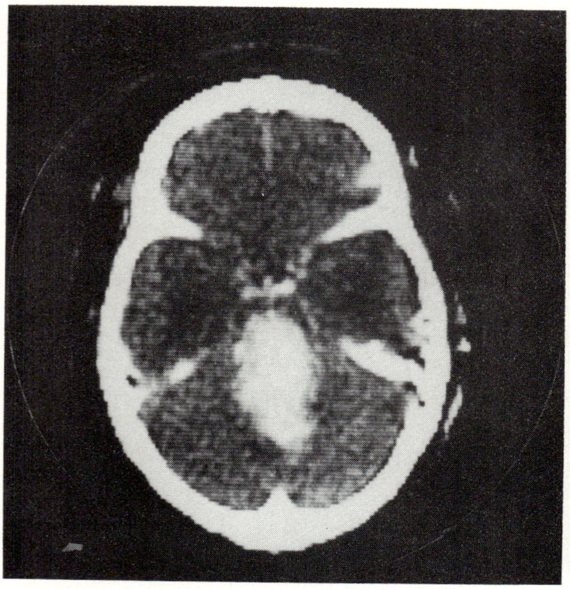

Figure 4–15a

2A

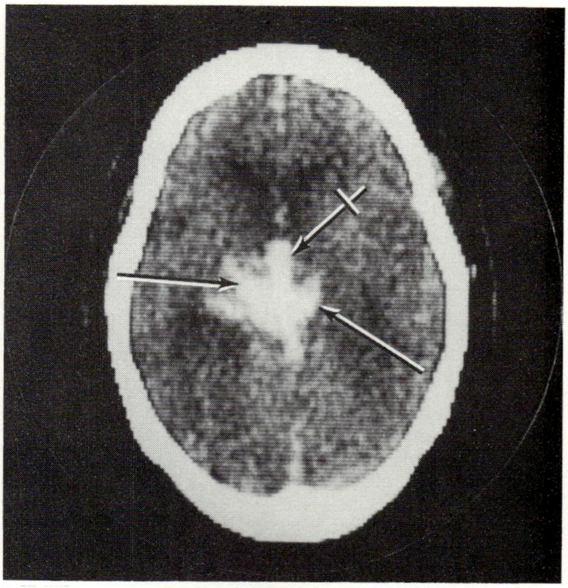

Figure 4–15b

SPONTANEOUS INTRACEREBRAL HEMORRHAGE IN A CHILD (Figure 4–16)

L. C., a 10 year old previously healthy female, developed a right hemiparesis and coma of sudden onset.

The routine CT scan reveals an irregular area of hemorrhage deep in the left parietal region, with slight shift of the lateral ventricles from left to right (arrow); density, from 54 to 82 u. The possibility of an occult arteriovenous malformation should be considered in such cases. The arteriogram did not reveal any evidence of an arteriovenous malformation. However, it appears that in many patients the hemorrhage can obscure or destroy the malformation. There was no change following the infusion of contrast material.

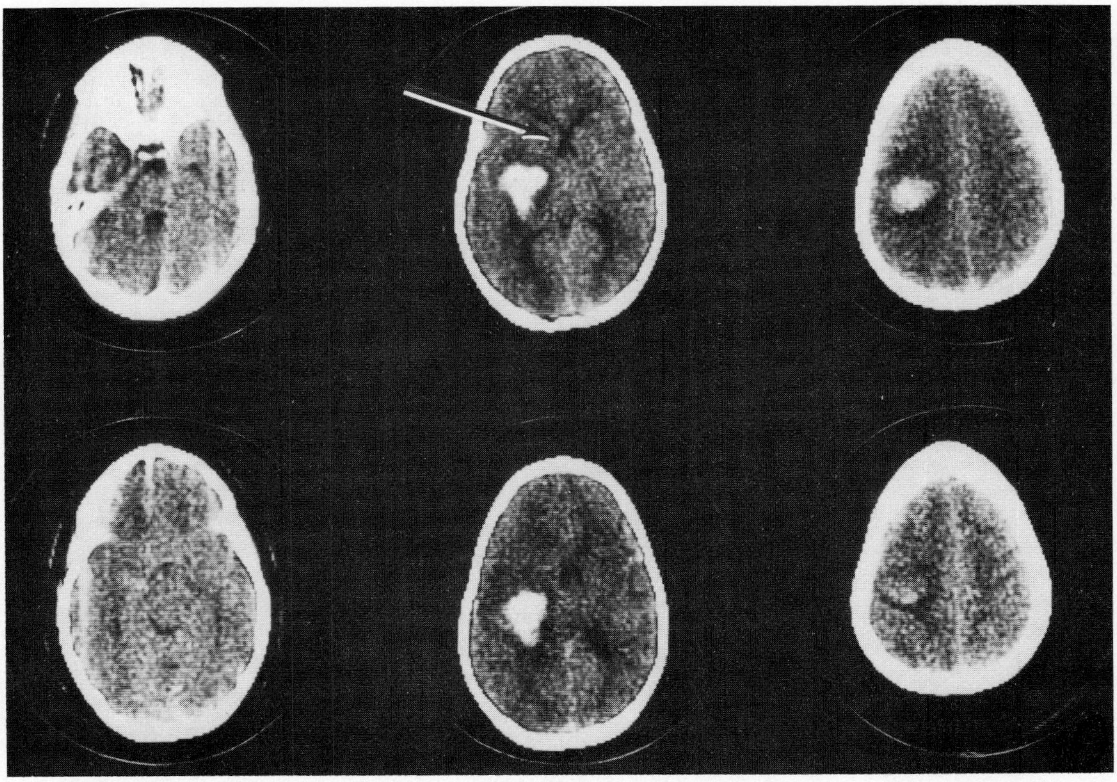

Figure 4–16

SPONTANEOUS INTRACEREBRAL HEMORRHAGE IN A CHILD (Figure 4–17)

This 4 year old male, who was previously healthy, first complained of a headache and then over a period of several hours became comatose and decerebrate.

The routine scan reveals a large irregular hematoma high in the right parietal region; density, 48 to 84 u. There was no change with contrast infusion. Notice how the configuration of the hematoma is similar to that in the preceding case. Also, these hemorrhages appear unlike the hypertensive hemorrhages that we see in the basal ganglia region. Cut 3A with electronic enhancement shows the hematoma to better advantage.

Autopsy and pathologic examination revealed an arteriovenous malformation surrounded by the hematoma.

2A 3A 4A

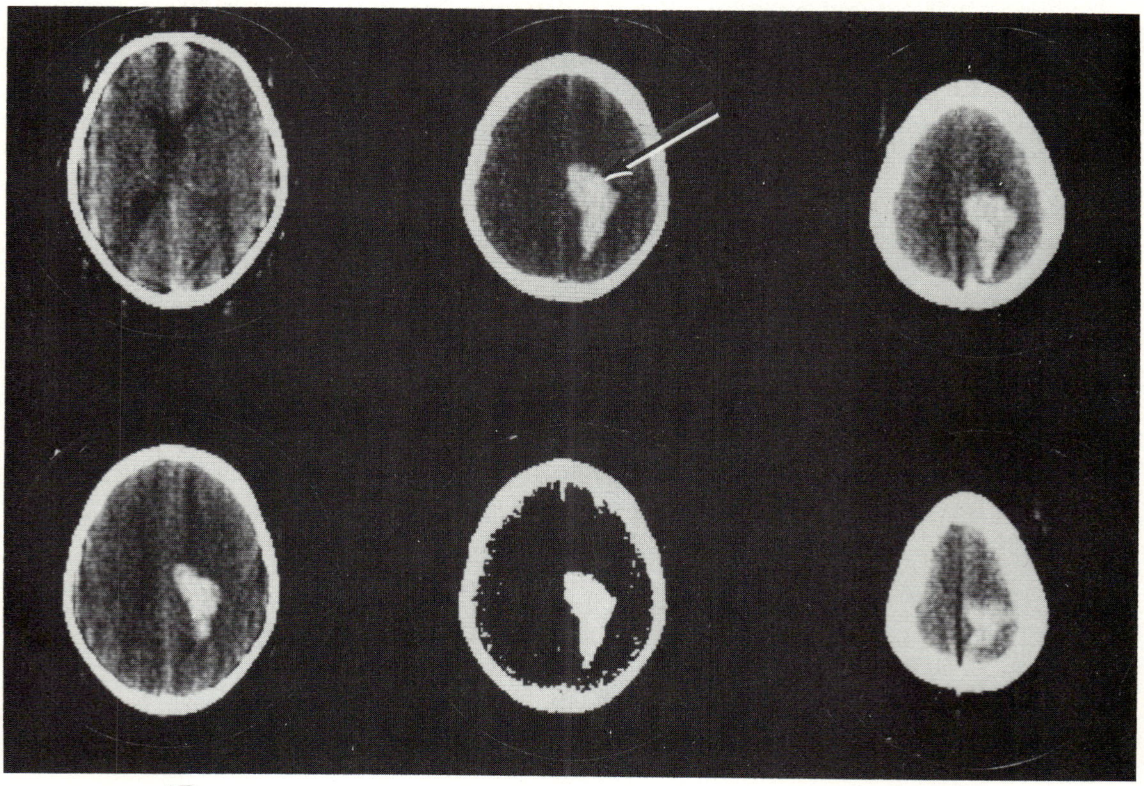

2B 3A 4B

Figure 4–17

SPONTANEOUS INTRACEREBRAL HEMATOMA (Figure 4–18)

C. B. is a 26 year old female with acute myelogenous leukemia and thrombocytopenia secondary to chemotherapy. Several hours prior to this study, she became aphasic, stuporous, and hemiparetic on the right side.

The routine scan reveals a moderate-sized, superficial frontoparietal hematoma with moderate shift of the lateral ventricles toward the right (arrow). Cut 3A with electronic enhancement shows the hematoma to better advantage.

The hematoma was evacuated and the patient gradually improved.

2A 3A

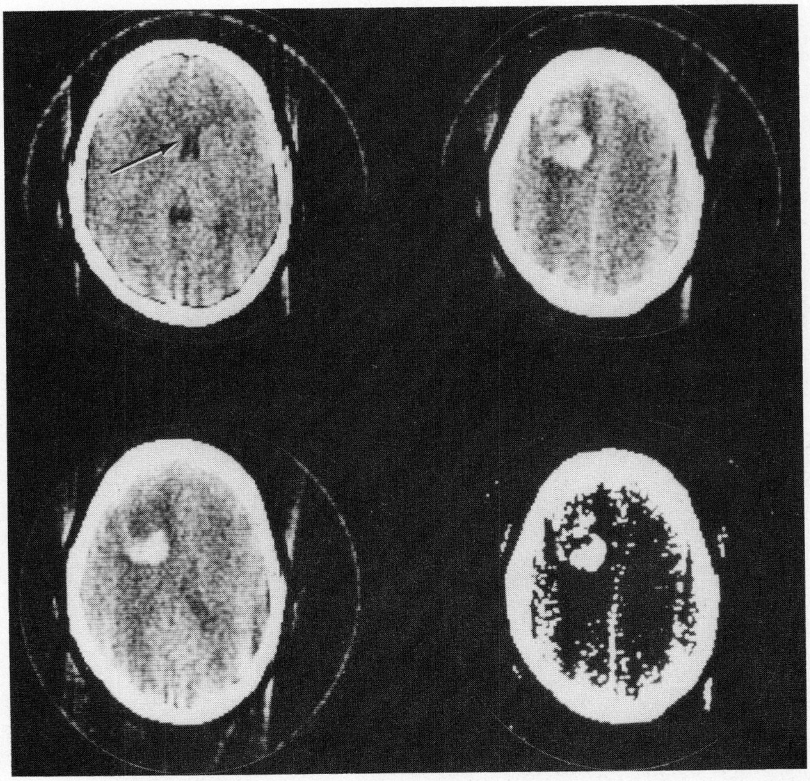

2B 3B

Figure 4–18

ANEURYSM WITH INTRACEREBRAL AND INTRAVENTRICULAR HEMORRHAGE (Figure 4–19)

M. G. is a 47 year old female who presented with severe headache, nausea, and vomiting. She then became disoriented and confused and gradually less responsive. Lumbar puncture revealed grossly bloody fluid. There were never any localizing signs. An arteriogram performed at another hospital revealed an anterior communicating artery aneurysm. There was associated vascular spasm.

a to c. The routine CT scan, obtained several days after admission here, reveals a moderate-sized hematoma in the right frontal lobe (arrows on a and b). Density, 50 to 66 u. There is a clotted blood cast of the left lateral ventricle (horizontal arrows on a and c) and a small clot in the dependent portion of the left lateral ventricle (crossed arrow on a and b). The pathologic specimen correlates well with the CT scan.

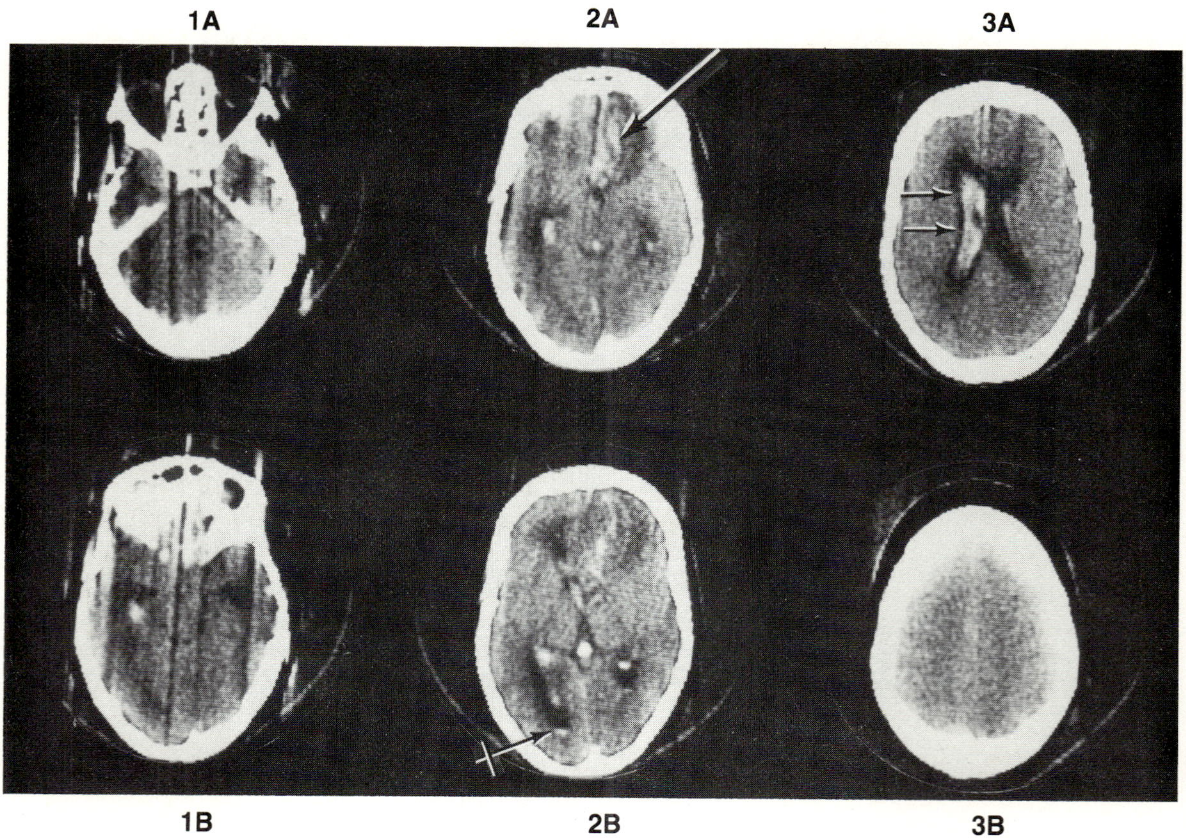

Figure 4–19a

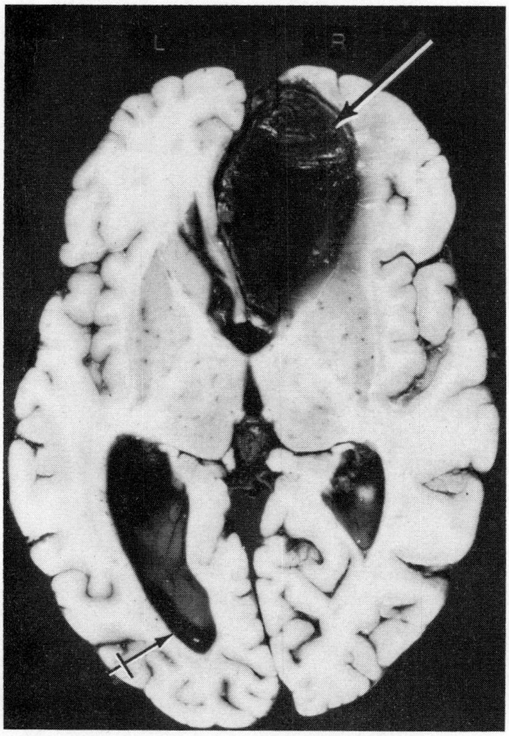

Figure 4–19b

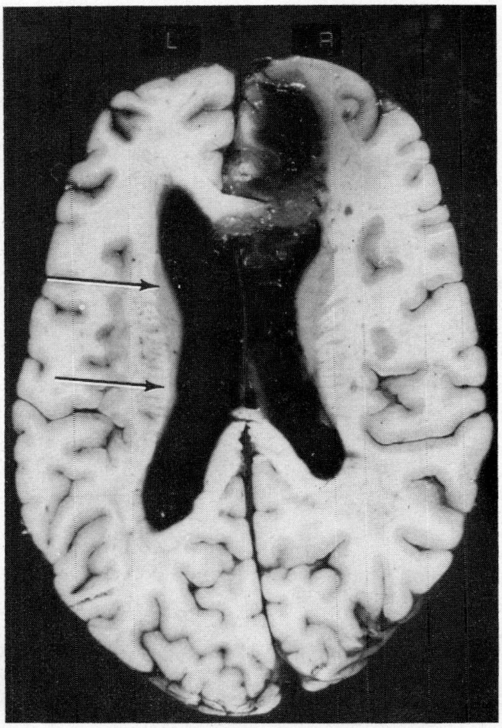

Figure 4–19c

SPONTANEOUS INTRACEREBRAL HEMATOMA (Figure 4–20)

P. H. is a 16 year old male who initially presented with 2 weeks of headache, nausea, and vomiting. He had previously been healthy.

a. The routine scan, obtained shortly after admission here, reveals an area of increased density in the left temporal lobe region that measured from 36 to 64 u. There is a moderate-sized area of surrounding lucency (arrow), along with a slight shift of the third ventricle to the right (short arrow).

b. The lateral view of the left carotid arteriogram shows elevation of several of the main middle cerebral artery branches (arrows).

c. The anteroposterior view in the arterial phase discloses a small distal shift of the anterior cerebral artery to the right side (see arrow), as well as a slight shift of the internal cerebral vein (not shown).

At surgery, a small partially resolved hematoma was evacuated. The large area of surrounding edema and lower than anticipated density on the CT scan are consistent with a partially resolved hematoma. The etiology remained obscure. Note that the CT scan outlines the character and position of the hematoma better than the arteriogram.

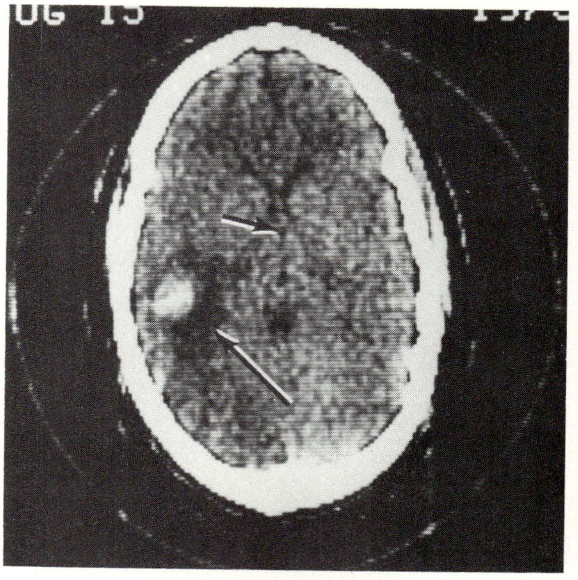

Figure 4–20a

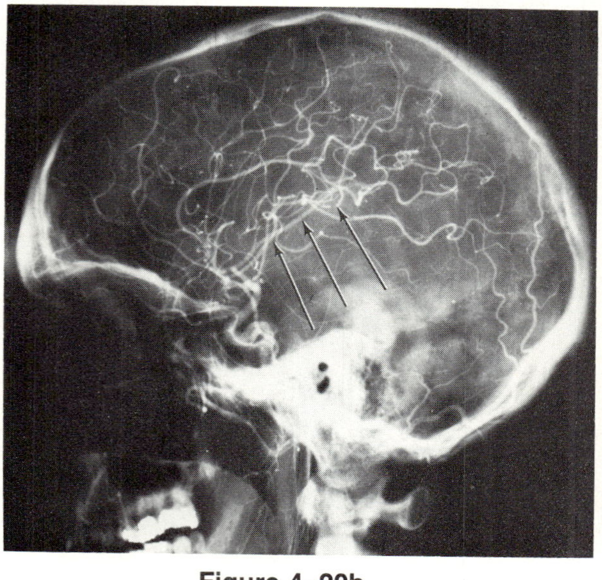

Figure 4–20b

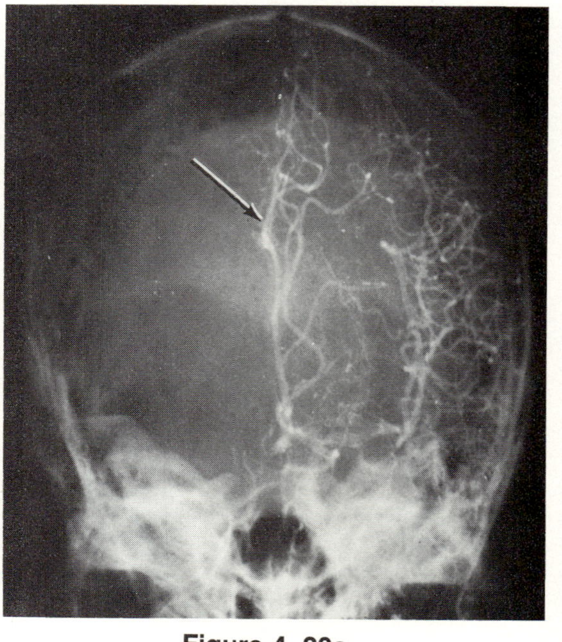

Figure 4–20c

CLASSIC BASAL GANGLIONIC HEMATOMA (Figure 4–21)

M. S. is a 47 year old male who presented with right-sided hemiparalysis and aphasia of sudden onset. Lumbar puncture revealed bloody spinal fluid.

a. The routine CT scan shows the classic picture of a large left basal ganglionic hematoma. This large, dense hematoma measured 50 to 84 u. There is shift of the midline to the right and obliteration of the left lateral ventricle. Although we cannot detect clotted blood in the ventricular system, some apparently has entered the subarachnoid space, resulting in the bloody cerebrospinal fluid.

b. In the lateral view of the left carotid arteriogram, elevation and forward telescoping of the sylvian triangle are seen.

c. The anteroposterior view reveals a distal shift of the anterior cerebral artery under the falx (crossed arrow) and lateral displacement of the sylvian point (long arrow) and the middle cerebral artery vessels. These are classic findings with a basal ganglionic hematoma.

d. The anteroposterior venous phase demonstrates a greater shift of the internal cerebral vein (arrows) than the artery. This finding is also quite typical of a basal ganglionic hematoma, and the venous shift may be the only arteriographic finding.

1A 2A

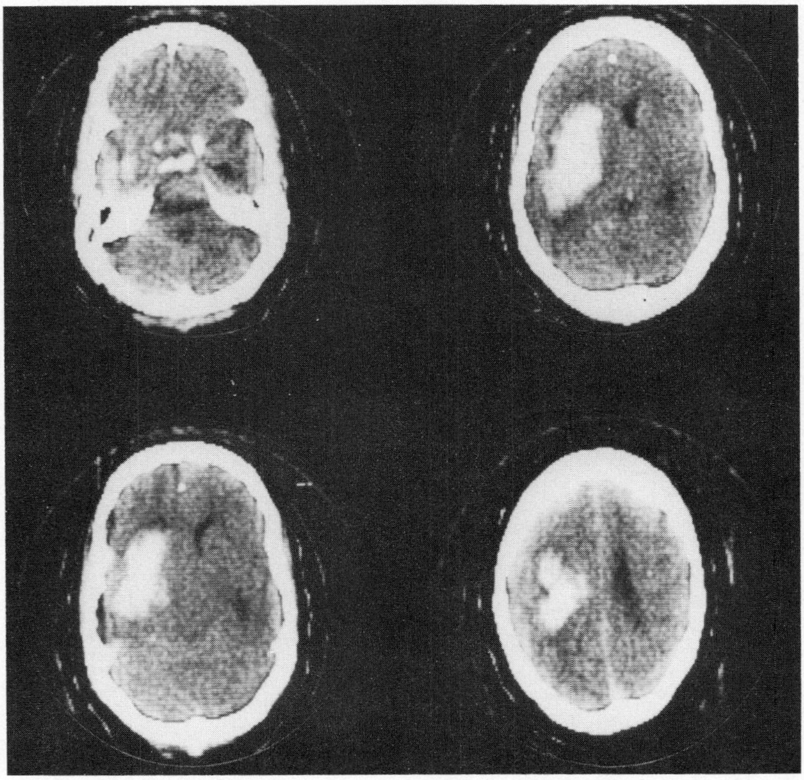

1B 2B

Figure 4–21a

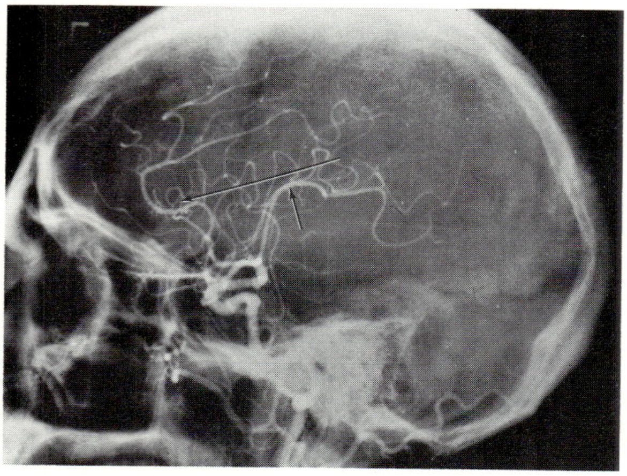
Figure 4–21b

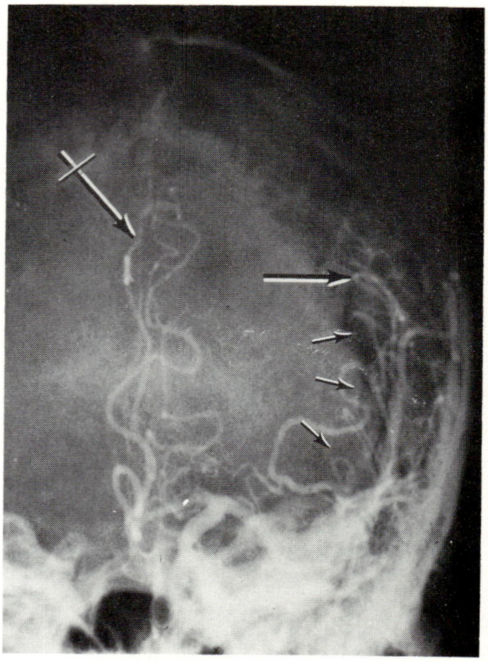
Figure 4–21c

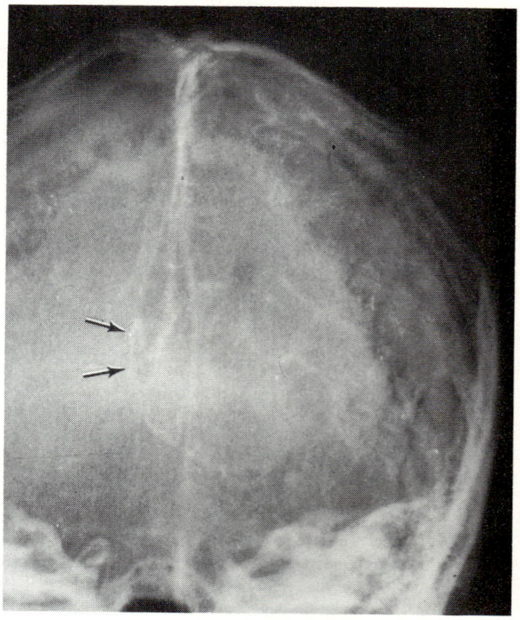
Figure 4–21d

BASAL GANGLIONIC HEMATOMA WITH INTRAVENTRICULAR COMPONENT (Figure 4–22)

N. S., an elderly female, entered with a mild right hemiparesis and marked obtundation. She was totally unresponsive even to painful stimuli. Lumbar puncture revealed bloody cerebrospinal fluid.

a. The routine CT scan reveals a small left basal ganglionic hematoma associated with a large intraventricular hemorrhage. There is a large accumulation of clotted blood in the left frontal horn and third ventricle (arrow on 2A) and a small accumulation in the dependent portion of the right lateral ventricle (arrows on 3A and 2B). There is a clot situated in the fourth ventricle as well (arrow on 1B). This blood in the ventricular system is responsible for the bloody cerebrospinal fluid found at the time of lumbar puncture. Note the moderate hydrocephalus secondary to obstruction of the normal cerebrospinal fluid pathways by clotted blood.

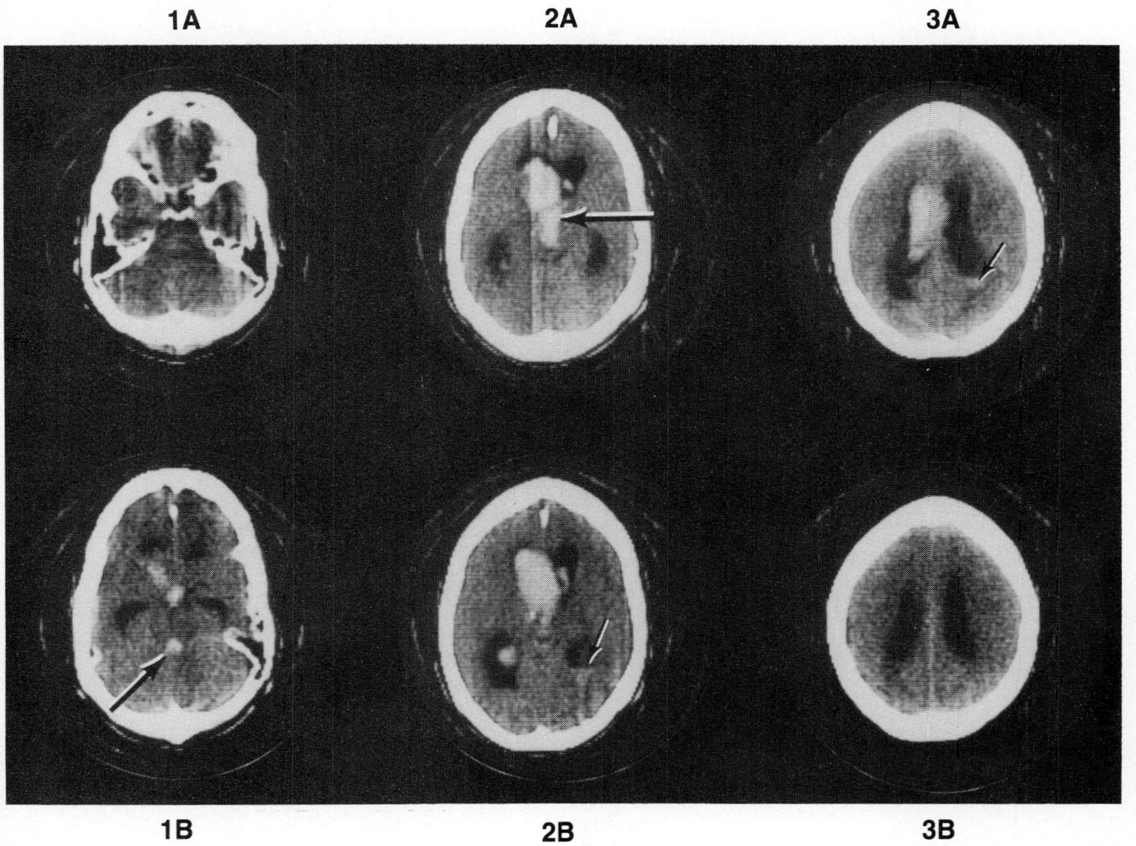

Figure 4–22a

b and c. The anteroposterior arterial and venous phases of the left carotid arteriogram demonstrate no shift of the anterior cerebral artery and a moderate shift of the internal cerebral vein (arrow on c), as well as hydrocephalus (small arrows on c are on the thalamostriate vein). The lenticulostriate arteries are noted to be displaced laterally (see arrows on b). Note: The lenticulostriate arteries may be displaced medially or laterally, depending on the position of the hemorrhage.

d and e. Arterial phase; the lateral view reveals mild spreading of the fronto-opercular branches of the middle cerebral artery but is otherwise unremarkable. On the lateral venous phase, however, there is evidence of massive ventricular enlargement, along with flattening of the internal cerebral vein and a wide open venous angle. The height of the lateral ventricle is outlined. These findings are quite typical of a basal ganglionic hematoma with intraventricular hemorrhage causing dilatation of the lateral ventricles.

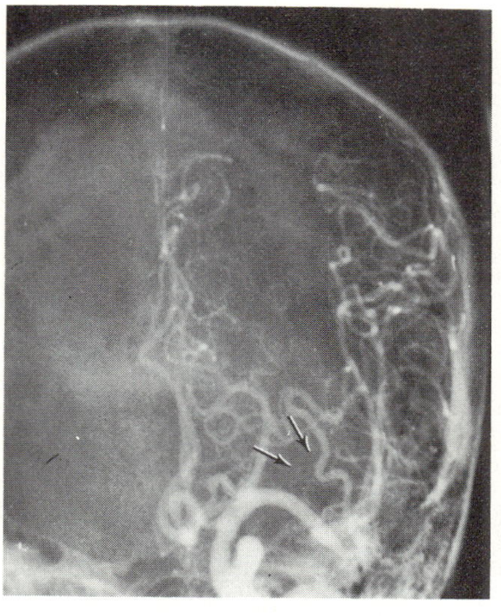

Figure 4–22b

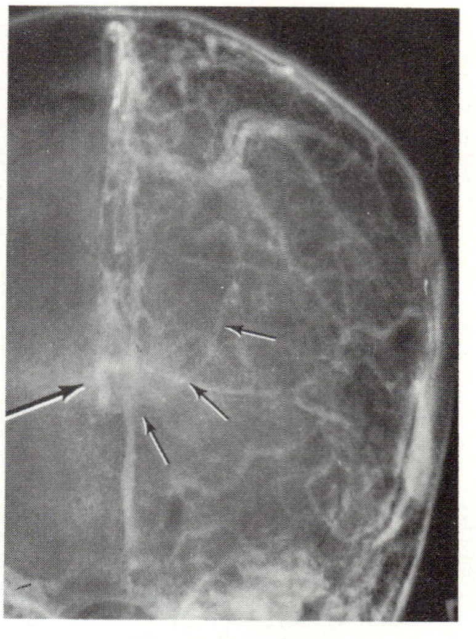

Figure 4–22c

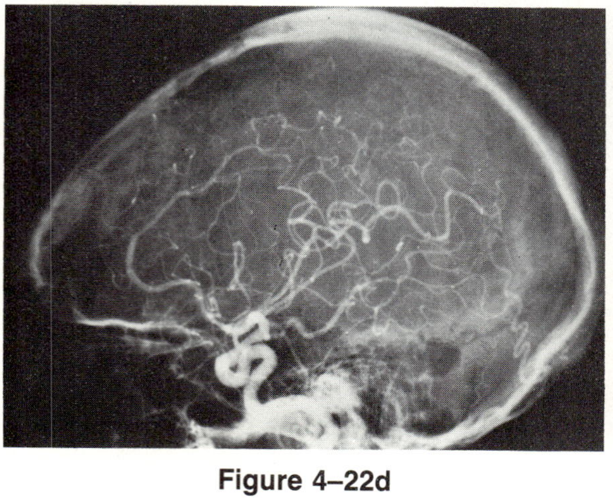

Figure 4–22d

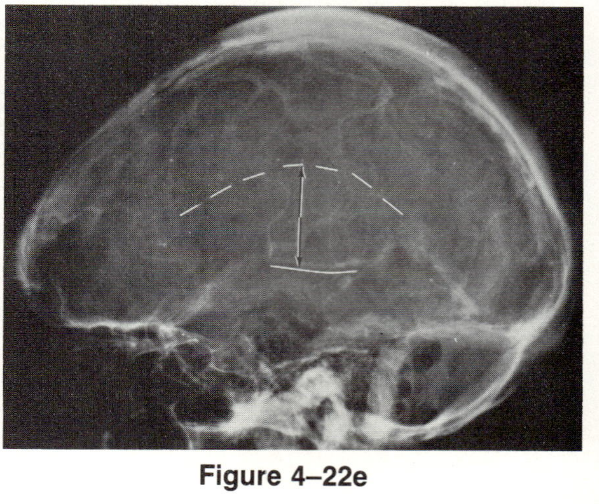

Figure 4–22e

VARIOUS APPEARANCES OF INTRACEREBRAL HEMORRHAGE (Figure 4–23)

The following are examples of the types of hemorrhages that may be studied by CT scanning.

a. A 21 year old woman with severe headache and blood in the cerebrospinal fluid. A small hema-

1A 1B

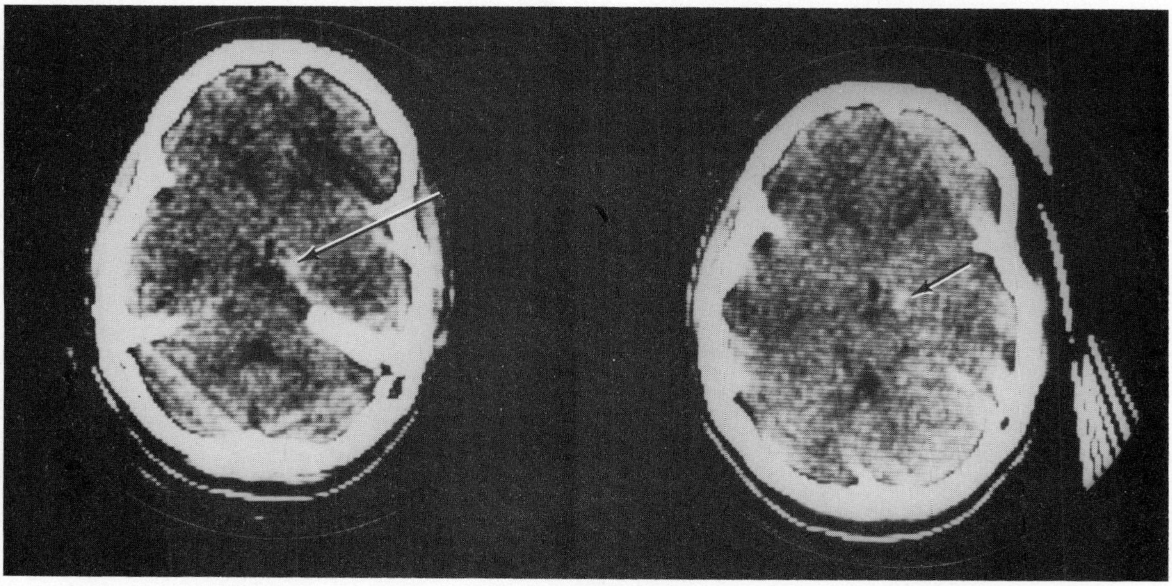

Figure 4–23a

1B 2B

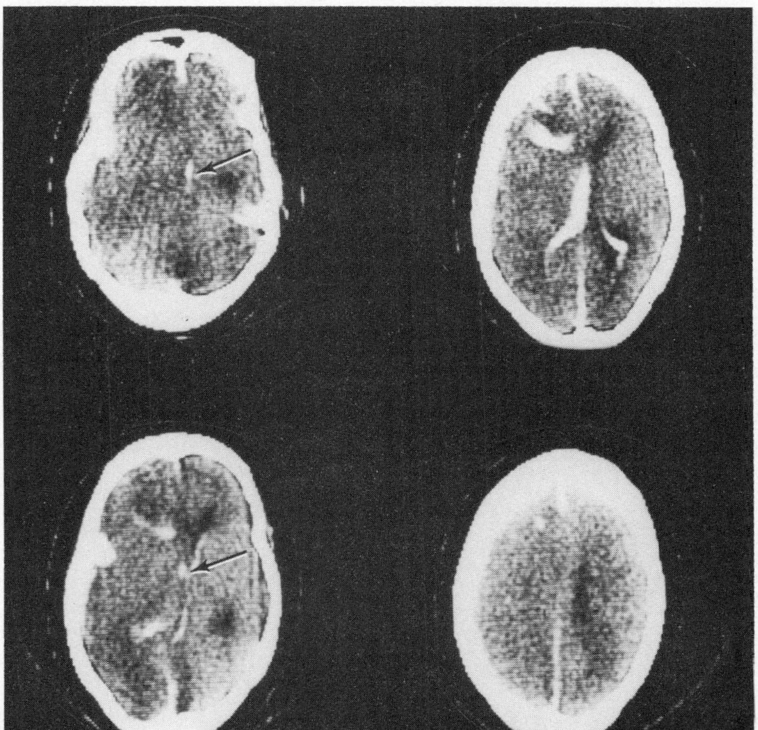

Figure 4–23b

2A 2B

toma, seen in the right thalamus, measured from 40 to 58 u (arrows). The arteriogram was essentially normal.

b. A 48 year old woman on renal dialysis developed headache and coma of sudden onset. The scan reveals a small left frontal hematoma with a density of 52 to 80 u. A large intraventricular component outlines the lateral ventricles. The third ventricle has shifted to the right and also contains clotted blood (arrow on 1B and 2A).

c. A 53 year old female hypertensive entered with mild right-sided weakness. There is a small left thalamic hematoma; density, 24 to 80 u (arrow).

d. This 47 year old hypertensive woman presented with sudden onset of somnolence and a right hemiparesis. The CT scan reveals a small to moderate left basal ganglia hematoma with a large intraventricular component. A clot can be seen in the fourth ventricle (arrow on 1B), and there is early obstructive hydrocephalus. The temporal horns are dilated

2B

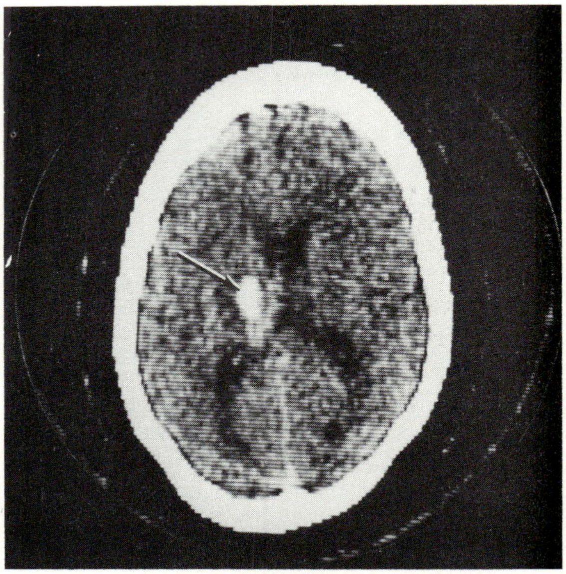

Figure 4–23c

1A 2A 3A

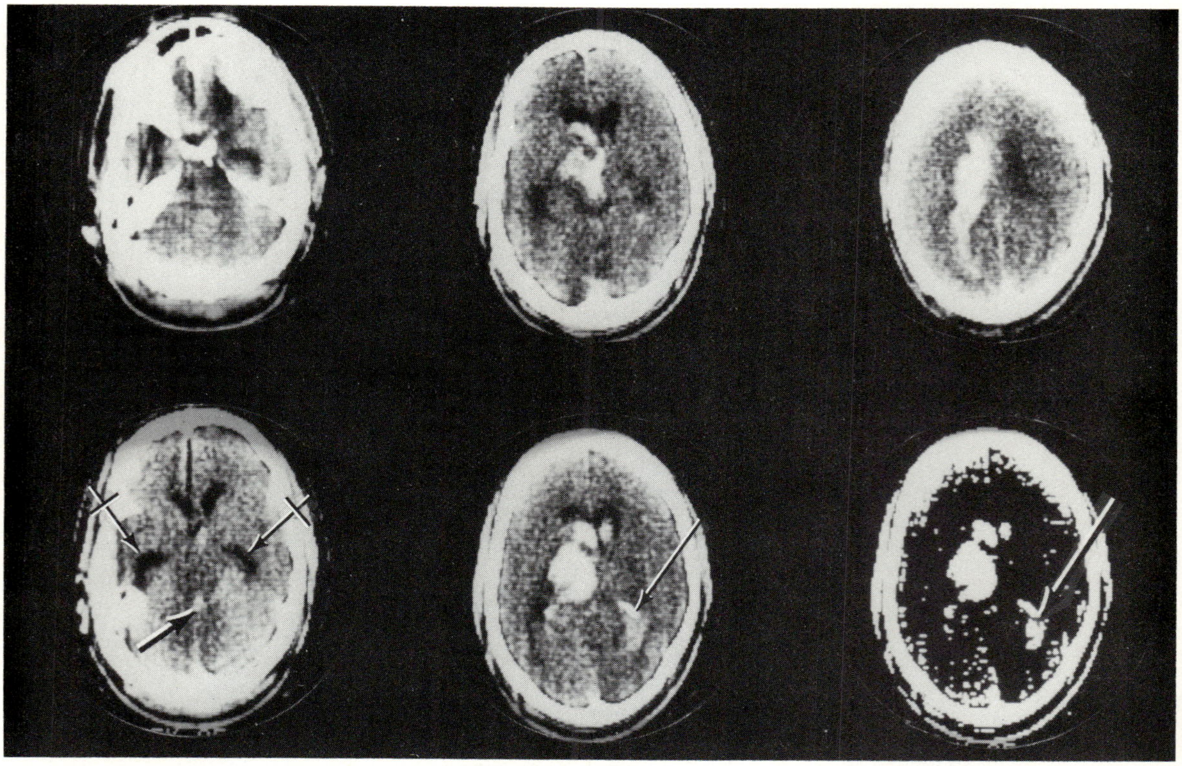

1B 2B 2B

Figure 4–23d

(crossed arrows on 1B), and there is blood in the dependent portions of the right lateral ventricle (arrow on 2B and on the 2B cut with electronic enhancement).

e. This 51 year old woman entered with right hemiparesis of acute onset. The routine CT scan reveals a large left frontoparietal hematoma, associated with marked shift from left to right. The density is 60 to 90 u.

f. A large left basal ganglionic hematoma with marked shift to the right. A small amount of blood can be seen in the compressed left lateral ventricle (arrow on 3A).

g. This 36 year old male had a previous surgical procedure for a left subdural hematoma 2 years prior to admission. At that time an incidental asymptomatic trifurcation aneurysm of the left middle cerebral artery was diagnosed at arteriography. The patient entered at this time with a mild right hemiparesis that ultimately became a dense paralysis associated with coma. The routine CT scan reveals the old craniectomy changes on the left side (arrows on 3A, but can be seen on all cuts) and a large left basal ganglionic hematoma with some blood in the lateral, third, and fourth ventricles. This hematoma is presumably secondary to rupture of the aneurysm.

h. This 49 year old man presented with coma of sudden onset and a dense right hemiparalysis. The scan shows a massive left basal ganglionic and intraventricular hemorrhage. The patient died shortly after this scan.

Most patients do not survive the catastrophic event of a large hemorrhage. It should be noted that these scans are relatively motion free because the patients are literally too obtunded and paretic to be able to move.

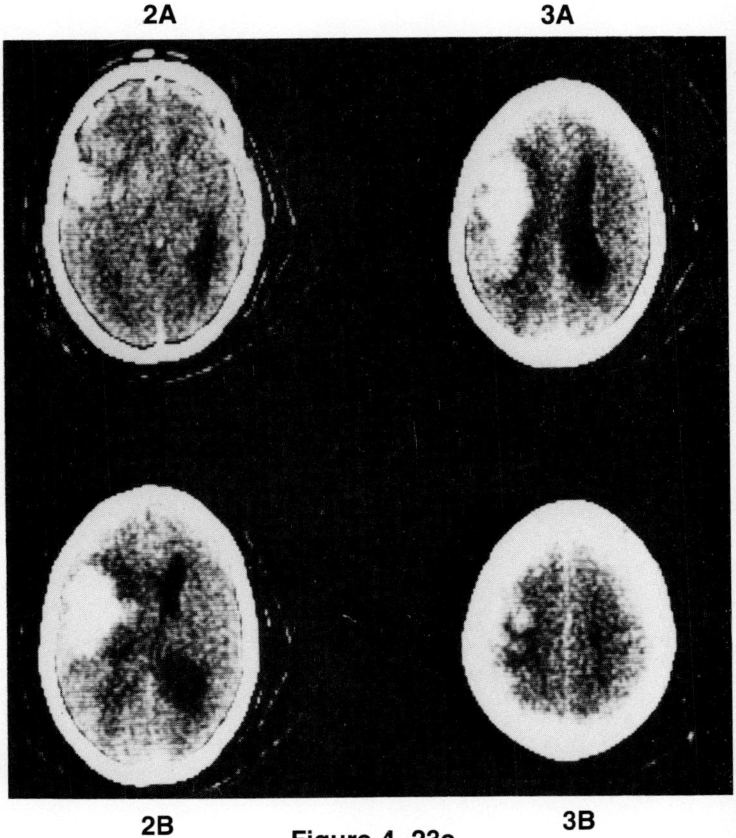

Figure 4–23e

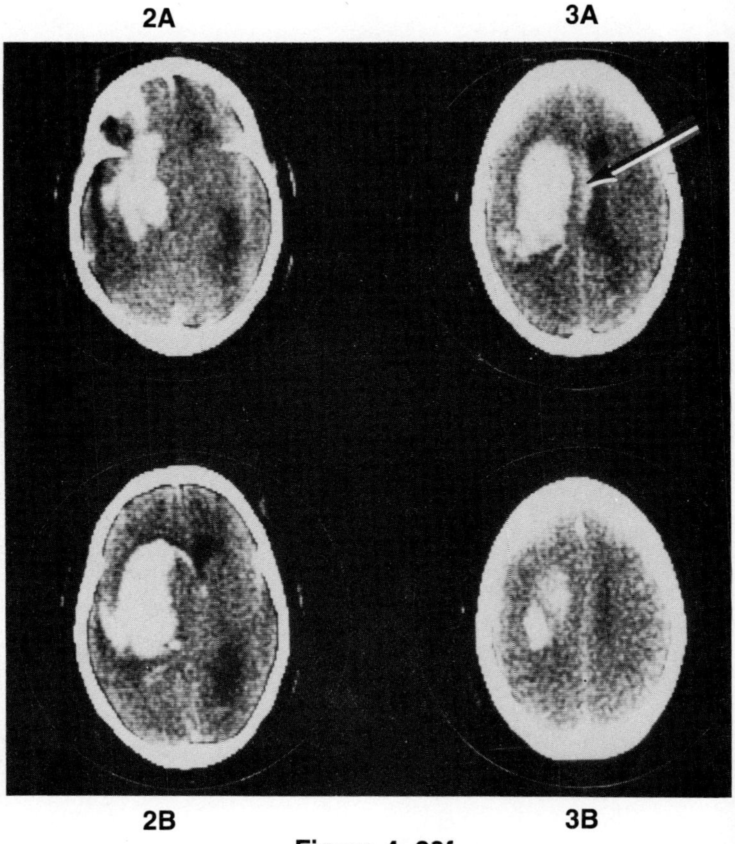

Figure 4–23f

1A 2A 3A

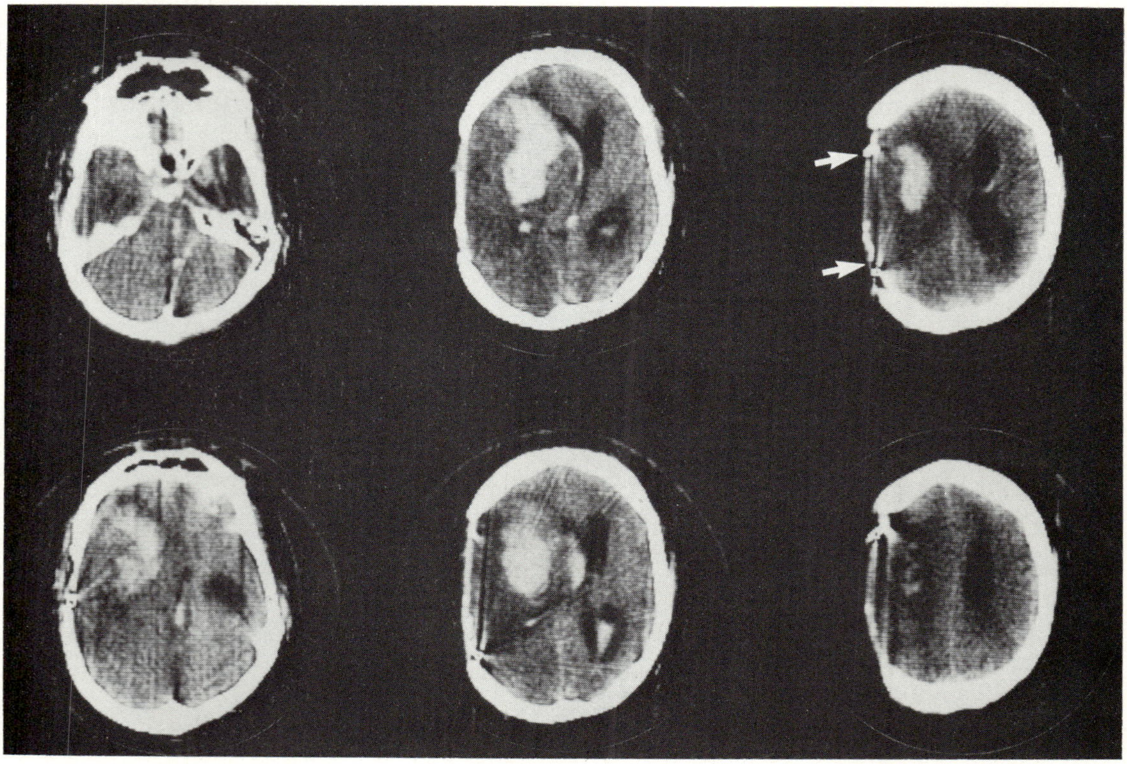

1B 2B 3B

Figure 4–23g

1A 2A 3A

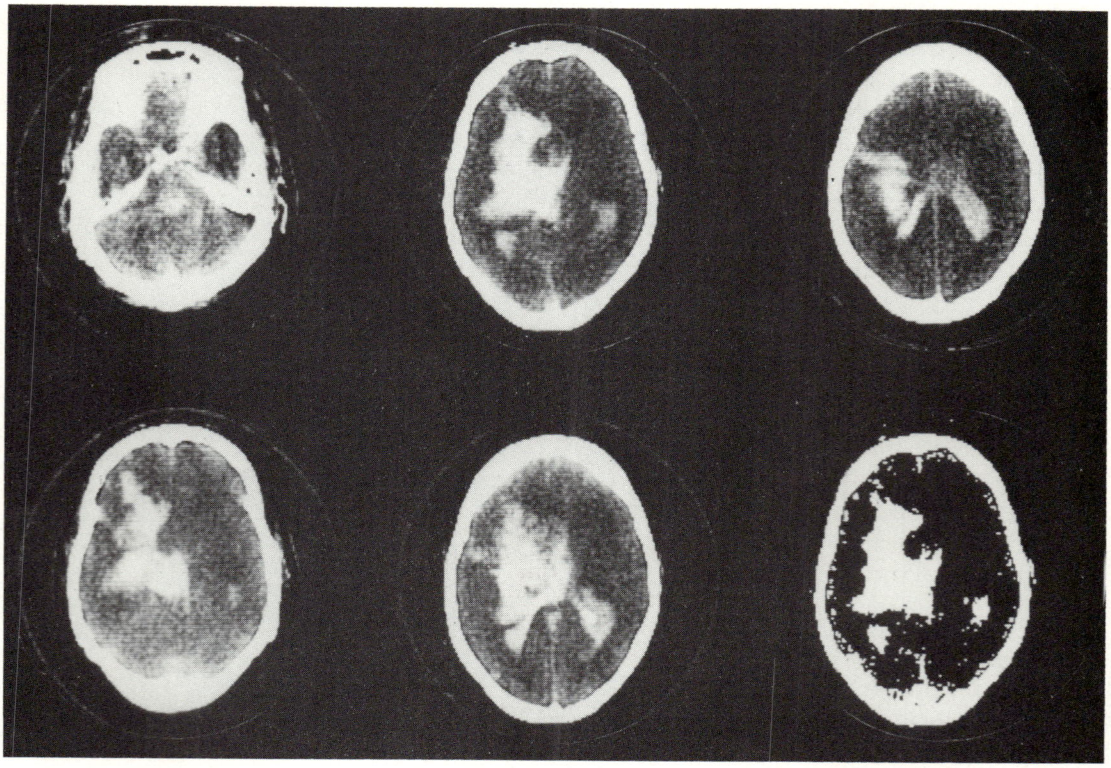

1B 2B 3B

Figure 4–23h

MODERATE-SIZED BASAL GANGLIONIC HEMORRHAGE (Figure 4–24)

J. W., a 47 year old hypertensive woman, was at her doctor's office when she collapsed. She was aphasic and had right-sided weakness. The initial scan was done within 1 hour after the original insult.

a. The initial scan reveals a moderate-sized left basal ganglionic hematoma with a density of 44 to 88 u, along with mild compression of the frontal horn of the left lateral ventricle.

Thirteen days later and after treatment with mannitol and Decadron, the arm and leg weakness had improved somewhat. She continued to have intermittent periods of hypertension.

A

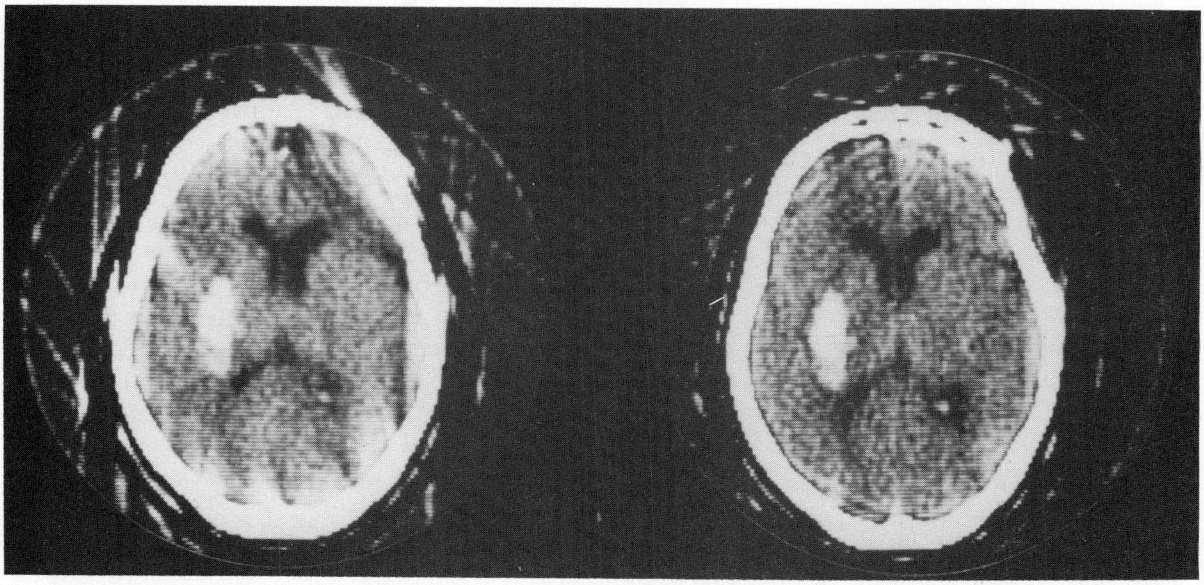

2B

Figure 4–24a

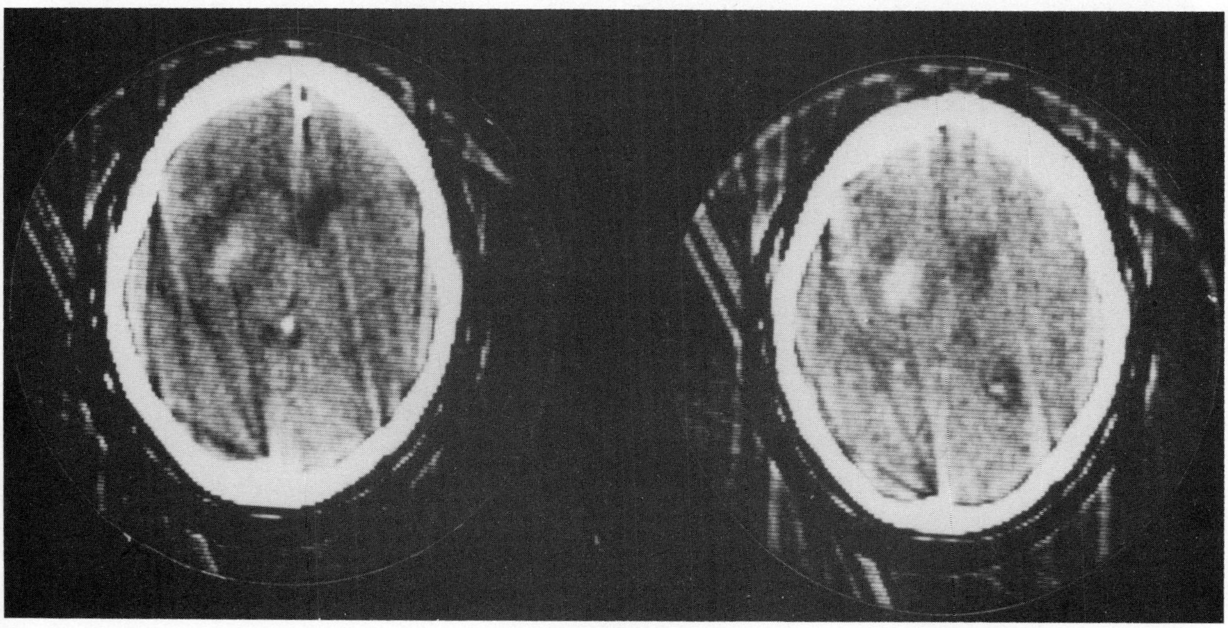

2B

Figure 4–24b

b. The follow-up scan reveals much more marked shift of the lateral ventricles than was noted previously. The hematoma, which has begun to resorb, is smaller and less dense—38 to 68 u—than on the initial study, and there is now a large area of surrounding edema. This type of insult could ultimately be expected to result in an area of porencephaly in the bed of the old hematoma.

BASAL GANGLIA AND INTRAVENTRICULAR HEMORRHAGE (Figure 4–25)

W. J., an elderly gentleman, was brought to the emergency room unconscious and unresponsive.

a. The routine CT scan discloses evidence of a small right basal ganglionic hemorrhage, a moderate-sized right parietal hematoma, and an extensive intraventricular hemorrhage. Because the patients are all scanned in the supine position, we can detect a fluid level between the clotted blood in the dependent portions of the lateral ventricles and the cerebrospinal fluid (arrows). The blood density was 54 to 84 u.

b. The pathologic specimen reveals excellent correlation with the scan findings. The hemorrhage in the right basal ganglia and right temporoparietal lobes can be readily identified (arrows).

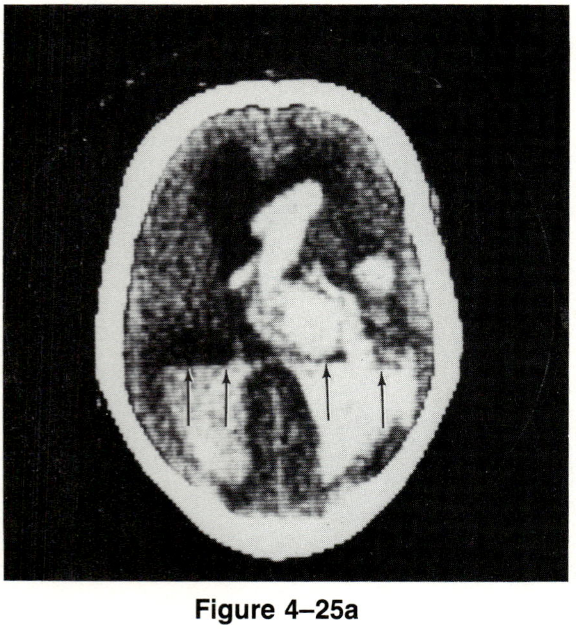

Figure 4–25a

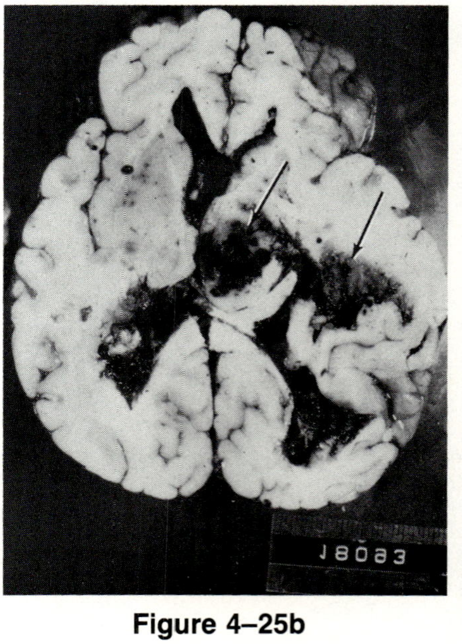

Figure 4–25b

Aneurysms

Although it has been shown that some large aneurysms can be visualized as dense areas even before the infusion of contrast material, more often these aneurysms are identified after the infusion of contrast material as small round areas of increased density. Again the index of suspicion must be high when studying an aneurysm, and infusion must be performed for complete evaluation. Unfortunately, it is difficult to identify aneurysms around the region of the sella because of their relatively small size and because these aneurysms are so closely associated with the bony density of the anterior and posterior clinoid processes. We can quite readily identify small areas of hemorrhage associated with these aneurysms; however, arteriography is again necessary to completely evaluate the presence and configuration of an aneurysm and to rule out additional aneurysms.

LARGE SUPRASELLAR ANEURYSM (Figure 4–26)

C. C. is a 39 year old female who presented with a left temporal hemianopsia.

a to d. The anteroposterior radionuclide angiogram demonstrates a focus of increased activity at the base of the brain (not shown). The early (see below) and delayed views both demonstrate an area of abnormal uptake in the suprasellar region that faded on the delayed views. This area corresponds to the area of uptake on the nuclide angiogram. The differential diagnosis is between suprasellar tumor, arteriovenous malformation, and aneurysm.

AP

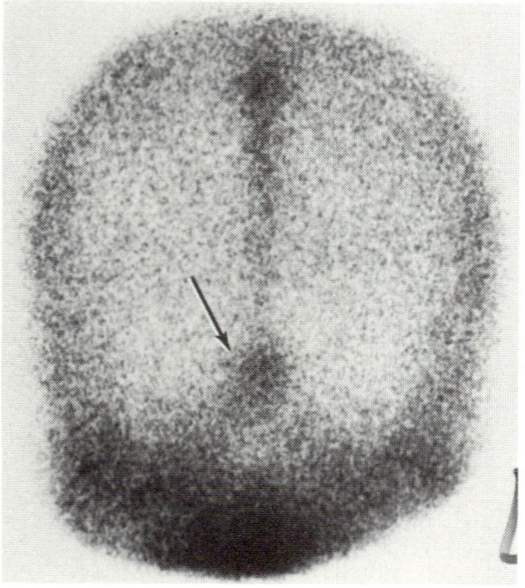

Figure 4–26a

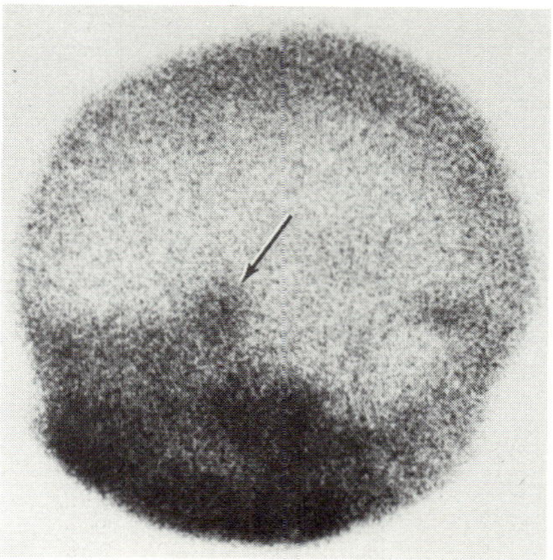

LT. LATERAL
Figure 4–26b

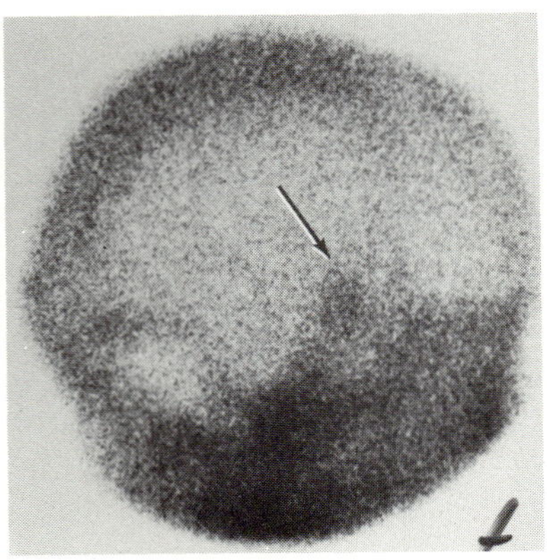

RT. LATERAL
Figure 4–26c

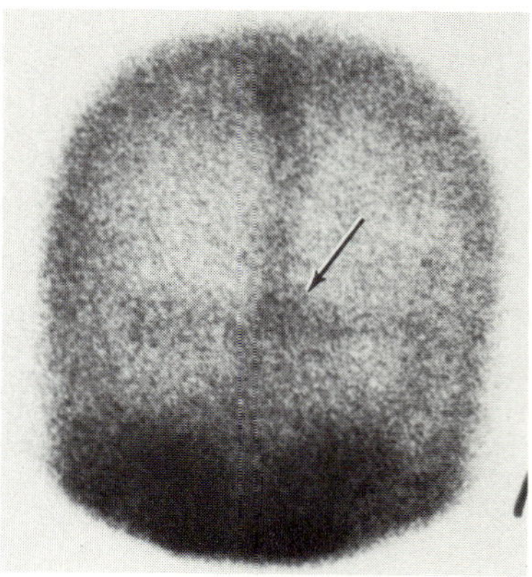

POSTERIOR
Figure 4–26d

e. The routine CT scan—without the infusion of contrast—discloses a round area of increased density in the midline in the suprasellar region that measures from 44 to 60 u. Subsequent arteriography reveals that this is a large aneurysm arising from the right internal carotid artery in the suprasellar area and extending medially. There is no evidence of thrombus formation, and the density apparently represents the normal density of flowing, unopacified blood!

f and g. The anteroposterior arterial and venous phases of the right brachial arteriogram reveal a large suprasellar aneurysm arising from the supraclinoid portion of the right internal carotid artery and extending medially. Note the hold-up of the contrast material in the aneurysm well into the venous phase.

1B

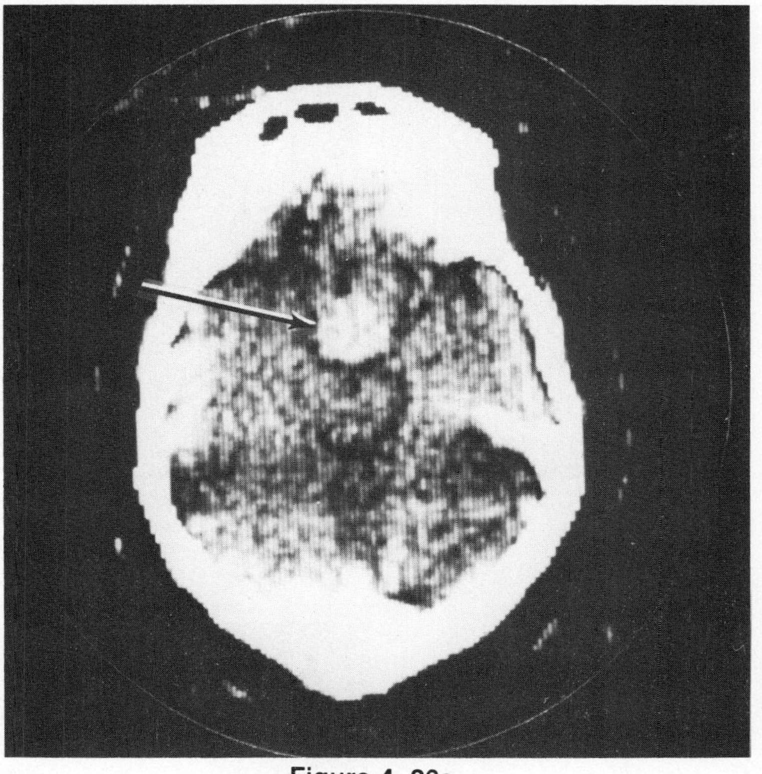

Figure 4–26e

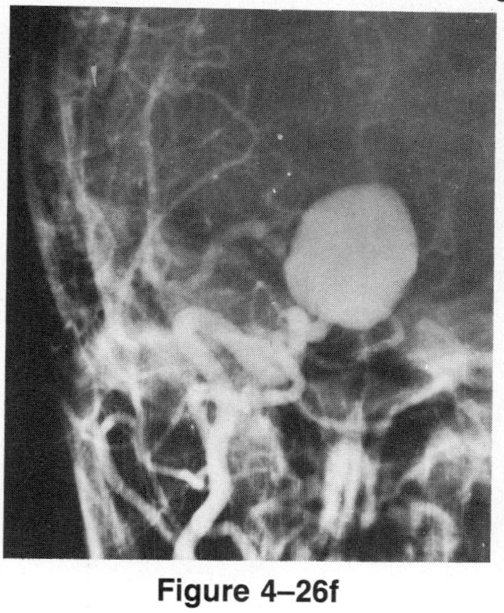

Figure 4–26f

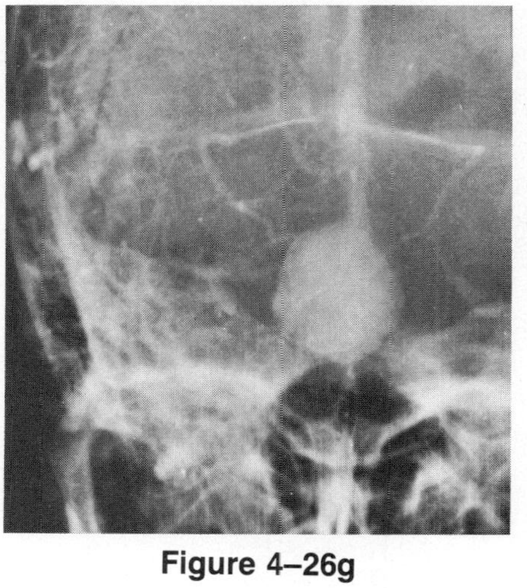

Figure 4–26g

h. The early arterial lateral view reveals the "jet stream" of contrast as it enters into the aneurysm (arrow), apparently through a rather small communicating channel.

i. A later arterial view shows the aneurysm completely opacified.

j. The venous phase reveals hold-up of the contrast in the aneurysm and layering of the contrast in the dependent portion of the aneurysm as the patient lies in the supine position (arrows).

Interestingly, after application of a Silverstone clamp on the carotid artery in the neck with partial occlusion of the common carotid artery, a subsequent right brachial arteriogram revealed that the aneurysm had thrombosed and excluded itself from the circulation.

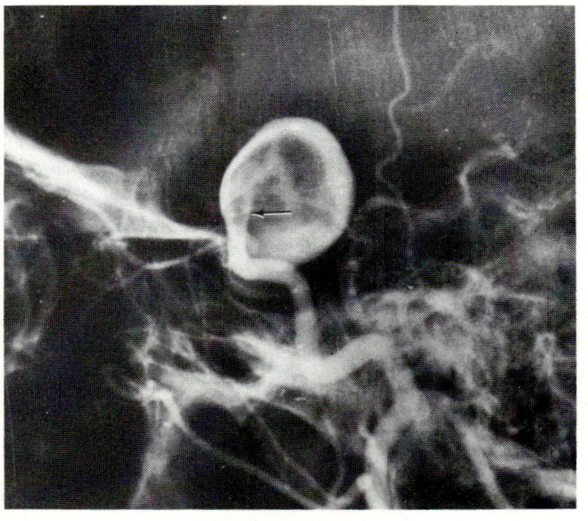

Figure 4–26h

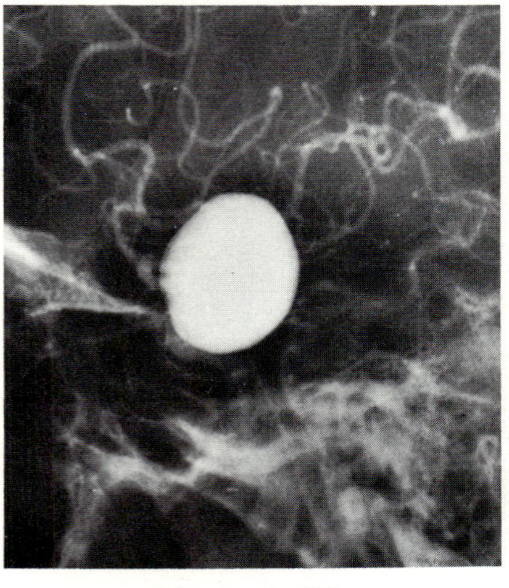

Figure 4–26i

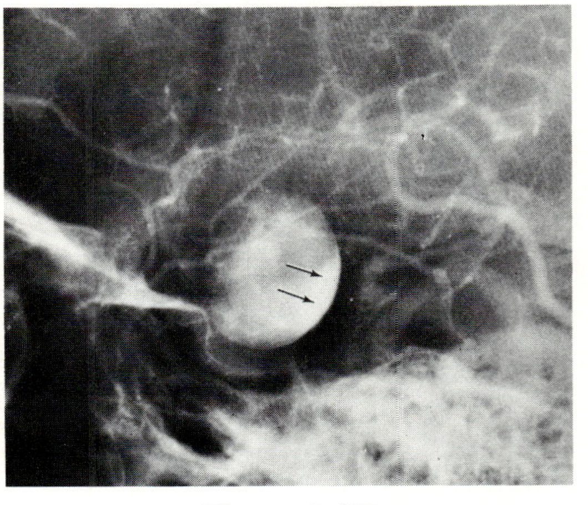

Figure 4–26j

MULTIPLE ANEURYSMS AND A TORTUOUS BASILAR ARTERY (Figure 4–27)

R. R., a 54 year old man, was admitted to our hospital following a subarachnoid hemorrhage. Outside arteriograms revealed multiple aneurysms.

a. The postinfusion CT scan shows a tortuous vertebrobasilar system (crossed arrow), and large aneurysms (arrows) in the region of the genu of the middle cerebral artery bilaterally. The one on the left measured 22 mm, and the one on the right measured 13 mm. An aneurysm of the anterior cerebral artery was not visualized, nor was a right posterior communicating artery aneurysm visualized. It has been our experience that aneurysms at the level of the sella have not been seen in many cases by CT scanning. Arteriography is certainly necessary for complete evaluation.

11A 12A

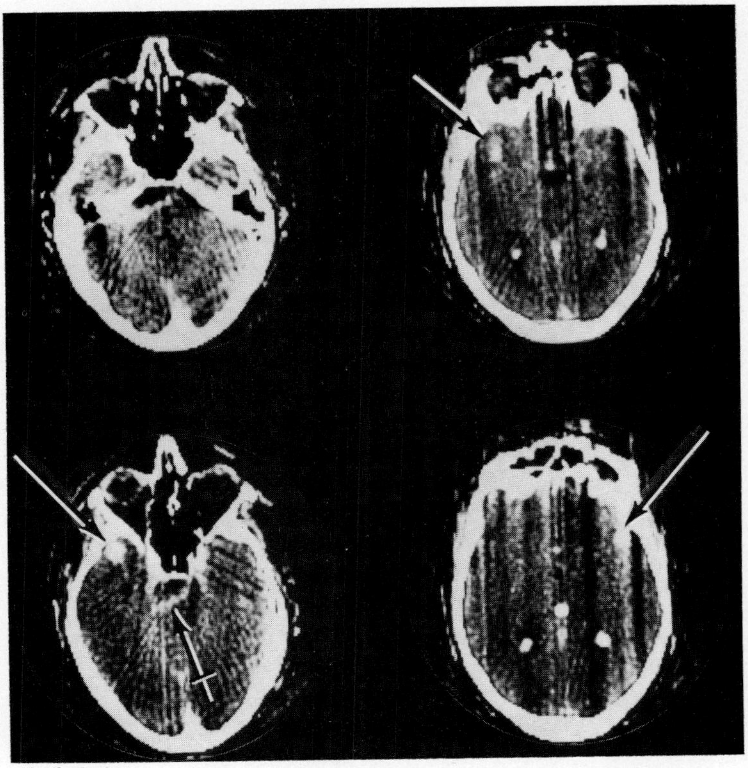

11B 12B

Figure 4–27a

b. The views with electronic enlargement show the aneurysms to better advantage.

c. The anteroposterior view, arterial phase, of the right brachial arteriogram reveals the very tortuous vertebrobasilar system (long arrows). The vessels also appear to be dilated, with the dilatation extending out to the right posterior cerebral artery (short arrows). The 13 mm aneurysm at the genu of the right middle cerebral artery is also filled (double crossed arrow).

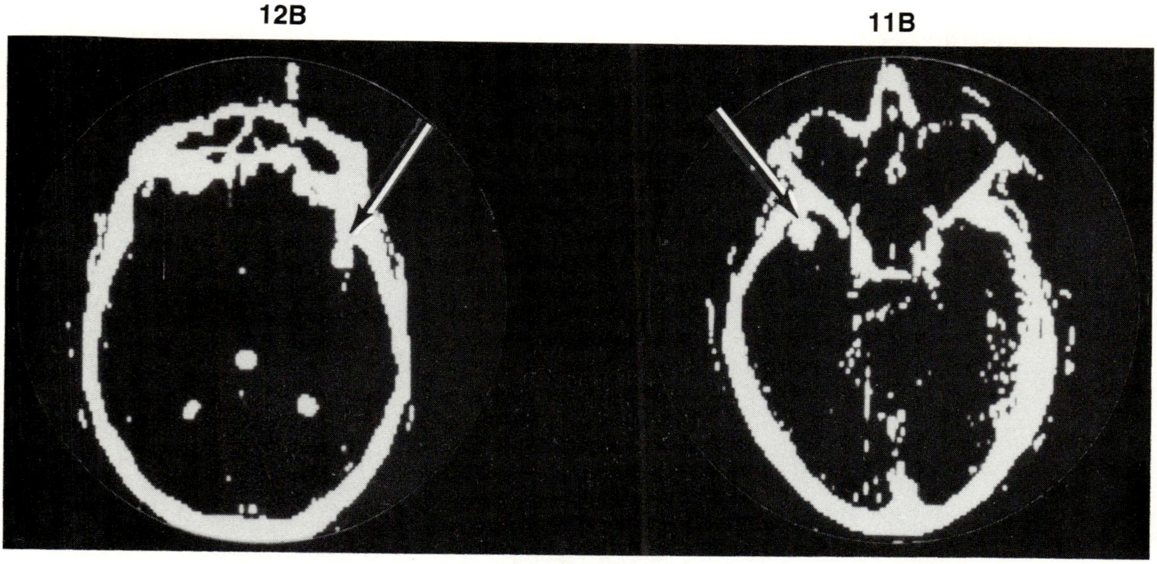

Figure 4–27b

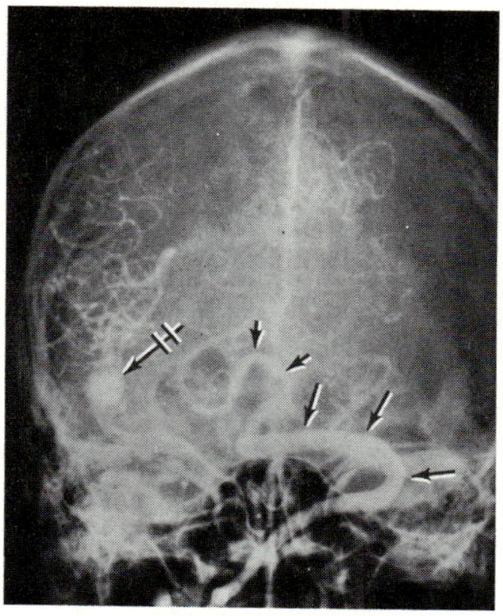

Figure 4–27c

d. The lateral view, arterial phase, of the right brachial arteriogram reveals the tortuous vertebrobasilar system (arrows), the aneurysm at the genu (double crossed arrow), a small aneurysm from the pericallosal artery at the level of a bifurcation (crossed arrow), and a lobulated right posterior communicating artery aneurysm (triple crossed arrow).

e. The anteroposterior view of the left carotid arteriogram, arterial phase, reveals a large 22 mm aneurysm at the genu of the left middle cerebral artery (long arrow), and the small aneurysm of the anterior cerebral artery (crossed arrow), which appears to protrude toward the left side. This aneurysm was noted to fill from the right side as well.

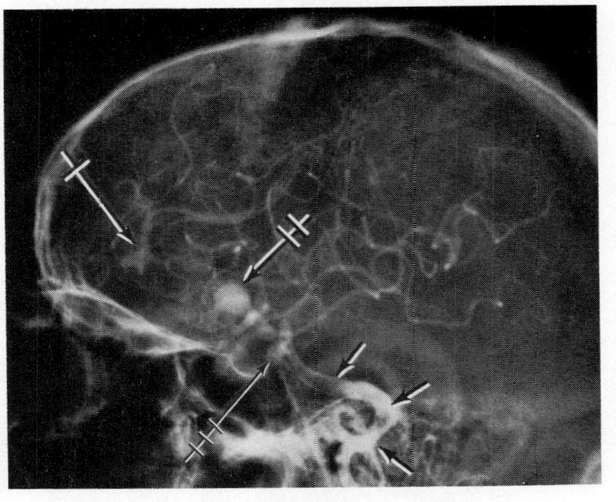

Figure 4–27d

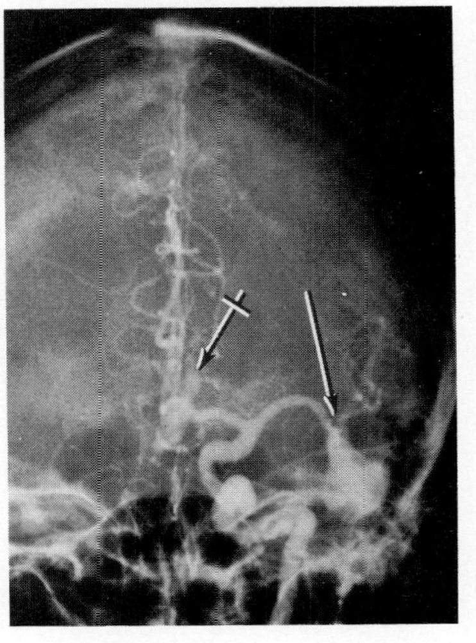

Figure 4–27e

ACUTE SUBARACHNOID HEMORRHAGE (Figure 4–28)

This 29 year old female presented with acute severe headache and lapsed into coma.

a and b. The two cuts in the region of the suprasellar cistern reveal blood—which appears white—surrounding the brain stem and extending posteriorly into the superior cerebellar cistern (arrowheads). There is also blood in the interhemispheric fissure (IF) and in the sylvian fissures bilaterally (SF). Note that the third ventricle appears as a lucent structure (arrow on b) surrounded by clotted blood in the interhemispheric fissure.

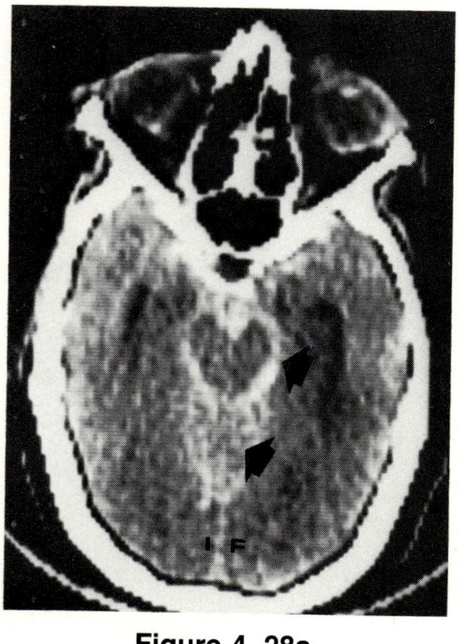

Figure 4–28a

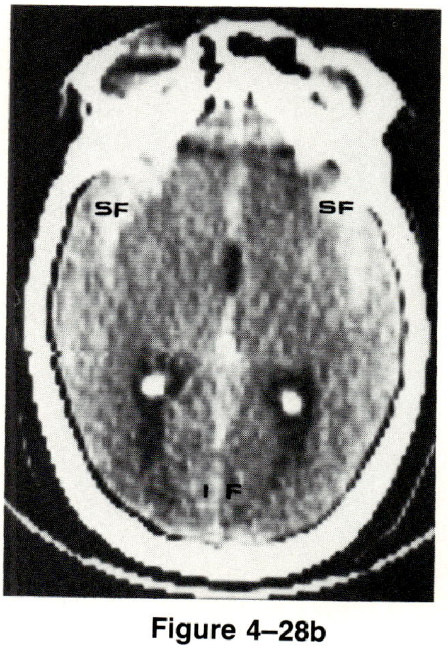

Figure 4–28b

TORTUOUS BASILAR ARTERY (Figure 4–29)

C. H. is a 50 year old woman with right hemiparesis of sudden onset.

The preinfusion CT scan was unremarkable with the exception of mild atrophy. After the infusion of contrast material, the tortuous basilar artery (arrow) appears as a well defined linear density across the pons. Close inspection reveals that the vessel makes a right angle turn just at the tip of the right petrous pyramid and returns to the midline just behind the dorsum sellae.

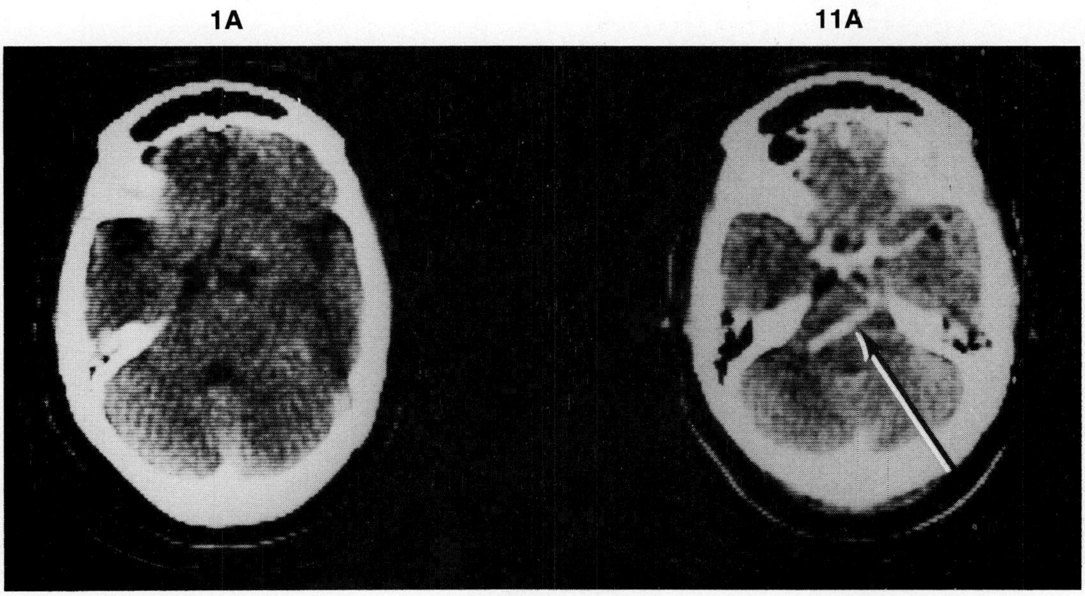

Figure 4–29

POSTERIOR COMMUNICATING ARTERY ANEURYSM (Figure 4–30)

D. G. is a 64 year old female with a right third nerve palsy.

This is an example of a right posterior communicating artery aneurysm that was not clotted, but was visible on the preinfusion CT scan as a density just lateral to the sella turcica (arrows). The density ranged from 44 to 56 u. The view with electronic enhancement shows the aneurysm to better advantage. On the arteriogram the aneurysm measured 12 mm.

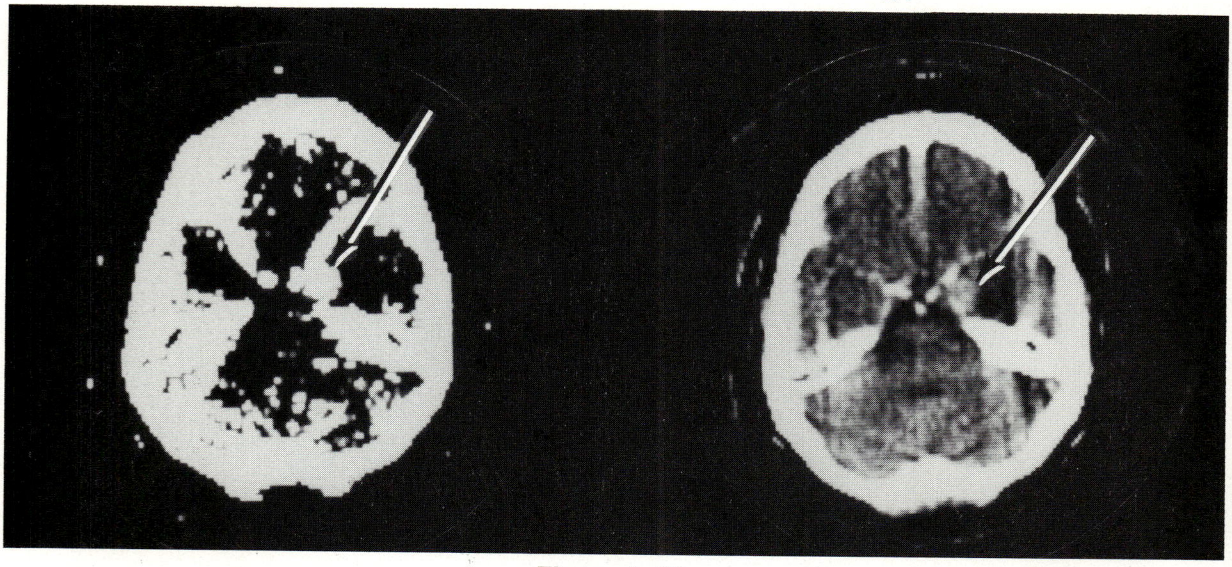

Figure 4–30

Arteriovenous Malformations

Since flowing blood is not picked up as such by the routine CT scan, an arteriovenous malformation may not be visualized with the preinfusion scan. Therefore the index of suspicion must be high, and a postinfusion scan should also be obtained in order to visualize the malformation. In some cases, perhaps because of shunting of blood away from the normal brain tissue, there may be a small area of lucency associated with the lesion because of local atrophy. In others, there may be areas of calcification that will be visualized on the preinfusion scan. After the infusion of contrast material, the remainder of the malformation will be readily visualized as, most often, a wedge-shaped area of increased density. Very often enlarged individual arteries and draining veins can be identified. Arteriography will confirm the abnormality and illustrate to better advantage the feeding arteries and the draining veins.

ARTERIOVENOUS MALFORMATION (Figure 4–31)

M. C. is a 51 year old female with a known right occipital arteriovenous malformation.

a to c. The posterior (a) and left (b) and right (c) lateral views reveal a wedge-shaped area of increased uptake in the right occipital pole that abutted the midline structures. This area of uptake faded on the delayed views. The findings are consistent with an arteriovenous malformation.

d. Cuts 2A and 2B of the routine CT scan reveal several patchy areas of increased density in the right occipital pole region. The density ranged from 44 to 84 u. This is consistent with the vascular calcification that is frequently seen with these malformations (arrows on 2A and 2B). Following the infusion of contrast material, there is marked enhancement of the arteriovenous malformation. The density has increased to 60 to 140 u, and there is an irregular area of enhancement that represents the feeding arteries, the draining veins, and the malformation itself. Arteriography is necessary to outline these abnormalities in more accurate detail.

POSTERIOR

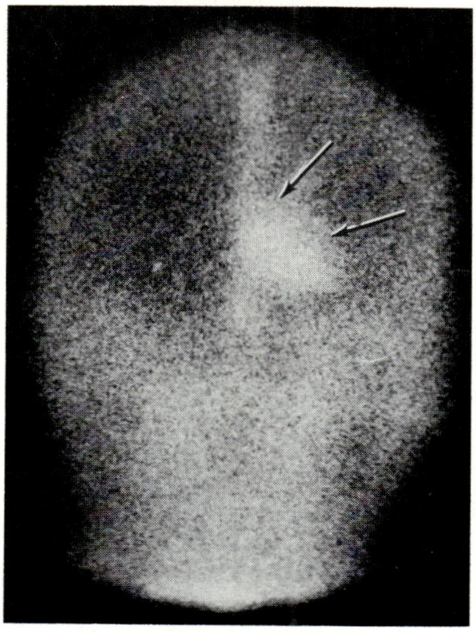

Figure 4–31a

LT. LATERAL

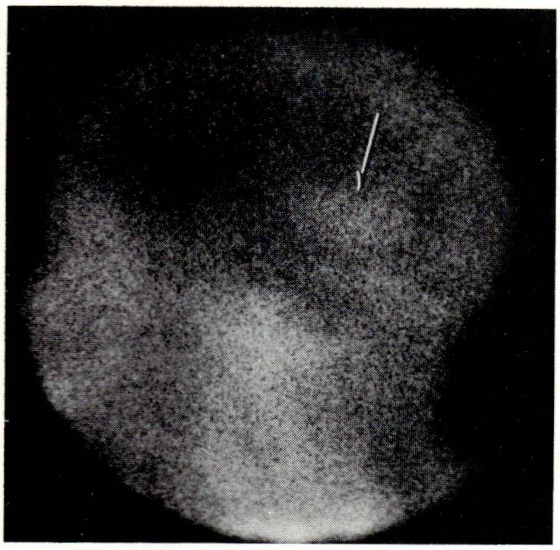

Figure 4–31b

RT. LATERAL

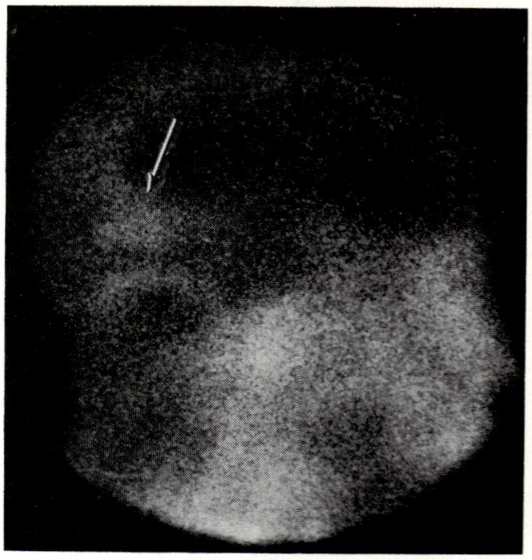

Figure 4–31c

e. The arterial phase of the left brachial arteriogram shows marked enlargement of the right posterior cerebral artery (arrows) as it feeds the malformation. Early filling veins have already obscured the malformation itself.

f. A later arterial phase discloses more venous filling and filling of the superficial veins (arrows) as they feed into the superior sagittal sinus.

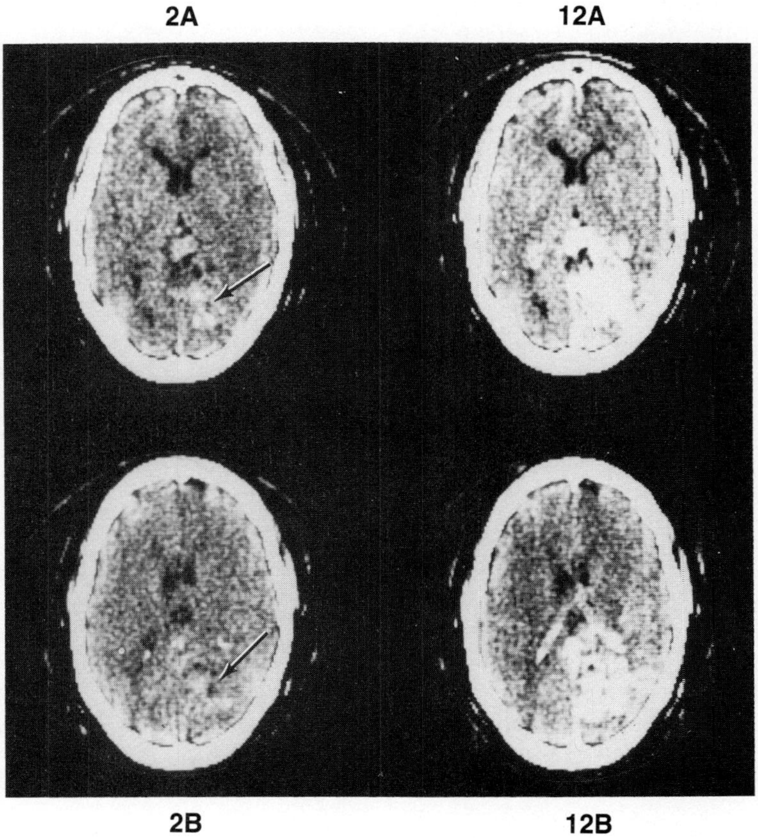

Figure 4–31d

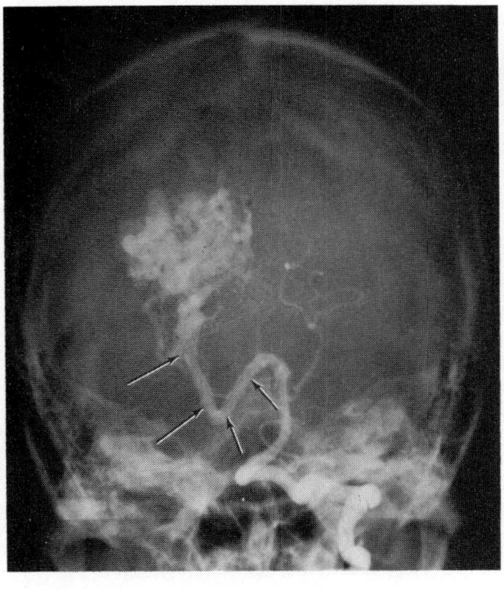

Figure 4–31e

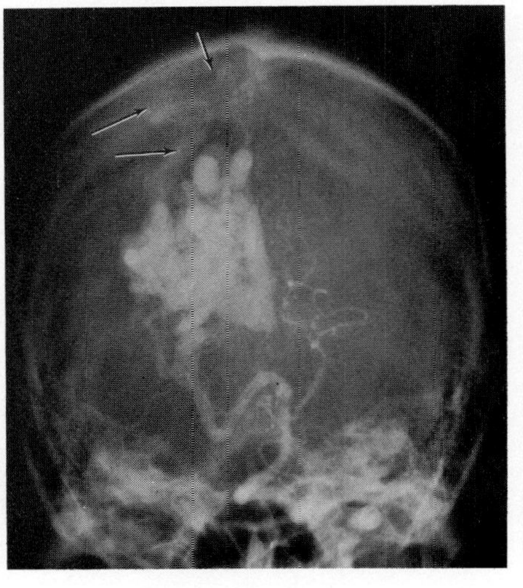

Figure 4–31f

g. The venous phase reveals that the arteriovenous malformation has emptied, leaving only the superficial veins (arrows), the superior sagittal sinus (crossed arrow), and the transverse sinus filled (lower arrows).

h. The lateral view of the right carotid arteriogram reveals enlargement of the feeding arteries of the middle cerebral artery (arrows). The enlarged draining veins have already obscured the malformation itself.

i. An early venous phase reveals filling of the great vein of Galen (arrows) and straight sinus (crossed arrows). The malformation can be faintly visualized (dashed line).

j. A late venous phase reveals only the tangle of draining veins.

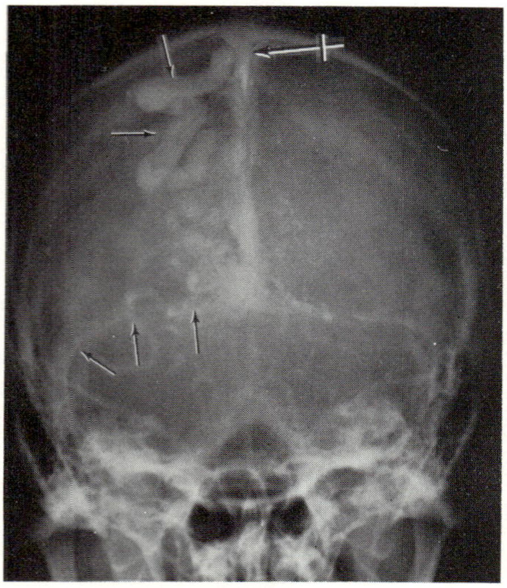

Figure 4–31g

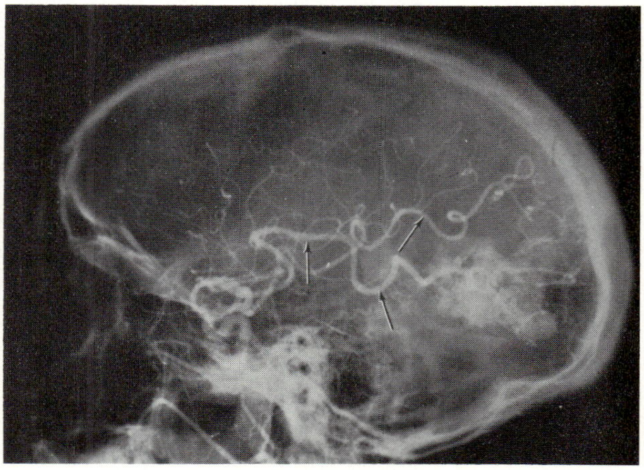

Figure 4–31h

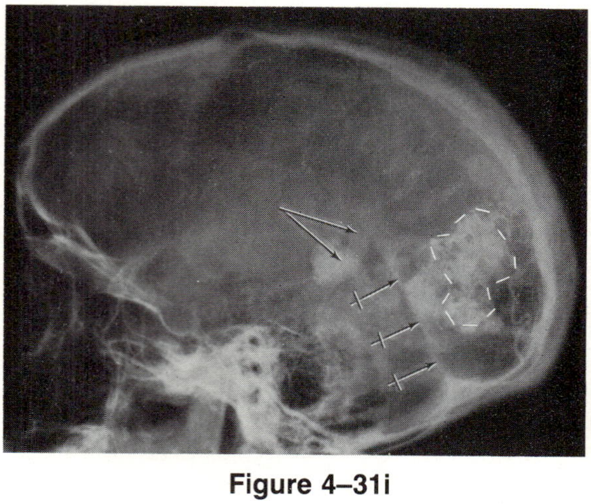

Figure 4–31i

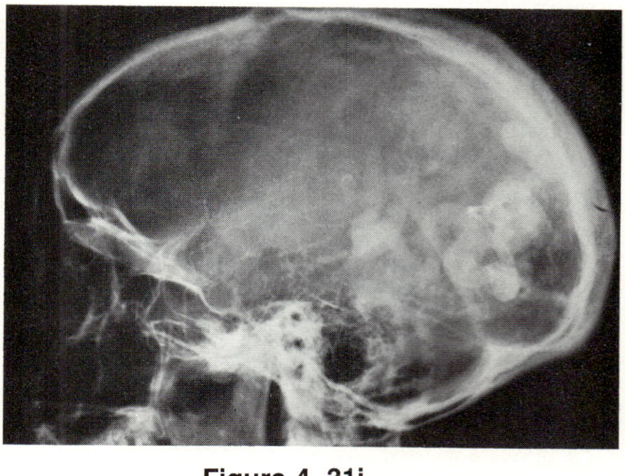

Figure 4–31j

ARTERIOVENOUS MALFORMATION (Figure 4–32)

P. A., a 59 year old male, was admitted following head trauma. He had previously been in good health.

a. The routine CT scan appears entirely within normal limits. After the infusion of contrast material, there was an area of enhancement in the high left parietal area just to the left of the midline. The area of enhancement had a rather serpentine appearance, and arteriovenous malformation was suggested.

b and c. The early and late lateral arterial views of the left carotid arteriogram reveal a small left parietal arteriovenous malformation. The malformation is fed by branches of the anterior cerebral artery and exhibits the classic early draining veins. Note how the large and small loops seen on the CT scan correspond with the large (long arrow) and small early draining veins (small arrow).

3A 13A

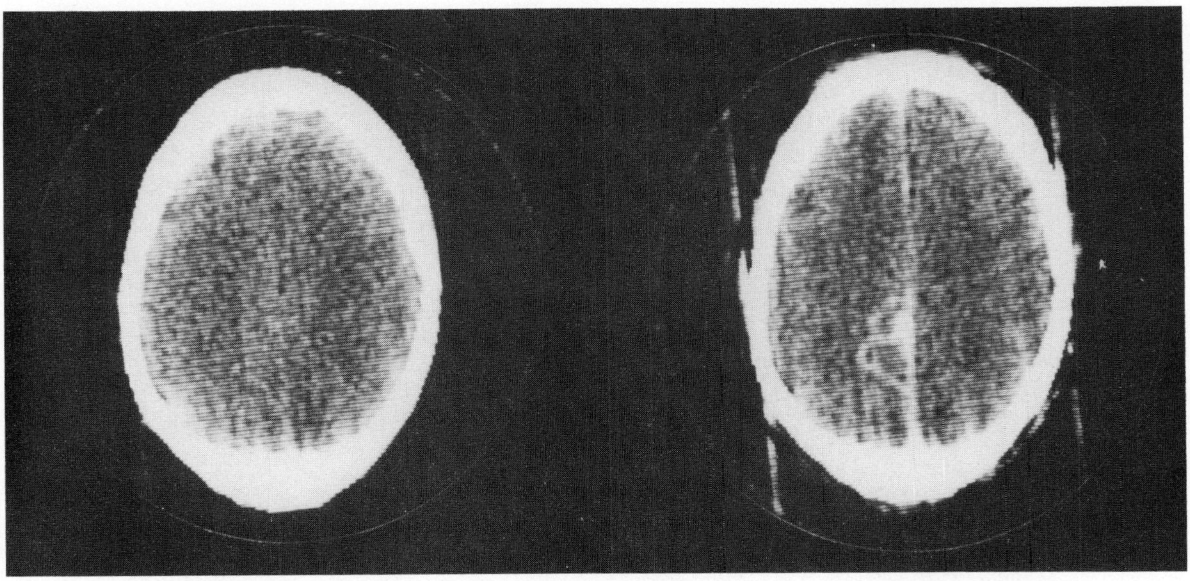

Figure 4–32a

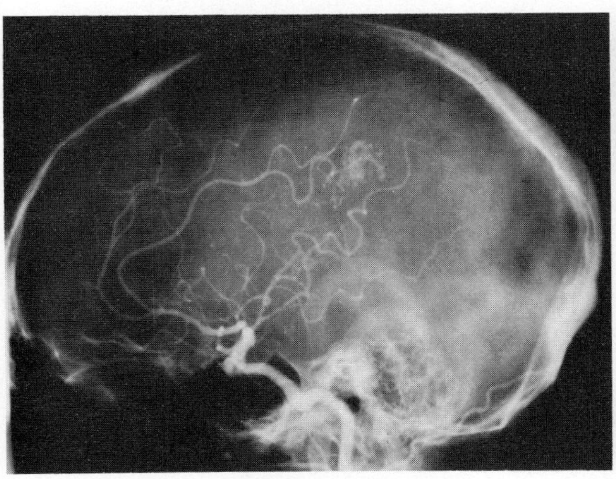

Figure 4–32b

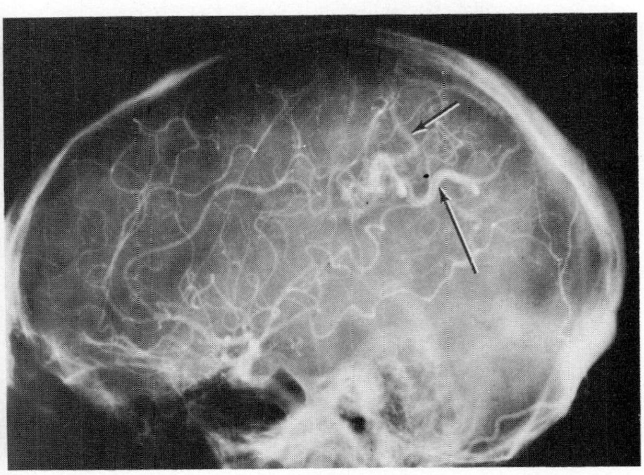

Figure 4–32c

d and e. The early and later anteroposterior views of the left carotid arteriogram again reveal the small arteriovenous malformation adjacent to the midline. The large draining vein (arrow) is again seen and correlates well with the CT scan findings.

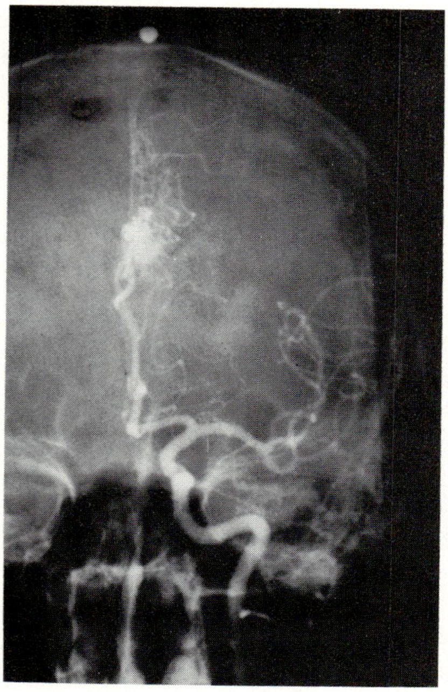

Figure 4–32d

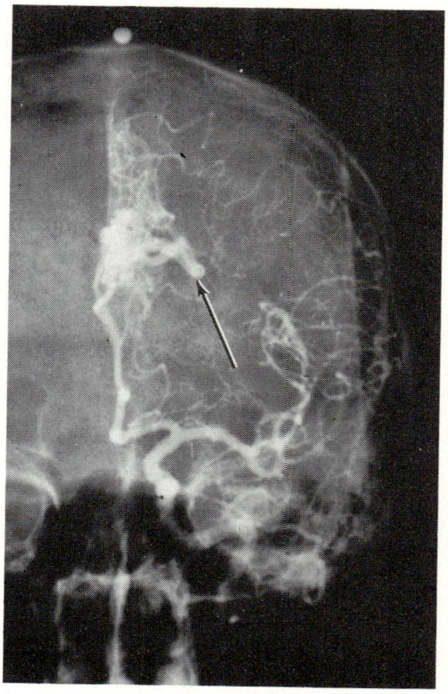

Figure 4–32e

Superior Sagittal Sinus Thrombosis

Thrombosis of the superior sagittal sinus (SSS) can be seen in a number of different clinical situations. It can develop following trauma, infection, dehydration, or childbirth, or it can be secondary to a combination of these factors. This lesion is not always fatal and is probably missed or misdiagnosed in a number of cases. It is more common in children. We have also seen examples of SSS thrombosis in the pediatric age group that lead to severe atrophy on follow-up examination.

At times this process is devastating and leads to the rapid demise of the patient, as seen in the next example.

Digital subtraction angiography (DSA) is very useful for evaluation of this problem. Contrast material is injected intravenously and the filming is performed over the cranial structures. The patient should be positioned for an oblique AP projection. The SSS will either be visualized or not, depending upon the absence or presence of thrombosis. Angiography may or may not confirm the presence of SSS thrombosis.

SUPERIOR SAGITTAL SINUS THROMBOSIS (Figure 4–33)

This 7 year old child was very lethargic when brought to the emergency room following 3 days of nausea and vomiting.

a. This initial study appears normal except for a small area of hemorrhage posteriorly in the temporal lobe area on the right side (arrow).

b. The postinfusion portion of the examination reveals a triangular-shaped area of lucency in the superior sagittal sinus (arrow). This appearance is very typical of SSS thrombosis. The small area of hemorrhage in the temporal lobe region is probably secondary to hemorrhagic infarction of the distribution of one of the cortical veins which drains into the SSS and is probably also clotted.

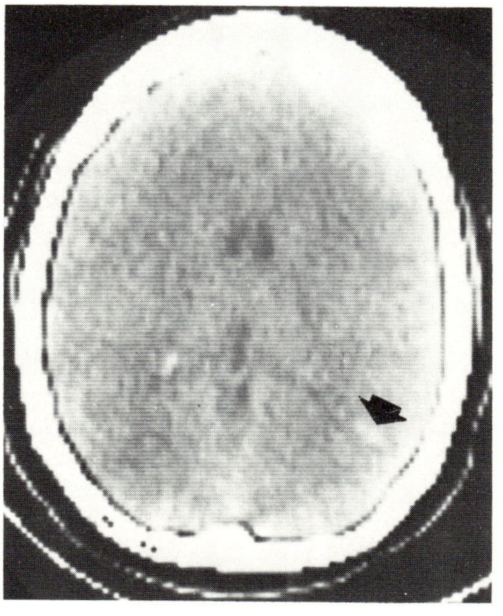

Figure 4–33a

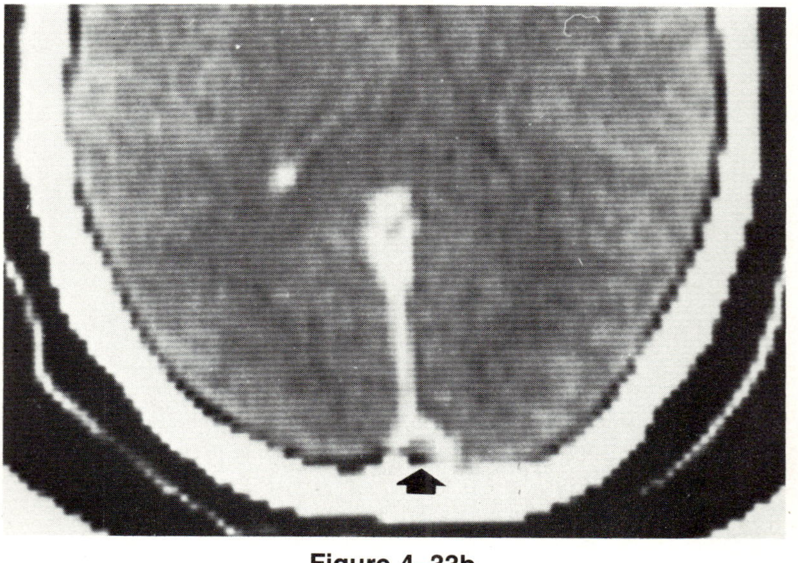

Figure 4–33b

SUPERIOR SAGITTAL SINUS THROMBOSIS (Figure 4–34)

G. J. is a 32 year old female with a history of Pott's disease and chronic schizophrenia who presented with sudden onset of dysphasia and loss of balance. Lumbar puncture revealed 10 mononuclear cells.

a and b. The anteroposterior (a) and left lateral (b) views of the radionuclide scan are suboptimal owing to poor cooperation; however, there does appear to be an area of increased uptake on the lateral view that parallels the superior sagittal sinus.

c. Cut 3A reveals multiple focal areas of hemorrhage. The densities ranged from a low of 50 to a high of 76 u. There was a slight change in the configuration of the areas after the infusion of contrast material (13A), and the densities increased to 44 to 120 u. The exact diagnosis remained obscure.

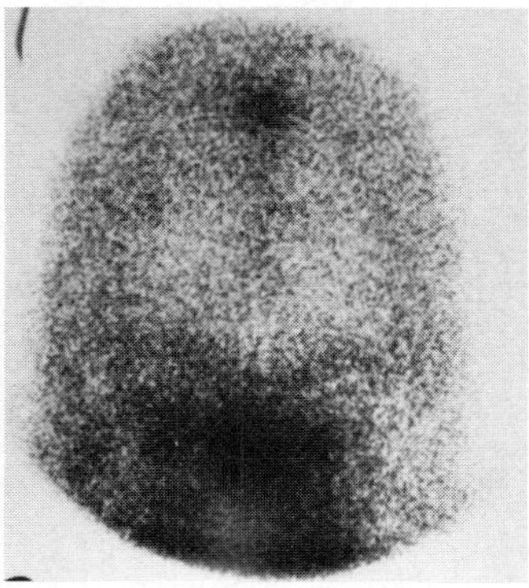

Figure 4–34a

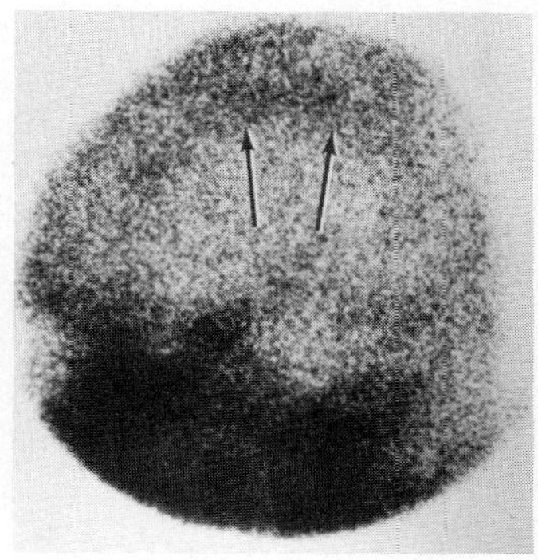

Figure 4–34b

3A 13A

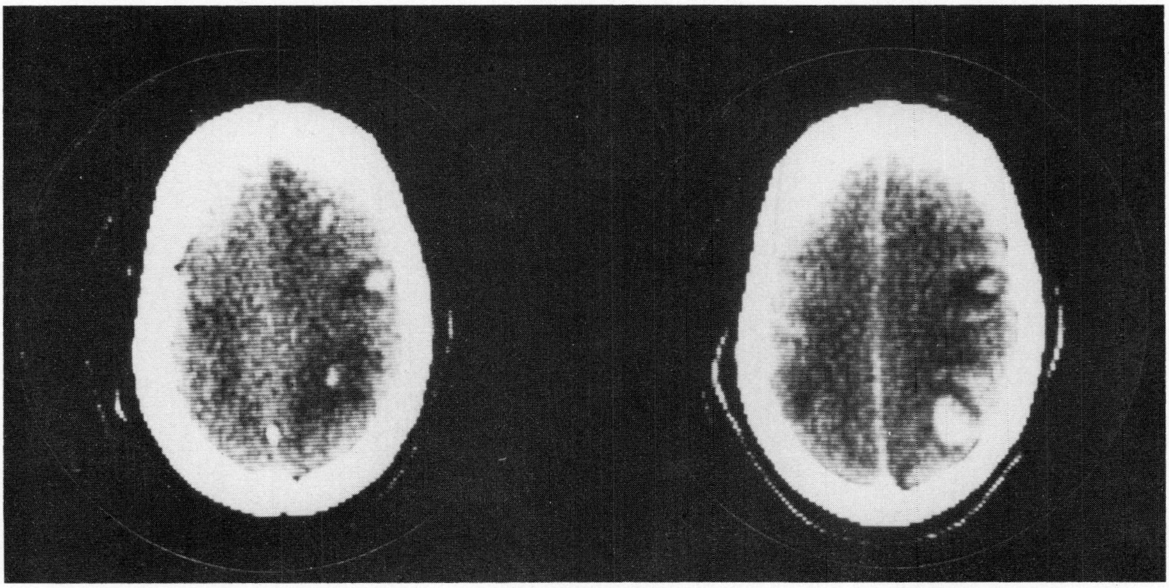

Figure 4–34c

d and e. Pathologic examination several days later reveals diffuse swelling of the brain, with thrombosis of the superior sagittal sinus and the superficial cortical veins (crossed arrow on e), as well as multiple scattered areas of intracerebral hemorrhage noted throughout the brain (arrows).

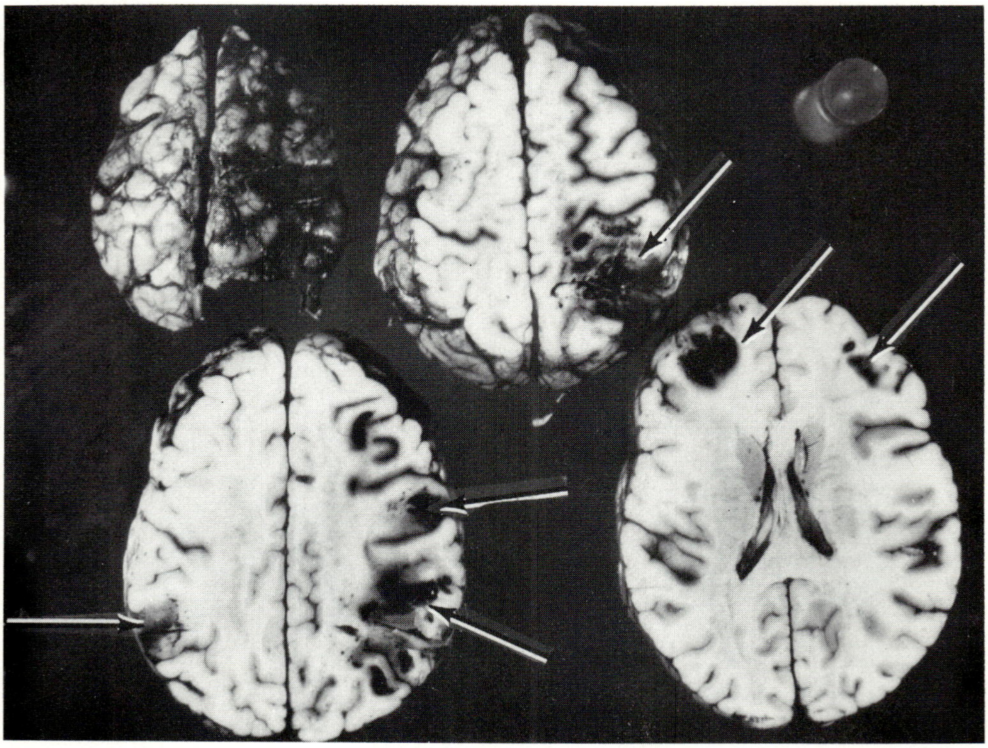

Figure 4–34d

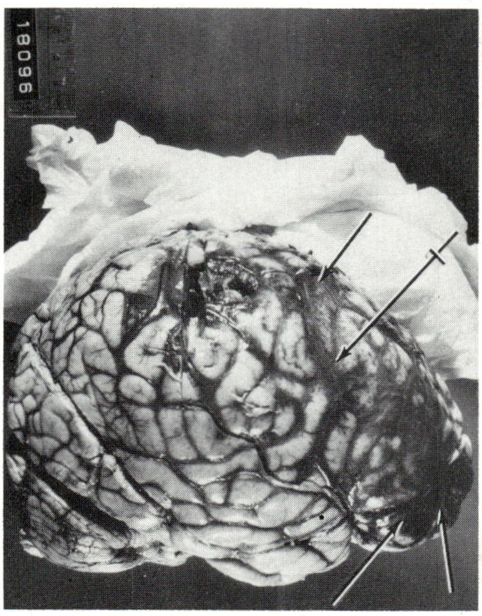

Figure 4–34e

CHAPTER 5

POST-TRAUMATIC ABNORMALITIES

A history of trauma, or external evidence of trauma, is present in a high percentage of cases of subdural hematoma. These subdural accumulations can have a variety of appearances. The acute subdural hematoma has the density of clotted blood and the appearance of an extracerebral accumulation of increased density over the abnormal hemisphere. In addition to the rim of increased density, there will be a contralateral shift of the lateral ventricles and the third ventricle. Occasionally one will be able to identify an associated skull fracture; infrequently there will be an associated intracerebral hematoma.

A somewhat different appearance is seen with a subacute or chronic subdural hematoma, in which there is an extracerebral accumulation of blood over the hemisphere measuring in a density range higher than cerebrospinal fluid but lower than clotted blood. This is consistent with a liquefied subdural hematoma with its highly proteinaceous fluid. Again, there will be a contralateral shift of the third and lateral ventricles.

The most troublesome appearance of a subdural hematoma from a diagnostic point of view is that in which the density of the extracerebral fluid accumulation is isodense with the normal brain tissue. In this situation the only abnormality that will be seen is the contralateral shift of the lateral ventricles. The index of suspicion must be high, and the pertinent clinical history is of the utmost importance. Incidentally, I have seen one case of bilateral subdural hemtomas which were isodense with the brain and showed simply that the lateral ventricles were more closely apposed than is normally seen; since the size of the subdurals was essentially equal, there was no shift of the midline.

Again, it should be emphasized that the index of suspicion must be high; when no history is available, the presence of a shift without an obvious intracerebral abnormality should increase the suspicion of a subdural hematoma.

RADIONUCLIDE SCAN OF A SUBDURAL HEMATOMA (Figure 5–1)

M. F. is a 49 year old woman who was brought to the emergency room after a 1-week history of headaches and confusion. Physical examination revealed a left pronator drift and bilateral papilledema.

a to c. The posterior (a), anterior (b), and vertex (c) views are shown here as the classic findings of a subdural hematoma. The nuclide angiogram demonstrates decreased perfusion to the left hemisphere, and the activity does not reach the convexity (not shown). This sign has been described in subdural collections. The routine scan reveals a diffuse increase in the activity over the left hemisphere with a crescentic appearance. This area of increased activity is seen on all three views.

The radionuclide studies will not be included with the following cases; this example represents the typical radionuclide findings seen with a subdural hematoma.

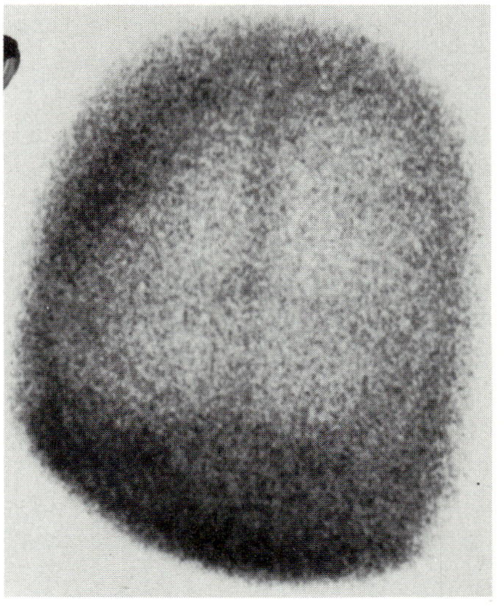

POSTERIOR
Figure 5–1a

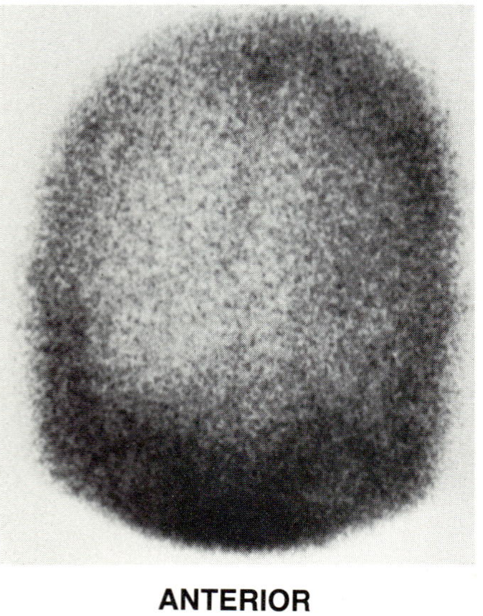

ANTERIOR
Figure 5–1b

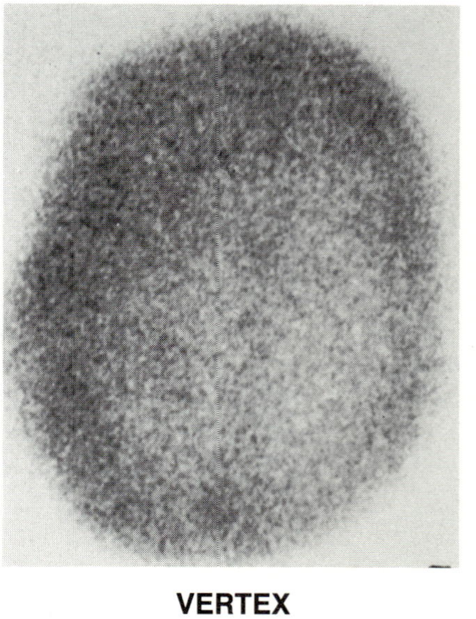

VERTEX
Figure 5–1c

LARGE LEFT SUBDURAL HEMATOMA (Figure 5–2)

M. K., an older male, was found unconscious and brought to the emergency room. He was decerebrate at the time of admission.

a. The emergency CT scan reveals a marked shift from left to right. There is a large left subdural hematoma. The appearance of this subdural accumulation, although not common, is classic. Unconscious patients are placed in the supine position soon after their arrival at the hospital; this results in a "settling" of the blood components and the appearance of a hematocrit level in the accumulated blood. Scattered droplets of Pantopaque are noted on the right side.

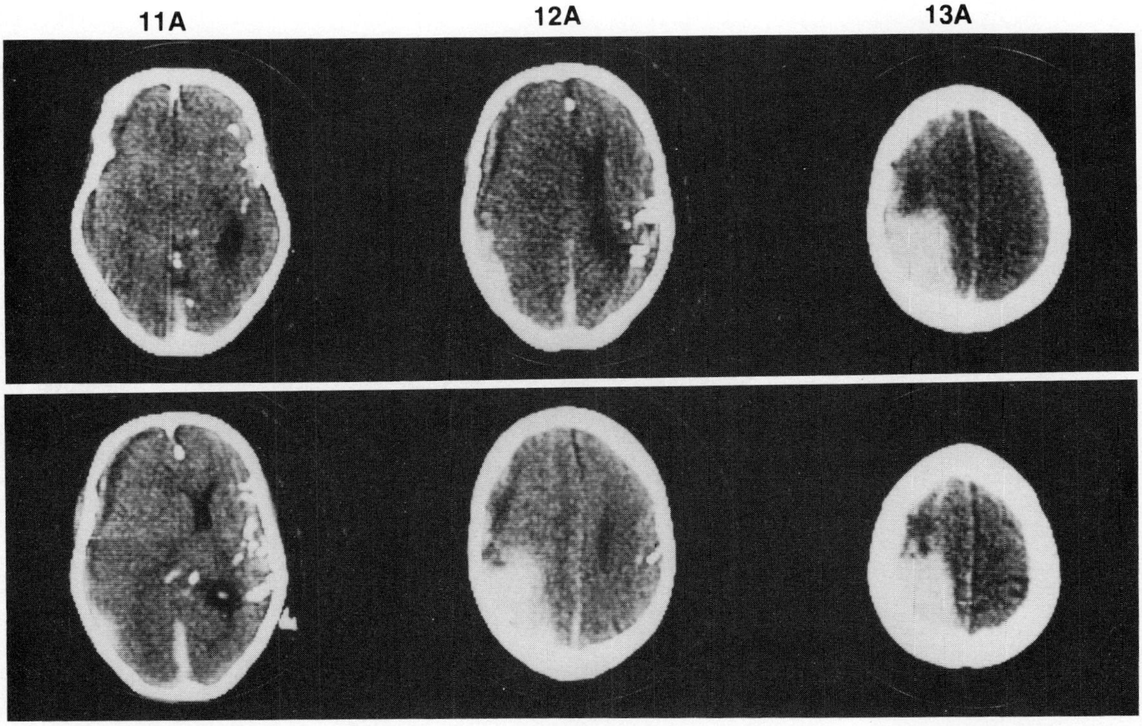

Figure 5–2a

Figure 5–2b

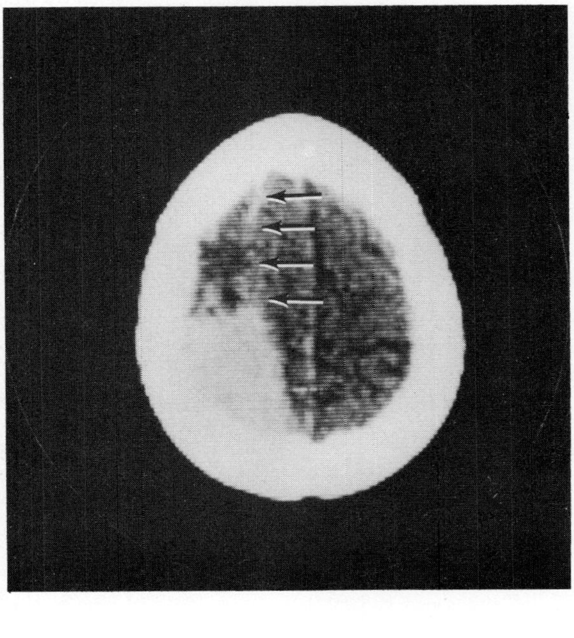

b. On the large picture of 13B, close inspection reveals that the medial border of the large subdural hematoma extends upward from the high density area (arrows) to the inner table anteriorly. The density in the more dependent portion of the subdural hematoma measures 48 to 84 u; in addition, the blood anterior to this large "settled" clot has a mottled increase in density.

A large clotted subdural hematoma was evacuated at the time of surgery. The appearance of the blood from the anterior and posterior portions of the hematoma was the same.

RIGHT SUBDURAL HEMATOMA (Figure 5–3)

L. C., a 47 year old woman, was brought to the emergency room with a history of seizures and coma. Further history revealed that she had been beaten by her boyfriend.

a. The emergency CT scan discloses an accumulation of fluid, density 16 to 36 u, over the right convexity in the frontal and parietal areas. Cut 12B reveals enhancement of a membrane of the subdural. A subacute subdural hematoma was removed at surgery. Cut 2B, obtained approximately 1 week after surgery, shows that the ventricles have returned to the midline; an extracerebral accumulation could no longer be detected.

b. The arterial phase reveals that the vessels did not extend to the cranial vault (short arrows), and that there was a proximal and distal shift of the anterior cerebral artery (arrows).

c. The lateral arterial phase shows downward displacement of the anterior cerebral artery as well as the sylvian triangle. The changes seen on the lateral view with subdural hematoma vary with the position of the hematoma.

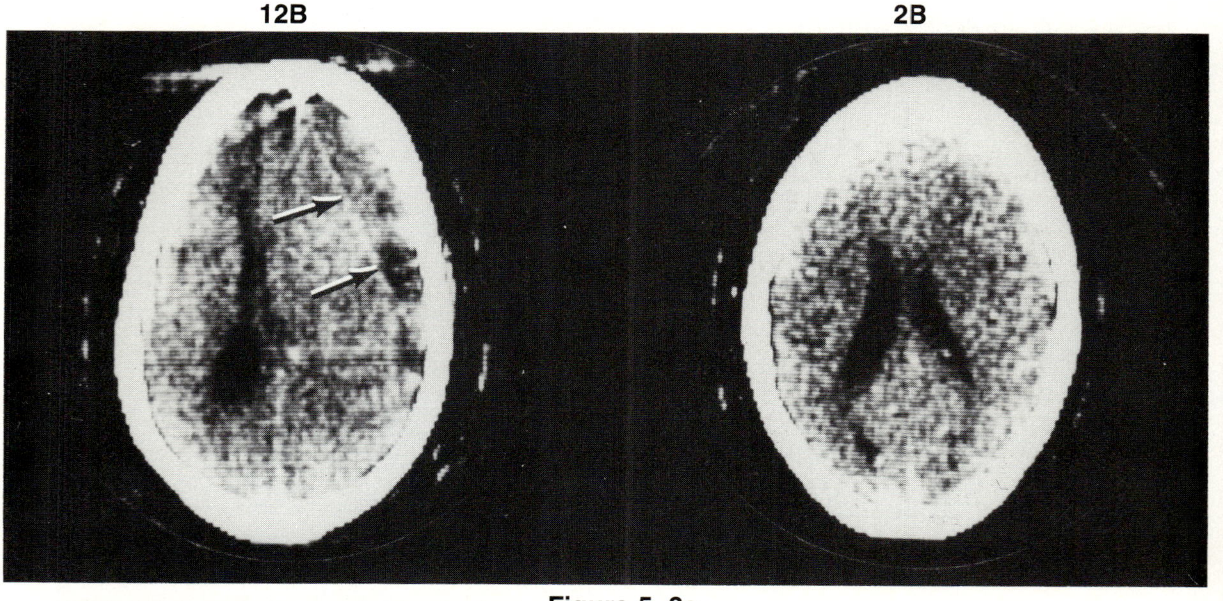

Figure 5–3a

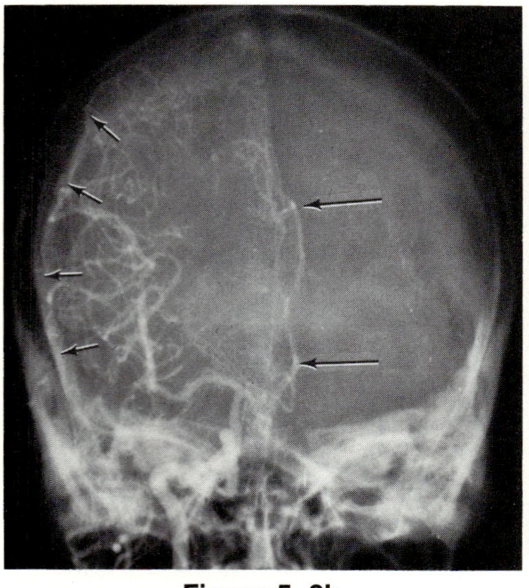

Figure 5–3b

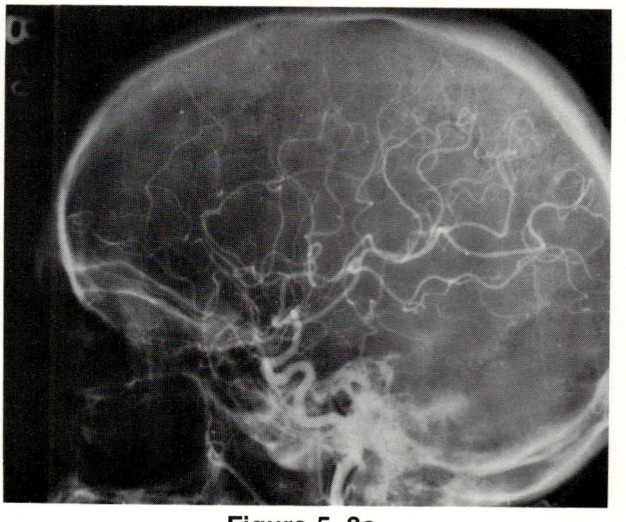

Figure 5–3c

ACUTE LEFT SUBDURAL HEMATOMA (Figure 5–4)

U. B. M. was found unconscious and was brought to the emergency room.

a. Cuts 2B and 3A reveal a small rim of extracerebral fluid, density 50 to 80 u, which appears to be clotted blood of an acute subdural hematoma. There is shift toward the right side, and obliteration of the left lateral ventricle on cut 3A.

b. Cut 2B, with electronic enhancement, emphasizes the subdural accumulation (arrows). The thin black line separating the subdura from the inner table of the skull is a computer artifact.

2B 3A

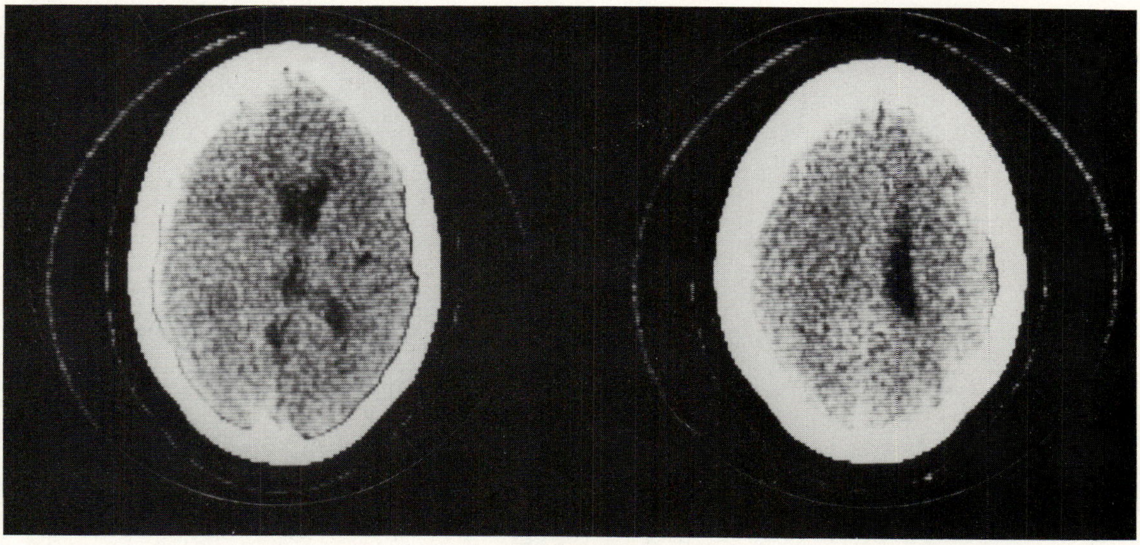

Figure 5–4a

2B

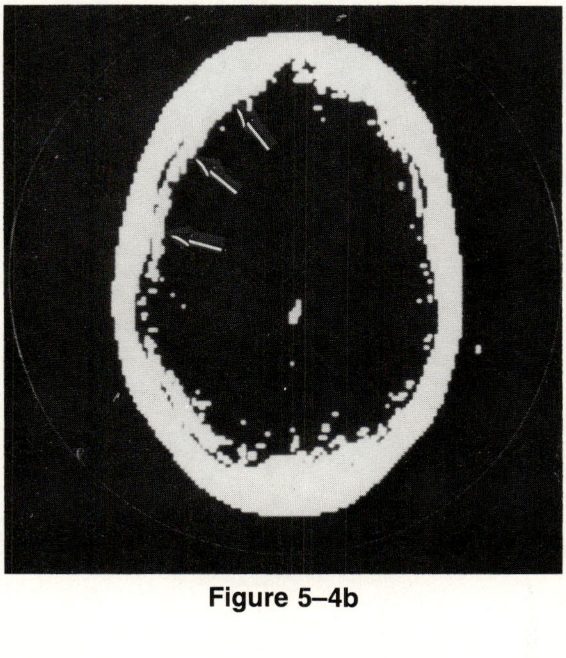

Figure 5–4b

SUBACUTE CHRONIC SUBDURAL HEMATOMA (Figure 5–5)

This 47 year old male was found unresponsive on the street.

a and b. The CT scan reveals a large crescentic extracerebral collection on the left side. There is marked shift from left to right and marked compression and distortion of the left lateral ventricle. In addition, the blood has settled in a "hematocrit" appearance (arrows) because the patient has been in the supine position for a prolonged period of time.

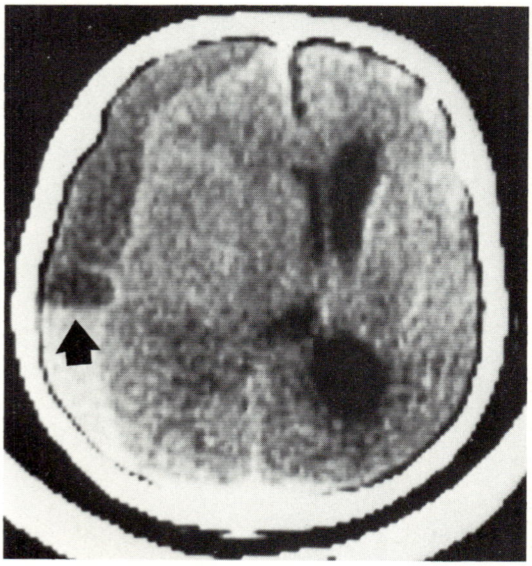

Figure 5–5a

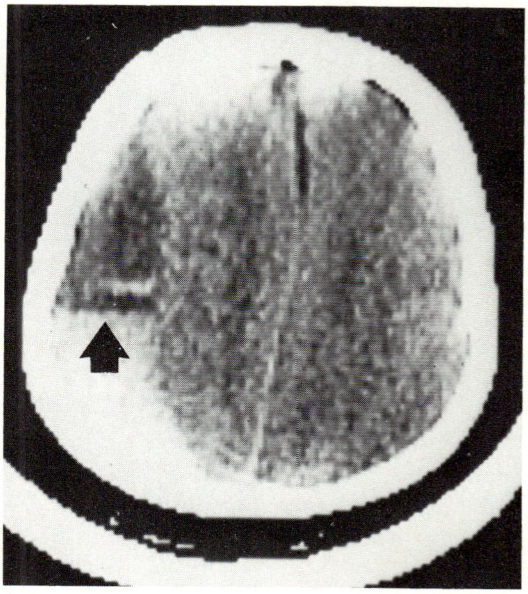

Figure 5–5b

ACUTE EPIDURAL HEMATOMA (Figure 5–6)

a and b. The epidural hematoma appears as a lentiform-shaped area of high density adjacent to the inner table of the skull. This occurs because the epidural collection must peel the dura (which forms the periostium of the inner table of the skull) away from the inner table of the skull. There is a marked shift to the contralateral side and compression of the ipsilateral ventricle.

These epidural hematomas may be associated with a fracture of the calvarium which crosses the middle meningeal artery groove. This fracture results in a shearing of the middle meningeal artery which causes arterial bleeding into the epidural space. Venous epidural collections may also occur.

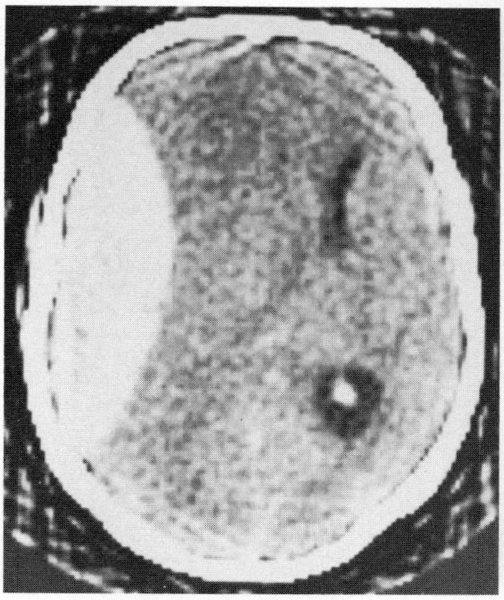

Figure 5–6a

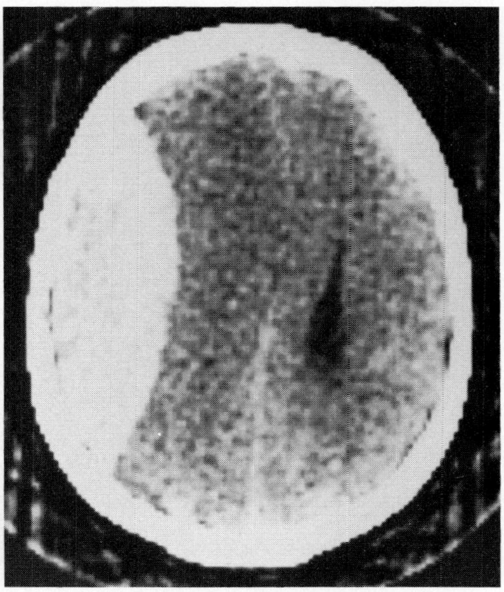

Figure 5–6b

ACUTE SHEARING INJURY (Figure 5–7)

This 52 year old male was in a motor vehicle accident and was thrown through the front windshield.

a and b. The preinfusion cuts reveal multiple small round intracerebral hematomas. In addition, there is blood in the subarachnoid space which causes increased density in the interhemispheric fissure posteriorly (arrows).

These shearing injuries result after a rapid deceleration injury because the gray and white matter are of different densities and therefore stop at different rates. This results in "shearing" at the gray matter–white matter junction. Histologically, there is also "balling up of the nerves" in the area of shearing. Thus the hematomas tend to occur at the gray matter–white matter junction.

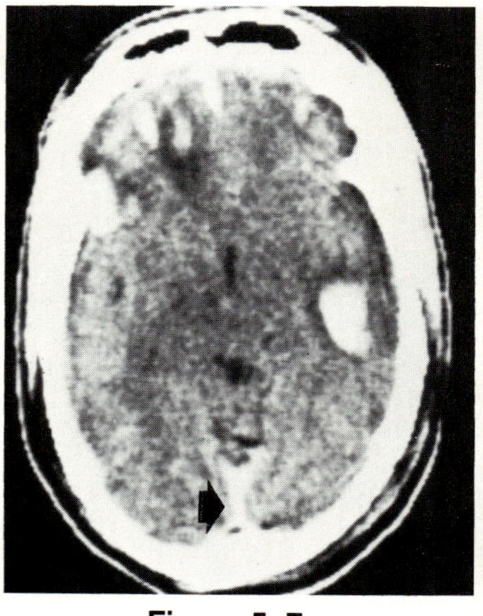

Figure 5–7a

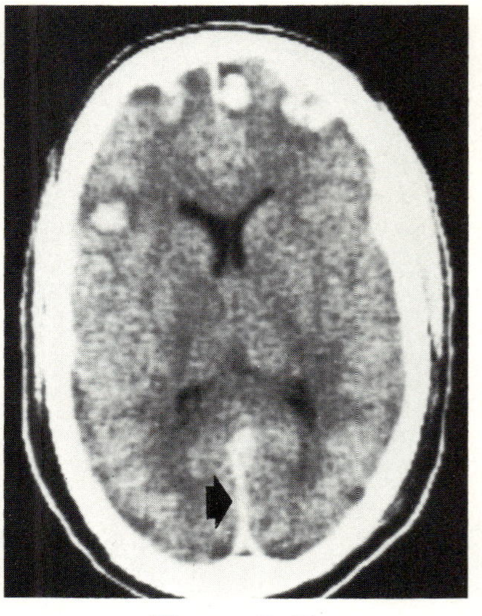

Figure 5–7b

SHEARING INJURY OF THE BRAIN FOLLOWING ACUTE HEAD TRAUMA (Figure 5–8)

Note that in these incidents the CT scan may appear surprisingly normal while the patient may be stuporous or even comatose.

a and b. The initial scans on this 7 year old patient who had been hit by an automobile could be mistaken as normal. Close inspection, however, reveals that there is blood along the free edge of the tentorium (curved arrow). There is also a very small amount of blood in the dependent portion of the lateral ventricles (arrowheads). The lateral ventricles are quite small.

c. While this may be normal in a 7 year old, the follow-up scan one week later showing slightly larger lateral ventricles sugests that the small ventricles may be secondary to diffuse edema.

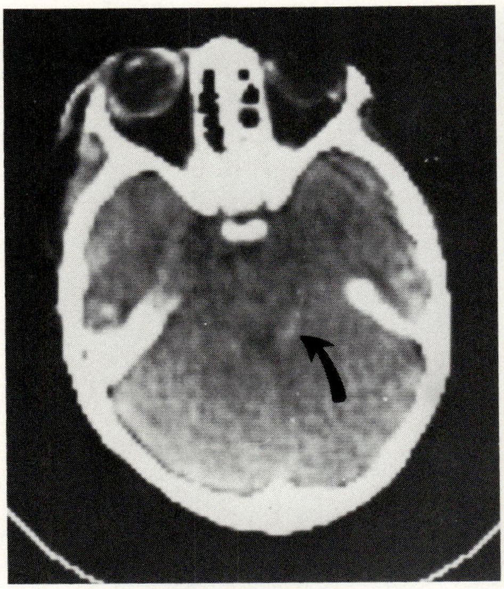

Figure 5–8a

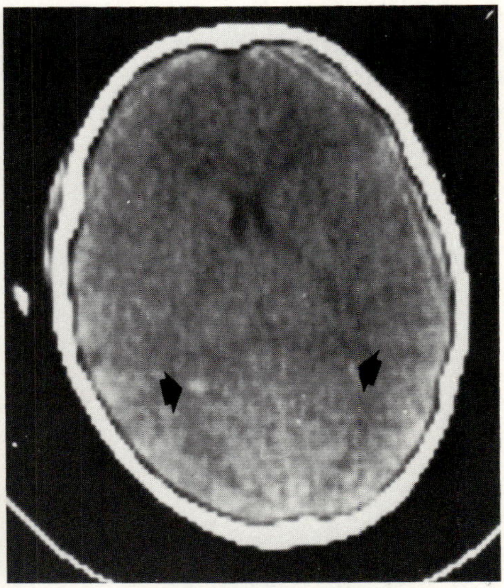

Figure 5–8b

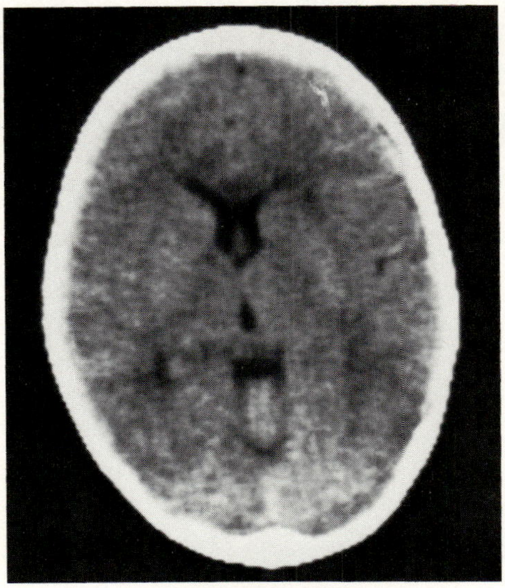

Figure 5–8c

d and e. Additional follow-up 6 weeks after the initial injury now reveals an appearance of diffuse atrophy. Acute or delayed hemorrhages may also be seen following rapid deceleration injuries. These hemorrhages occur at the gray matter–white matter junctions and are secondary to varying density of the cerebral tissues, resulting in shearing of the nerves at this level.

The small area of lucency in the right frontal area is secondary to placement of an intracranial pressure monitoring device.

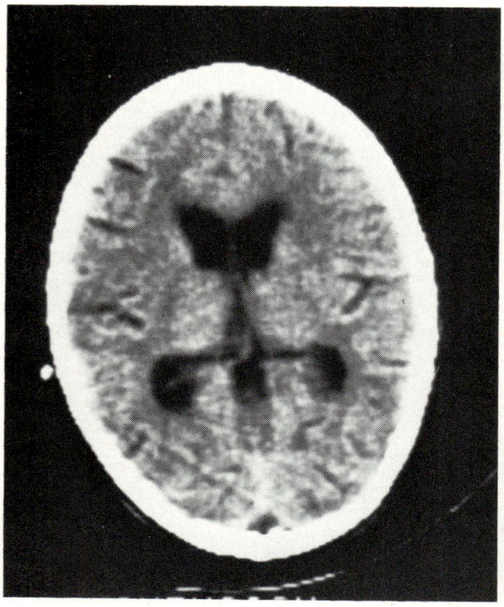

Figure 5–8d

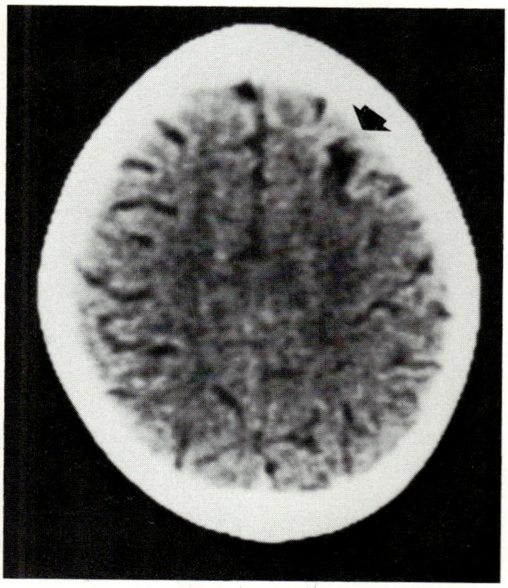

Figure 5–8e

DEPRESSED SKULL FRACTURE (Figure 5–9)

This 7 year old male was hit by a car.

a. The CT scan on a window width appropriate for bone reveals a depressed skull fracture in the left parietal region (arrow). Note the associated extracranial soft tissue swelling.

b. The routine CT scan reveals the depressed skull fracture. The intracranial contents are normal. Note that this could have the appearance of a small epidural hematoma. Therefore, appropriate density measurements must be made to determine if this is, in fact, bone or blood density.

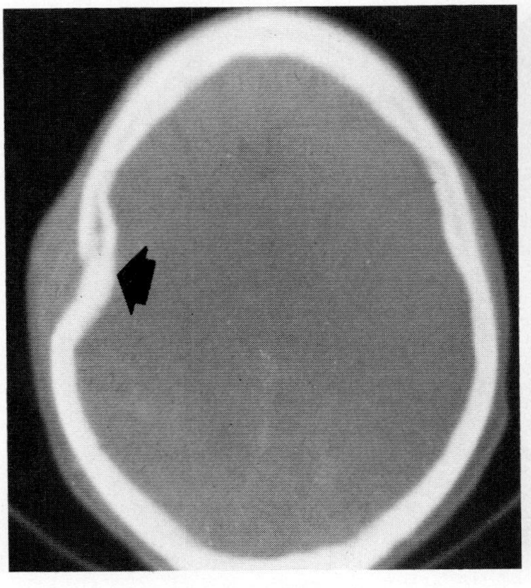

Figure 5–9a

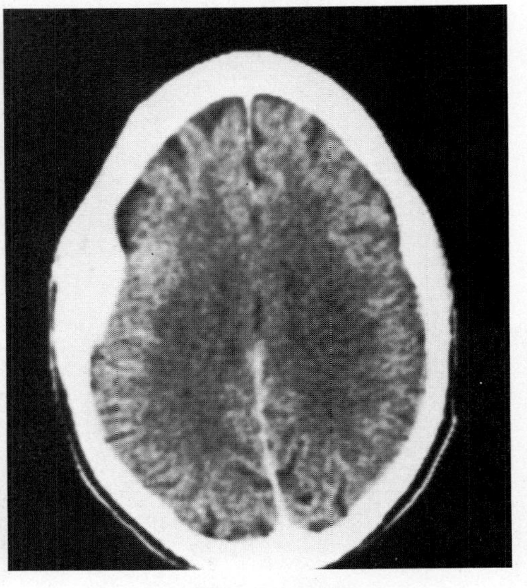

Figure 5–9b

BATTERED CHILD SYNDROME (Figure 5–10)

A. M., a 1½ year old female, was brought to the emergency with a history of "falling down" a flight of stairs. The child had multiple soft tissue injuries and a severe occipital scalp laceration.

a and b. Routine skull series reveals a long irregular occipital bone fracture that crosses the lamboid suture and extends into the sagittal suture as well (arrows). There is diastasis of the coronal suture.

c. A routine chest series shows a normal heart and lungs, but multiple bilateral rib fractures with callus formation. The rib fractures were obviously not sustained at the time of the acute injury, raising the very strong possibility of child abuse. A long bone survey was obtained but was negative for additional fractures.

d. On emergency CT scan the intracranial structures appear nor-

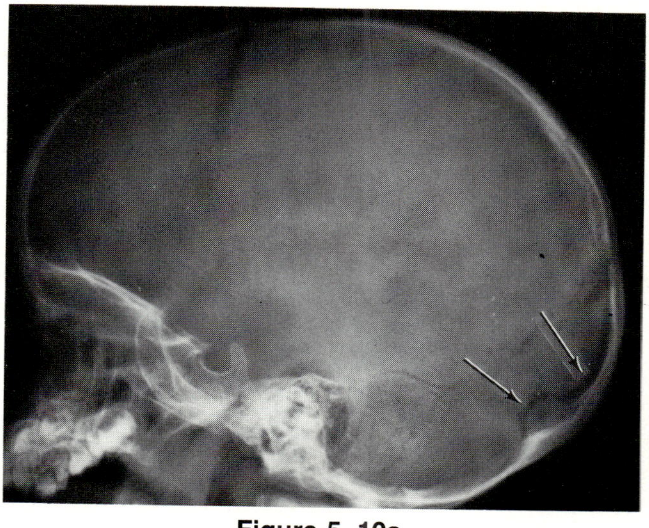

Figure 5–10a

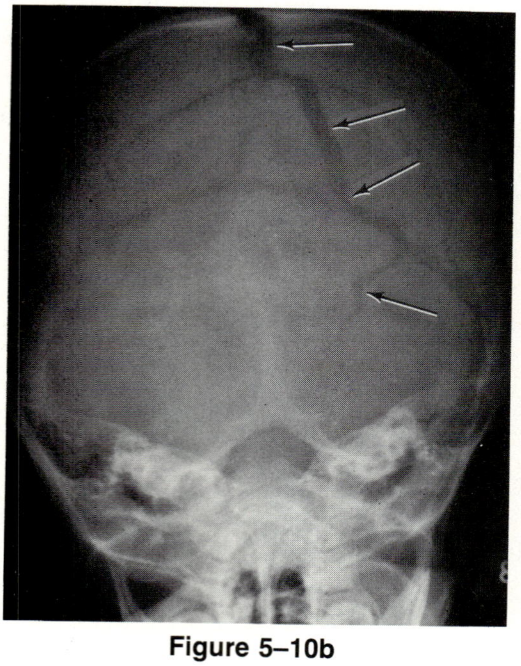

Figure 5–10b

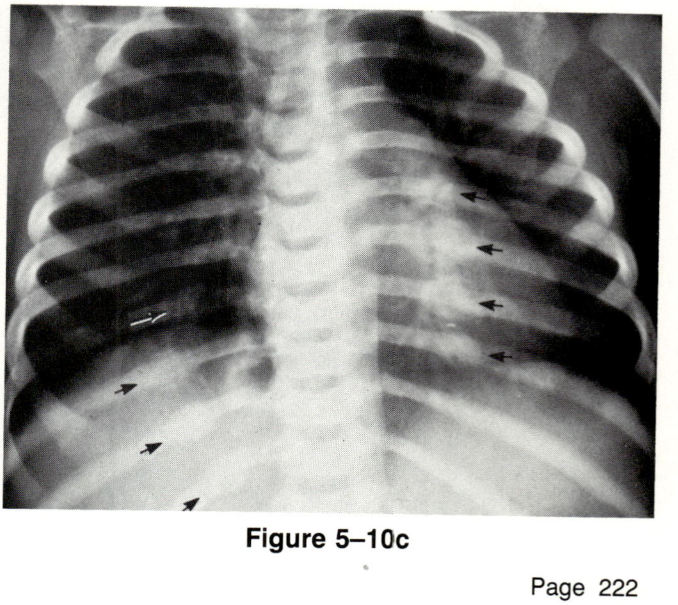

Figure 5–10c

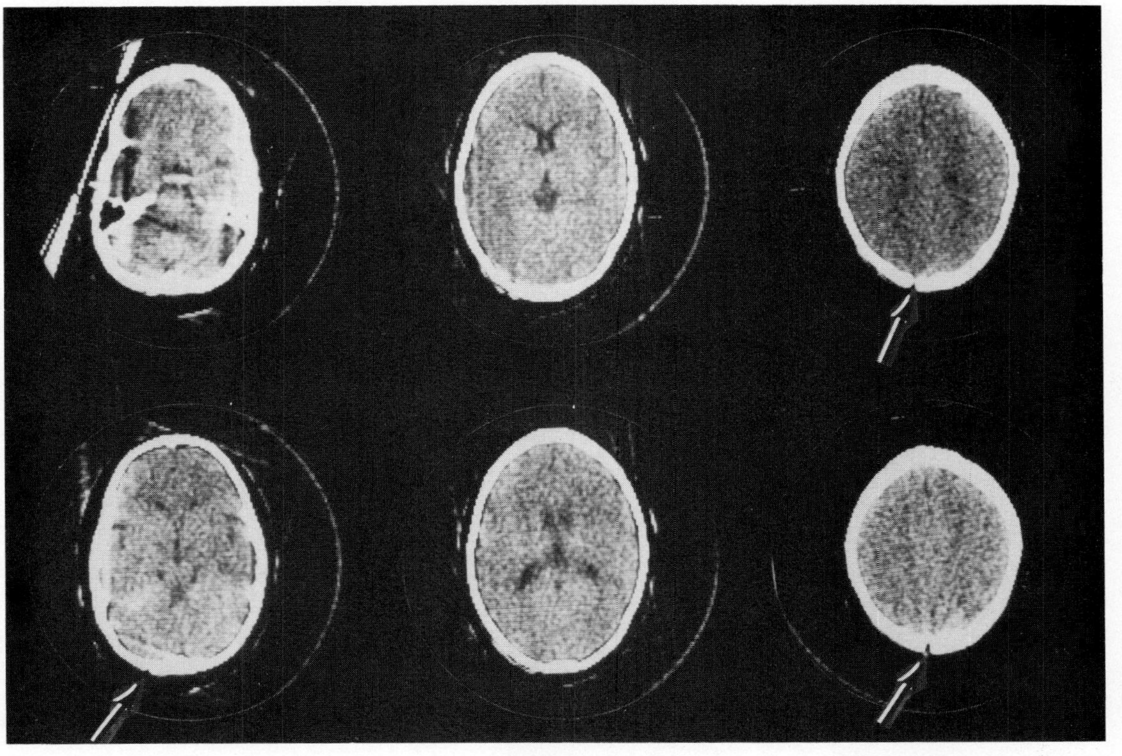

Figure 5–10d

mal—the occipital bone fracture can be identified on multiple cuts (arrows).

e and f. Because of persistent right arm weakness and a right leg limp, a left carotid arteriogram was done. There was no shift. The sagittal sinus is noted to be displaced away from the inner table from the coronal suture to the torcular, raising the possibility of a small epidural accumulation of fluid. The patient improved, and no surgery was done.

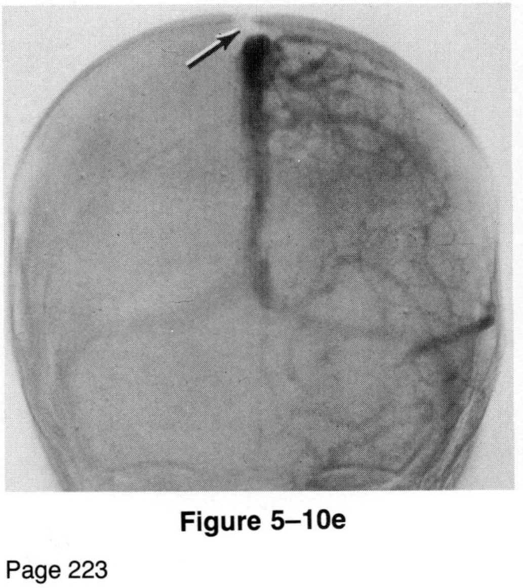

Figure 5–10e

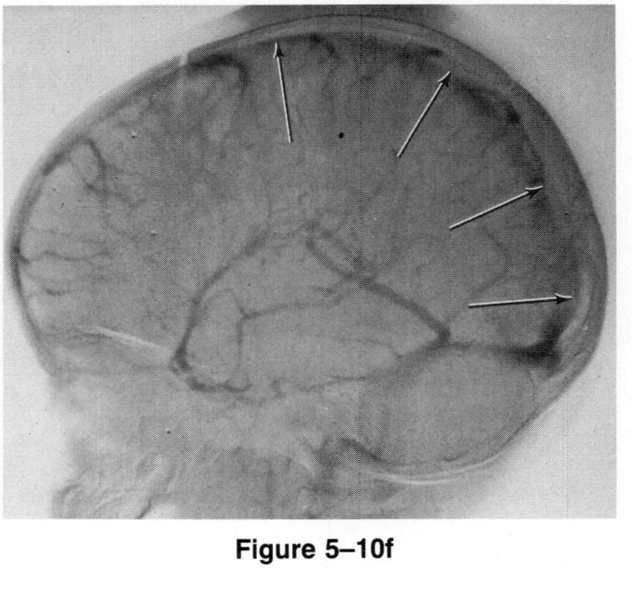

Figure 5–10f

TETRAPOLAR TRAUMA (Figure 5–11)

C. B., a 6 year old girl, was hit by a passing car as she disembarked from the school bus. She sustained severe body and head trauma and was brought to the emergency room unconscious.

a and b. Routine skull series shows several fractures in the right parietal and occipital regions. A ventricular pressure monitoring catheter is in place anteriorly.

c. The emergency computed tomogram reveals evidence of tetrapolar trauma. Soft tissue hematoma and the right parietal skull

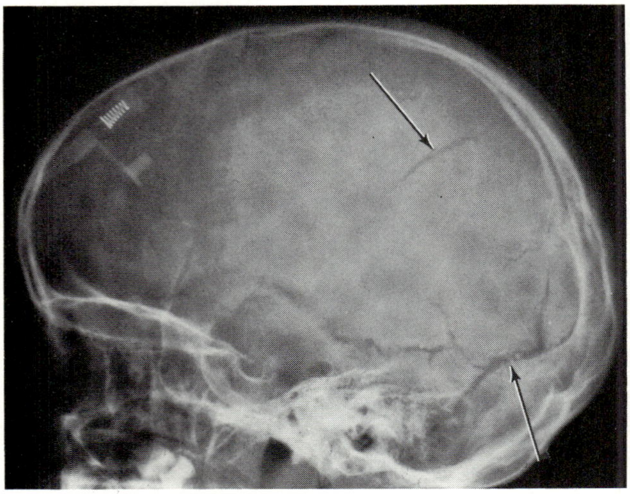

Figure 5–11a

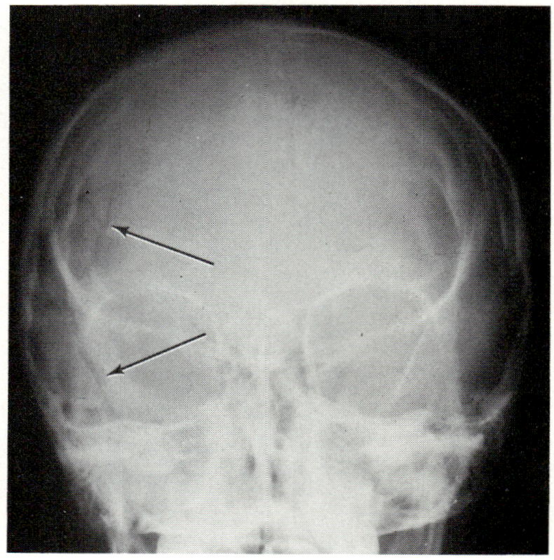

Figure 5–11b

1A 2A 3A

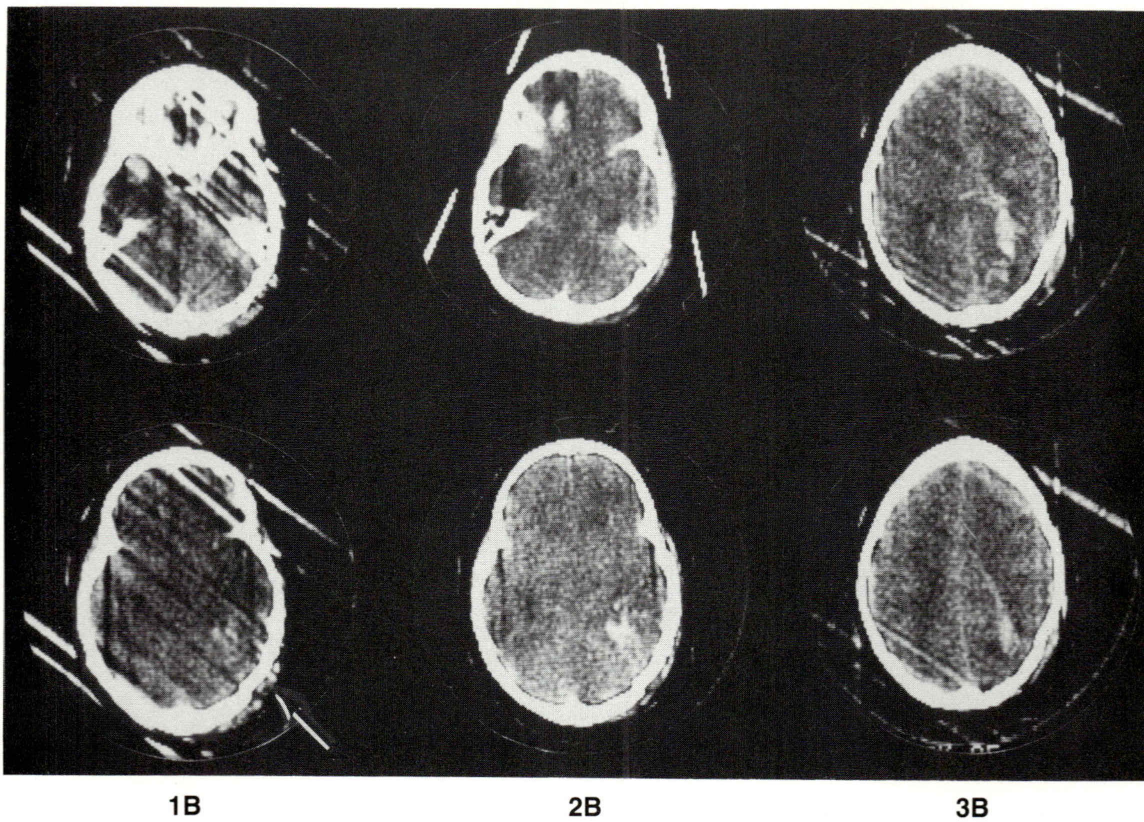

1B 2B 3B

Figure 5–11c

fracture are noted. There is a small left temporal hematoma (1A), as well as a left frontal intracerebral hematoma (2A) surrounded by an area of edema. There is a small irregular hematoma in the right parietal region deep to the scalp injury and skull fracture, with a small amount of blood in the occipital horn of the right lateral ventricle (cuts 3A and 3B). The densities ranged from 48 to 78 u.

In spite of aggressive medical management the patient never came out of shock, developed renal failure, and died 3 days after admission.

LEFT SUBFRONTAL EPIDURAL HEMATOMA (Figure 5–12)

V. P. is a 44 year old female who sustained severe head trauma 7 days prior to admission. A left carotid arteriogram revealed minimal shift toward the right side.

The routine CT scan shows an area of markedly increased density superior to the roof of the left orbit (best seen on cut 1B). The density is 62 to 100 u, and there is a mild shift of the frontal horns toward the right side (arrow on cut 2A). A low density area in the left frontal horn (cut 2A) represents contusion or edema surrounding the hematoma. Note that an intracerebral hematoma of this size is unlikely because of the rather minor shift compared to the size of the clot.

A left subfrontal subdural hematoma was felt to be most likely. However, surgery revealed a left subfrontal epidural hematoma.

1A 2A

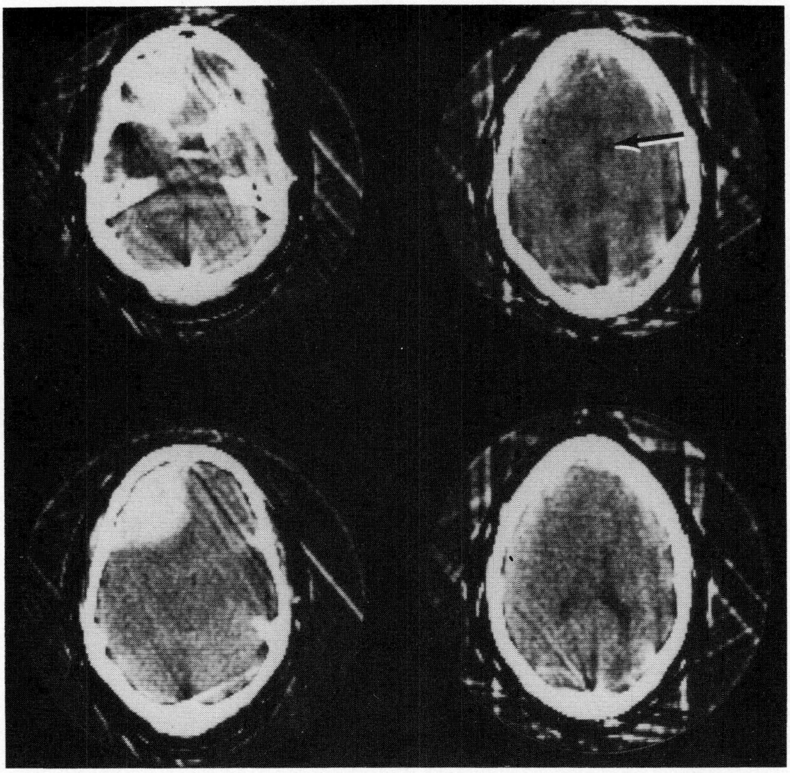

1B 2B

Figure 5–12

POSTSURGICAL INTRACEREBRAL HEMATOMA (Figure 5–13)

L. P. developed the onset of grand mal seizures following insertion of a ventricular pressure monitoring catheter into the right frontal horn.

The routine scan reveals the shunt tip in place in the right frontal horn (arrow) and an iatrogenic right frontal hematoma along the shunt tract from the right frontal horn to the frontal convexity.

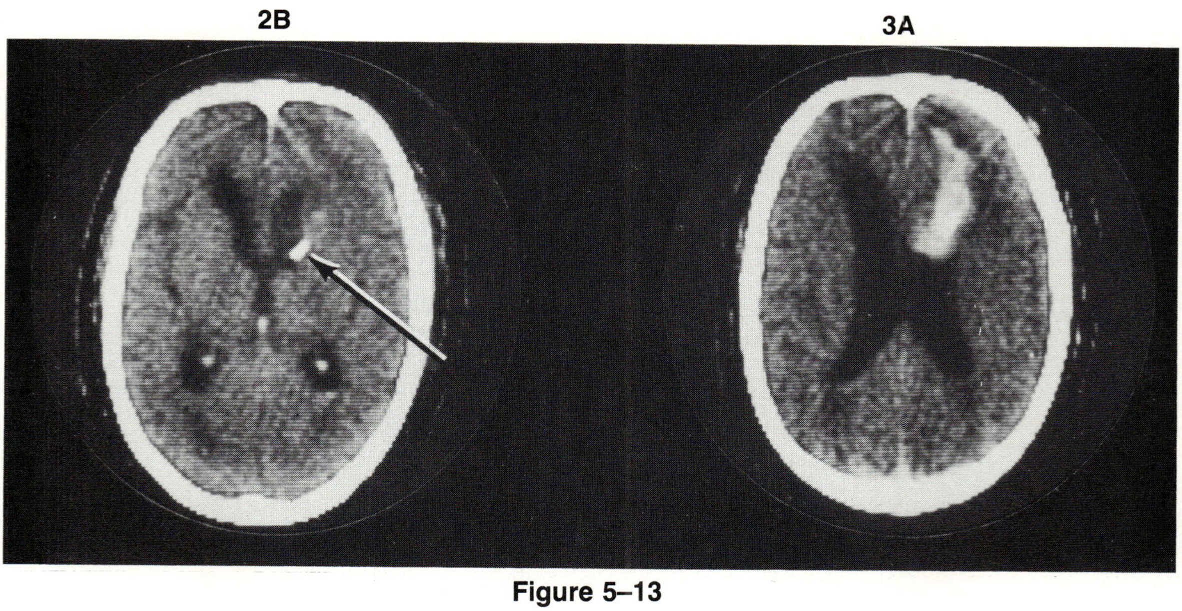

Figure 5–13

INTRACEREBRAL HEMATOMA AND RESULTING PORENCEPHALIC CYST (Figure 5–14)

W. S. is a 47 year old man who sustained a severe blow to the left side of his head. The routine skull series disclosed a small depressed skull fracture in the left temporal bone.

The initial scan (top row), obtained at the time of the acute injury, reveals the soft tissue swelling in the temporal region, as well as the depression of the bone associated with the depressed skull fracture. There is a small irregular intracerebral hematoma—density, 40 to 64 u—just beneath the skull fracture (arrow on 2A). A slight mass effect with compression of the left frontal horn is best seen on cut 2B (arrow). The second scan (bottom row), obtained as a follow-up examination 5 months after the first study, reveals a small porencephalic cyst occupying the previous position of the hematoma (arrows). The density was the same as the cerebrospinal fluid. There is now no shift of the lateral ventricles. Note that the depressed skull fracture can still be identified (crossed arrow).

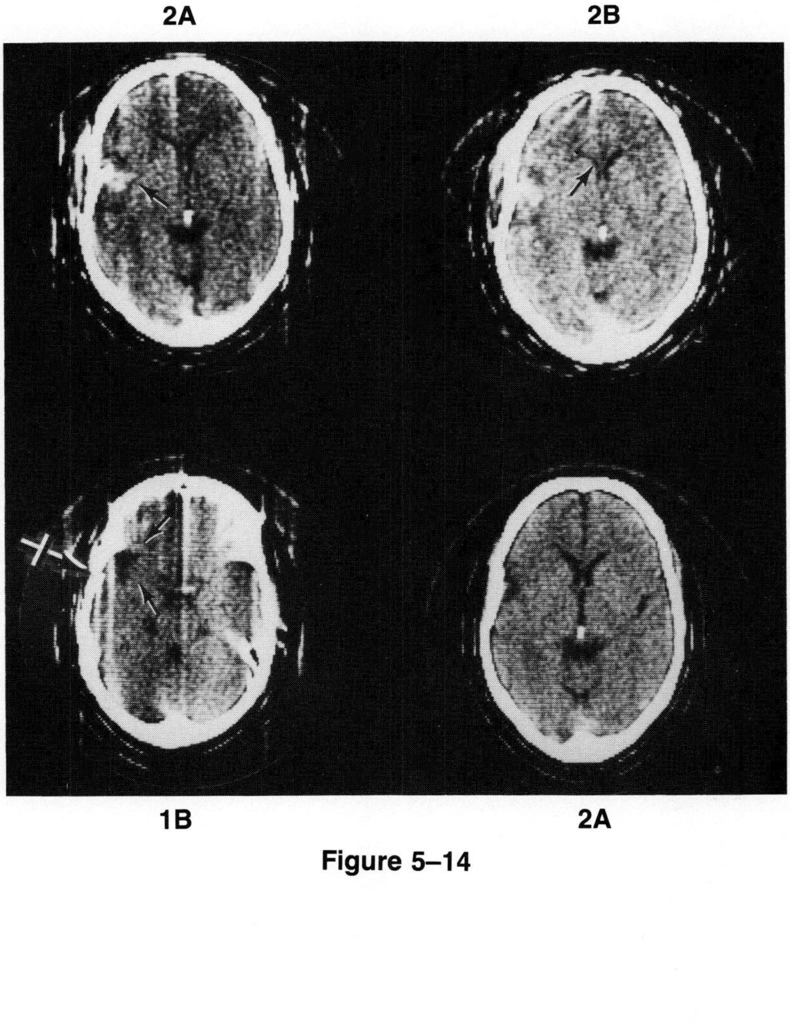

Figure 5–14

CHAPTER 6

ACQUIRED ABNORMALITIES

Atrophy

Figures 6–1 and 6–2 show the classic findings in atrophy. There is enlargement of the lateral ventricles, as well as enlargement of the cortical sulci. The sylvian fissures (arrows) are also noted to be enlarged bilaterally. Computed tomography is an ideal method for evaluating the presence or absence of atrophy; pneumoencephalography, with its attendant discomfort and morbidity, can most often be omitted. It should be noted, however, that there is an apparent normal increase in the size of the ventricles with age, and so the age of the patient should be considered when deciding if the ventricles and cortical sulci are pathologically enlarged. Generalized atrophy is a common finding; however, small or focal areas of atrophy may also be seen. These focal areas of atrophy usually develop as a result of a cerebrovascular accident, although focal atrophy does not follow every cerebrovascular accident. Pontocerebellar atrophy can be seen in association with various degenerative diseases; vermis atrophy may be seen in association with alcoholism.

1A 2A 3A

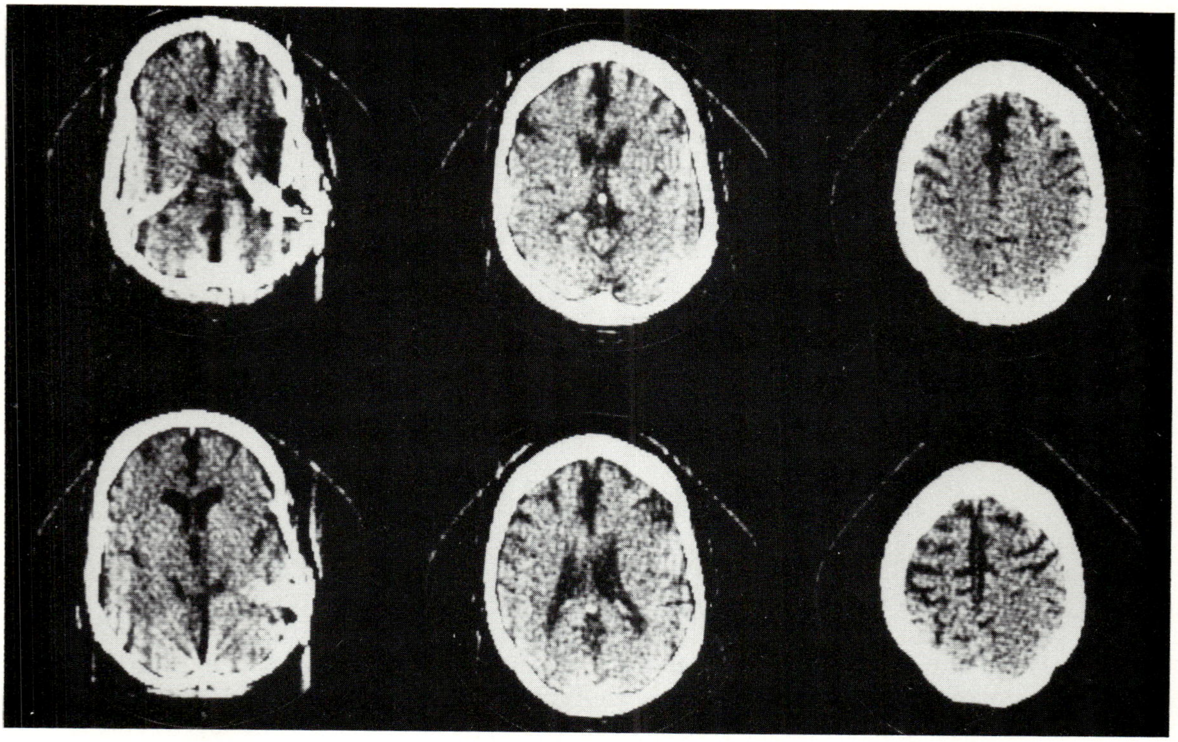

1B 2B 3B

Figure 6–1

1A 2A 3A

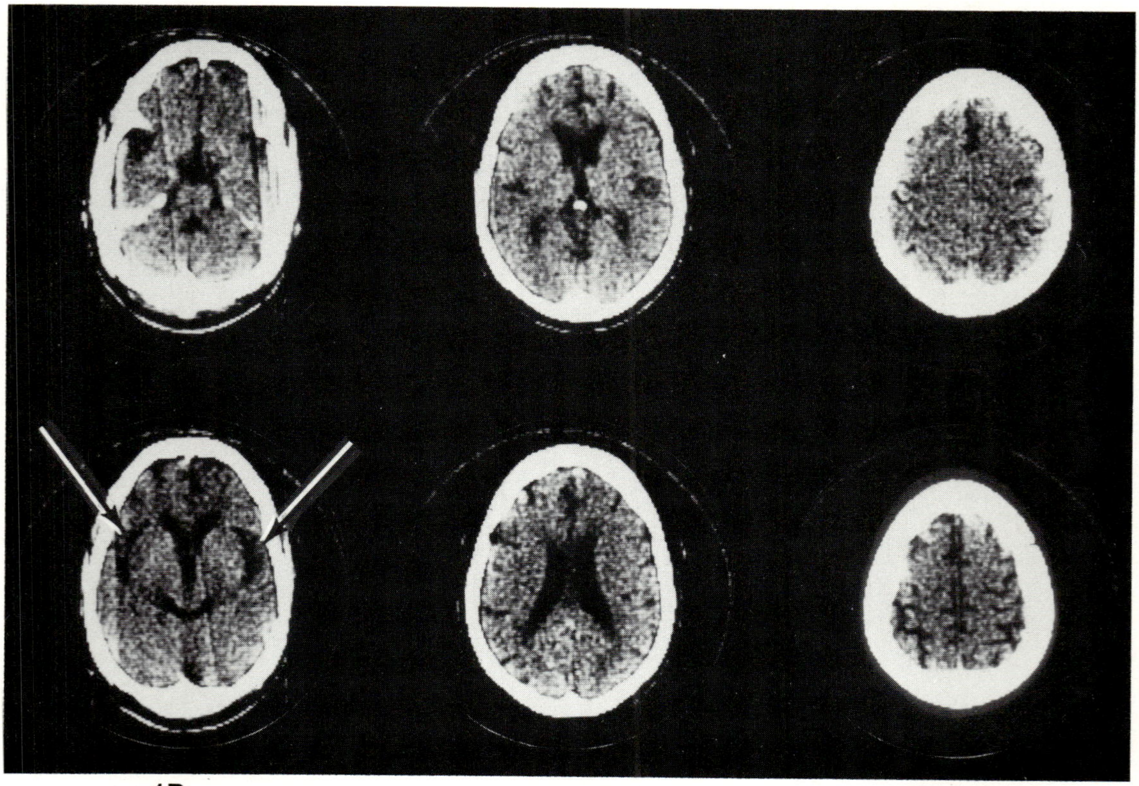

1B 2B 3B

Figure 6–2

ATROPHY SIMULATING SUBDURAL ACCUMULATIONS (Figure 6–3)

N. L. is a 9 month old female infant with failure to reach the normal milestones.

a. The routine CT scan reveals moderate enlargement of the lateral ventricles, as well as enlargement of the interhemispheric fissure. Multiple areas of decreased density are noted over the cerebral convexities bilaterally. Many of these areas have a semilunar configuration, suggestive of the possibility of chronic subdural accumulations, in addition to atrophy.

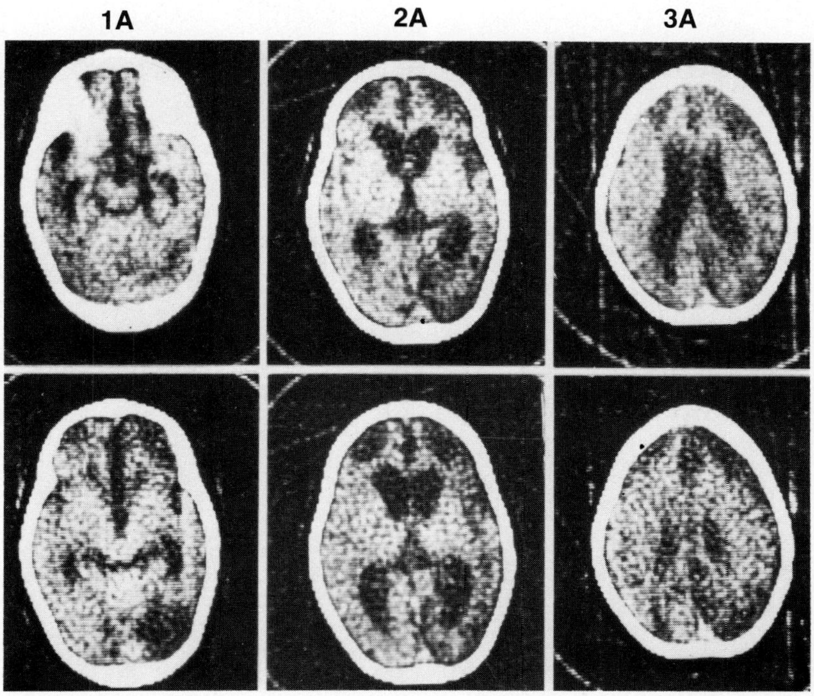

Figure 6–3a

b. The right brachial arteriogram demonstrates displacement of the vessels from the cranial vault (arrows). Note also the blush of the choroid plexus in the temporal horns bilaterally (small arrows).

c. The lateral arterial view also shows downward displacement of the vessels from the inner table of the skull (arrows). Note the blush from the choroid plexus of the temporal horn as it is supplied by the anterior choroidal artery (lower arrow).

Surgical exploration revealed atrophy without evidence of subdural accumulations.

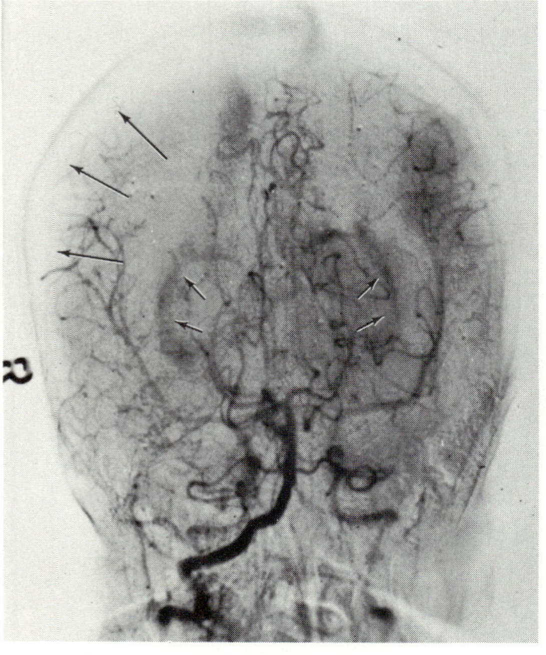

Figure 6–3b

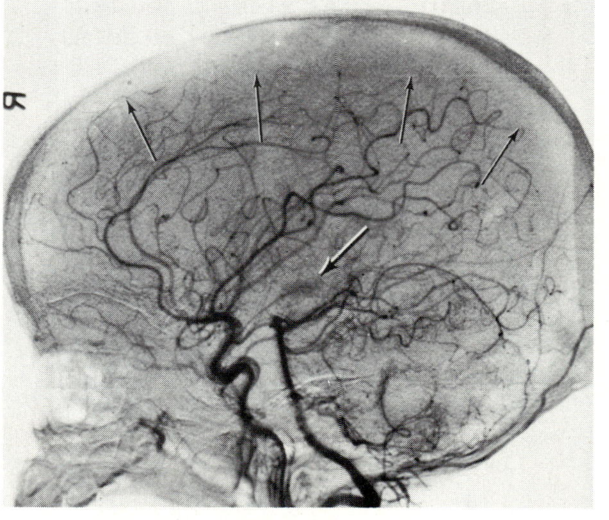

Figure 6–3c

Other Acquired Abnormalities

COMMUNICATING HYDROCEPHALUS (LOW PRESSURE HYDROCEPHALUS) (Figure 6–4)

a. Scan of a patient with mental confusion several weeks after an episode of subarachnoid hemorrhage. Note that the lateral ventricles are moderately enlarged without evidence of cortical sulcus enlargement. This pattern of ventricular enlargement can be seen following meningitis or a subarachnoid hemorrhage. There is no obstruction to the ventricular system, but rather a failure of normal absorption of cerebrospinal fluid.

b. Scan of a patient with the primary diagnosis of idiopathic communicating hydrocephalus. The lateral ventricles and the fourth ventricle (arrow) are all noted to be large. There is no evidence of cortical sulcus enlargement. The shunt device was placed 1 day prior to this study in the hope of effecting clinical improvement.

1A 2A 3A

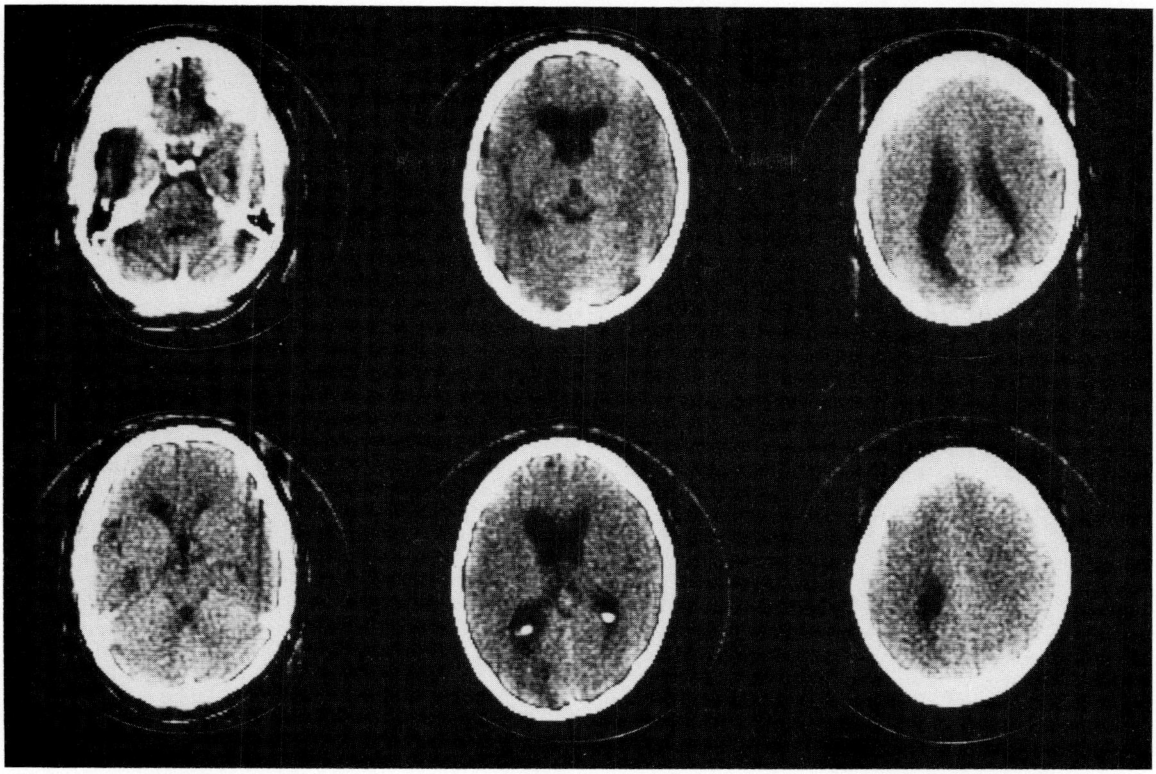

1B 2B 3B

Figure 6–4a

1A 2A 3A

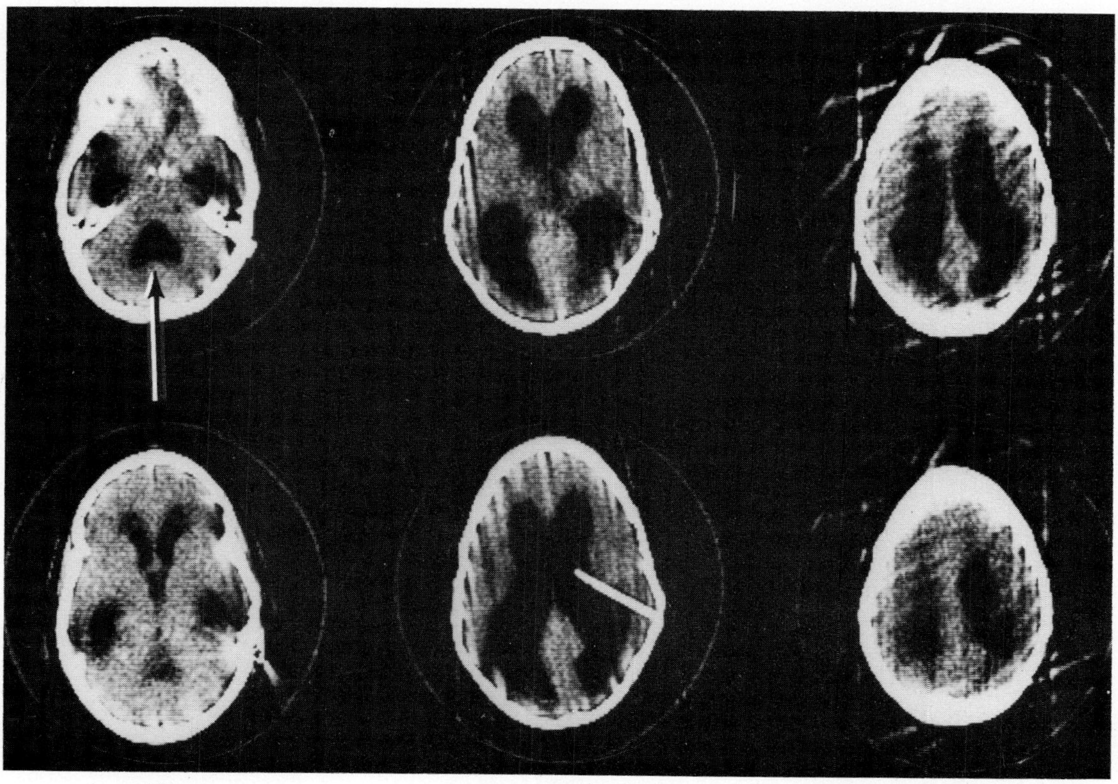

1B 2B 3B

Figure 6–4b

Multiple Sclerosis

The CT scan of patients with multiple sclerosis may be normal. Some patients show an appearance of diffuse atrophy beyond what would be anticipated in a patient of that age. On the other hand, one may be able to identify areas of lucency surrounding the lateral ventricles secondary to the demyelinated plaques so typical of multiple sclerosis. At times these areas of plaque formation may enhance following the infusion of contrast material. This is felt to be secondary to the acute phase of the demyelination process. Plaques which do not enhance are thought to be older.

At other times the enhancement of these plaques may not become apparent until after the infusion of twice the normal amount of contrast material and a scan performed following a ½ hour delay.

MULTIPLE SCLEROSIS (Figure 6–5)

a to d. Both the pre- and postinfusion portions of the examination are normal.

e and f. After the infusion of twice the normal amount of contrast material (80 gm of iodine, or 600 ml of 30 per cent solution of contrast material) and a delay of 30 minutes prior to scanning, periventricular plaques are visible (arrows).

The absence of these plaques does not rule out the diagnosis of multiple sclerosis.

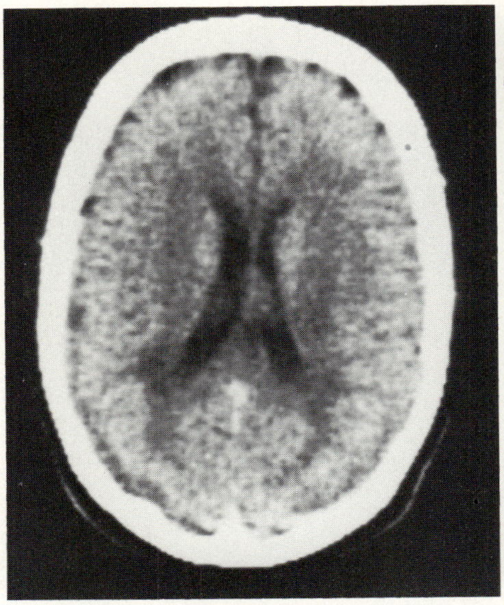

Figure 6–5a

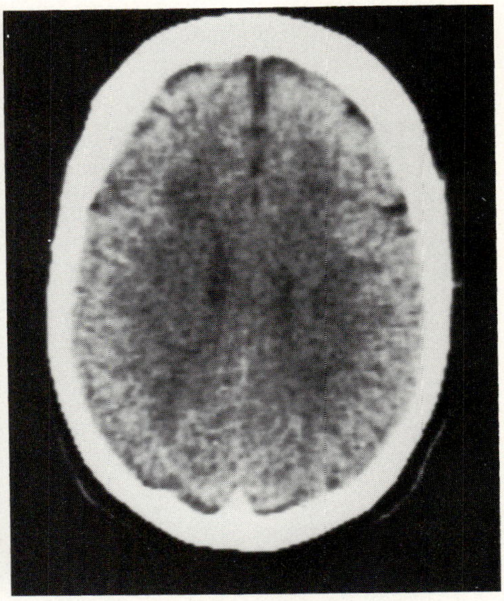

Figure 6–5b

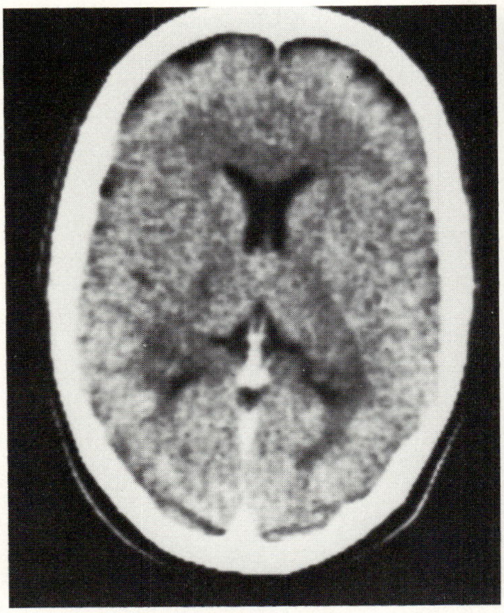

Figure 6–5c

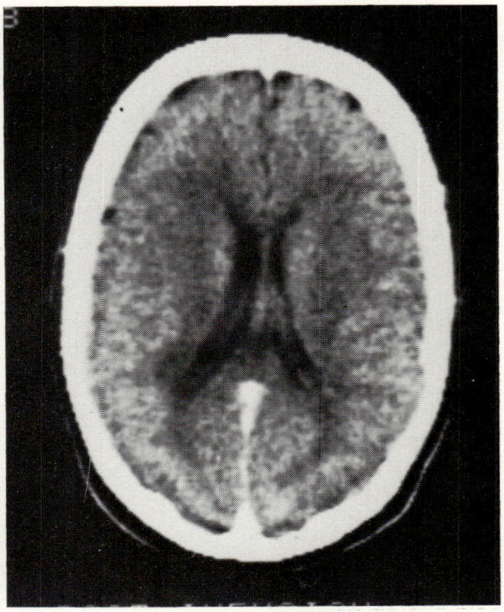

Figure 6–5d

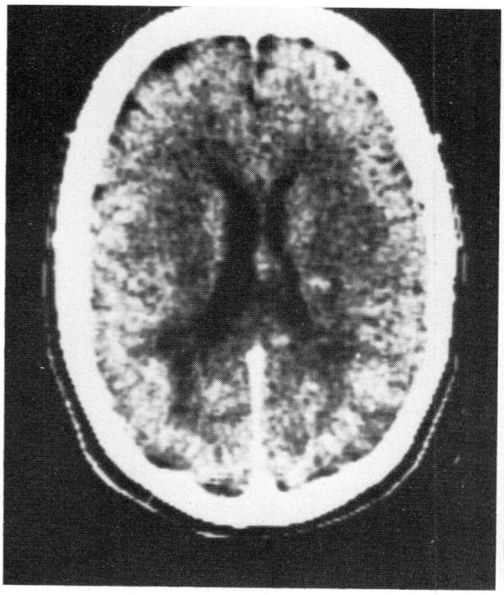

Figure 6–5e

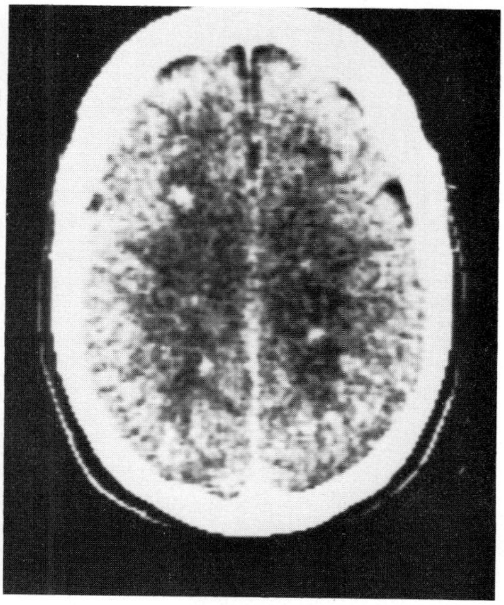

Figure 6–5f

CHAPTER 7

CONGENITAL ABNORMALITIES

CHIARI MALFORMATION WITH POST-OPERATIVE CHANGES (Figure 7–1)

This patient was born with a myelomeningocele and a gradually enlarging head size.

a. The lowest cut in the initial scan demonstrates that the fourth ventricle is never seen. There is a large cisterna magna present posteriorly.

b. The upper cut reveals the greatly enlarged lateral ventricles.

This appearance is quite typical of the Chiari malformation. The fourth ventricle is not seen because it is displaced inferiorly into the cervical canal region because of the abnormal hind brain.

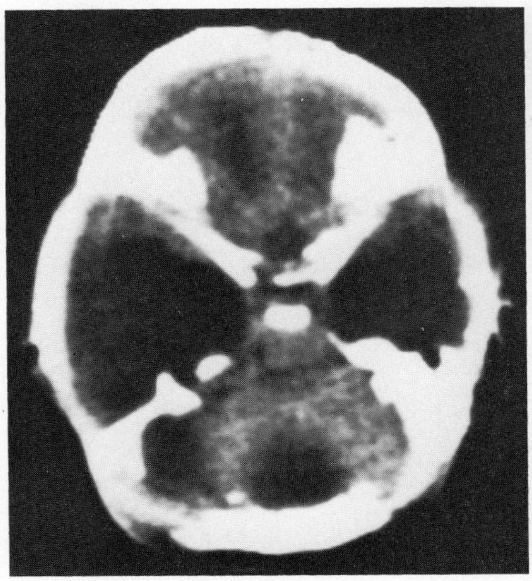

Figure 7–1a

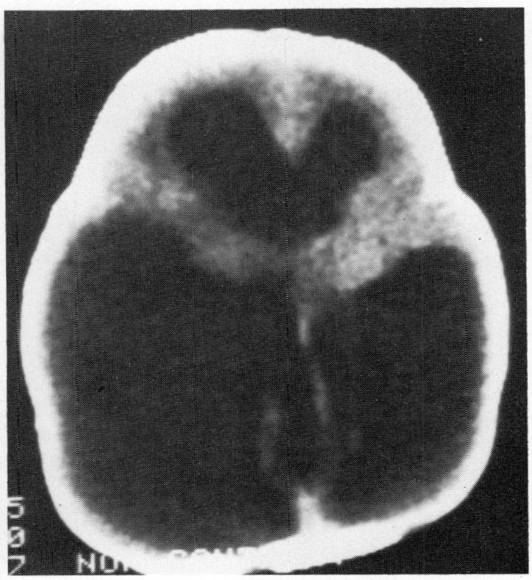

Figure 7–1b

c and d. Following the placement of the shunt device the lateral ventricles have decreased in size. However, there are now bilateral extracerebral collections of fluid which accumulate when the brain falls away from the inner table of the skull.

These bilateral "hygromas" are fairly common following shunt tube placement in patients who have marked ventricular dilatation.

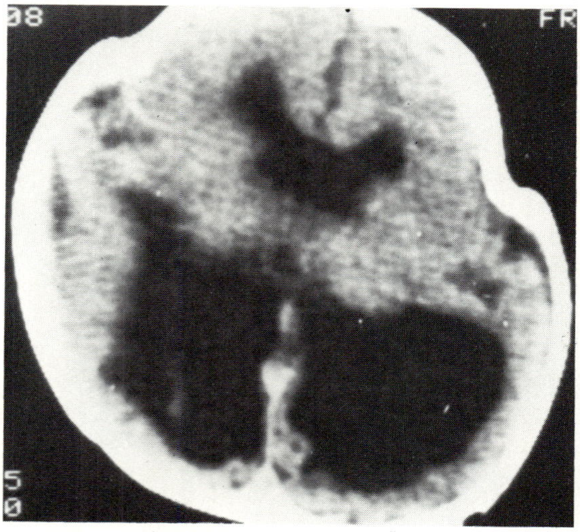

Figure 7–1c

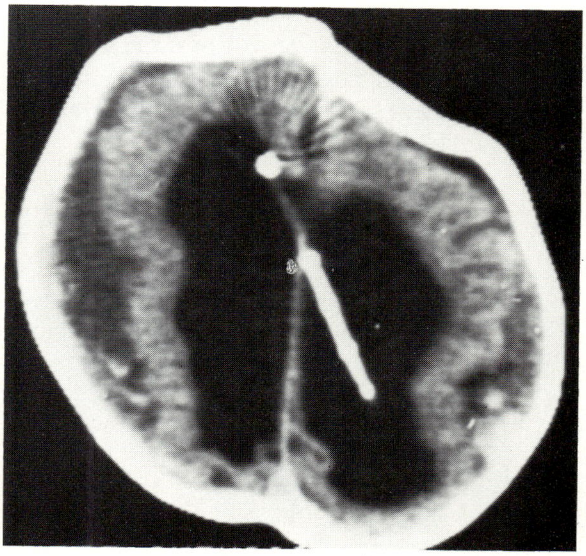

Figure 7–1d

CHIARI MALFORMATION (Figure 7–2)

This 1 year old patient was born with a myelomeningocele and hydrocephalus. The patient had undergone 3 shunt revisions since the time of birth.

a. The lowest cut reveals a small rounded cerebrospinal fluid–containing structure which is actually a dilated cerebral aqueduct and *not* a small fourth ventricle (arrow). The fourth ventricle is actually displaced inferiorly into the cervical area because of the kinking of the hind brain. Note also the large abnormal "towering" vermis surrounding the aqueduct, which is also characteristic of the Chiari malformation.

b. The upper cut demonstrates the large lateral ventricles with differential enlargement of the occipital horns, as compared to the frontal horns, a finding seen in the Chiari malformation. There has been partial relief of the hydrocephalus by the shunt device.

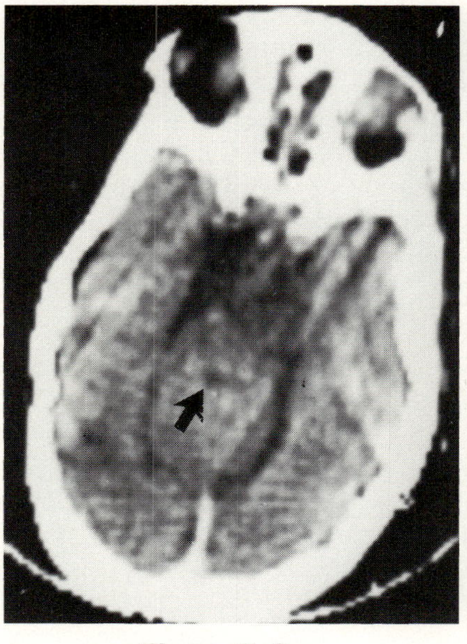

Figure 7–2a

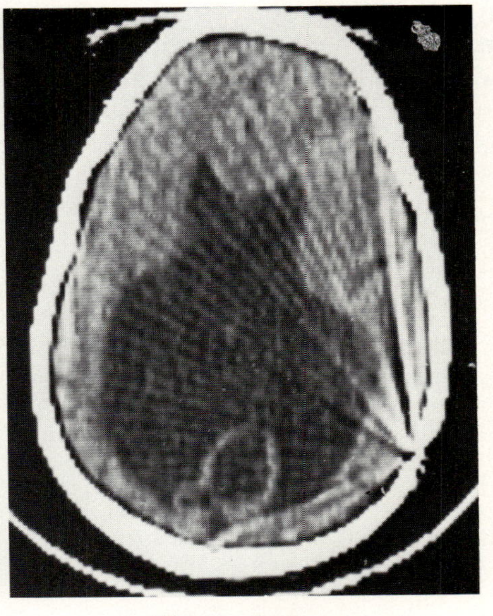

Figure 7–2b

Porencephalic Cysts

The CT scan is an ideal method for diagnosing porencephalic cysts. These lesions usually have a well-defined border, are readily apparent, and contain fluid that is of cerebrospinal fluid density. In many of these patients there is a history of birth trauma or of trauma in adult life. These patients may have permanent focal neurologic deficits and/or a seizure disorder; they may, however, be entirely asymptomatic and neurologically intact. There are a variety of causes other than trauma, ranging from infection to cerebrovascular accident to repeated spasm. Areas of "closed porencephaly" are thought to be secondary to cerebrovascular accidents and do not communicate with either the lateral ventricles or the subarachnoid spaces. It is significant in regard to this later type of abnormality that by any other neuroradiologic technique the appearance is that of a space-occupying lesion, whereas with the CT scan the porencephalic cyst can be diagnosed for what it is. As noted above, the cyst is usually well defined and contains fluid of cerebrospinal fluid density; in addition, after the infusion of contrast material there is no change in the appearance of the cyst and no evidence of either a mass or a vascular rim of enhancement. It has been our experience that in these cases the radionuclide scan either has been negative or, occasionally, has shown areas of relatively decreased uptake. Angiography reveals displaced vessels correlating with the position of the cyst and no evidence of a tumor blush. In summary, the CT scan has proved to be the nearly ideal method of studying this type of problem and is in fact the only examination necessary in many cases.

CEREBELLAR PORENCEPHALIC CYST (Figure 7–3)

A. C. is a 6 month old male infant who entered with failure to reach the normal milestones. The radionuclide scan was within normal limits. Pneumoencephalography revealed that the fourth ventricle was displaced to the right, but no air entered into the cystic lesion. The lateral and third ventricles were mildly dilated, but otherwise unremarkable.

a. The routine CT scan reveals a large, well defined area of cerebrospinal fluid density in the left posterior fossa. The fourth ventricle is shifted markedly to the right (see arrow on electronic enhancement view of cut 1A). The lateral ventricles are mildly enlarged and there is enlargement of the sylvian fissures and extracerebral fluid space over the frontal lobes. There appears to be mild atrophy of the supratentorial structures.

b. On the postinfusion scan, the straight sinus is displaced to the right. The cyst itself appears unchanged.

c. After surgical drainage, the biopsy reveals a cerebellar cyst associated with markedly hypoplastic cerebellar tissue. The large arrow identifies a markedly hypoplastic cerebellar gyrus, and the small arrows identify the collapsed lining of the cyst.

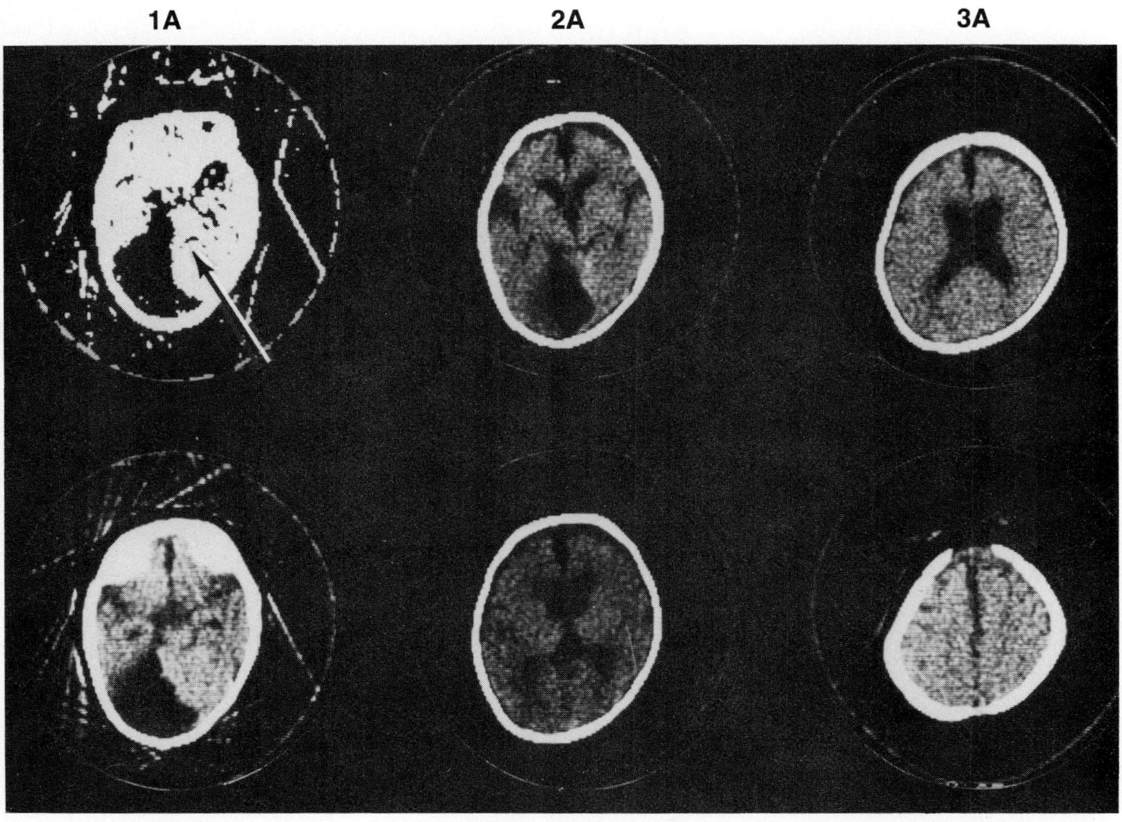

Figure 7–3a

11A 11B

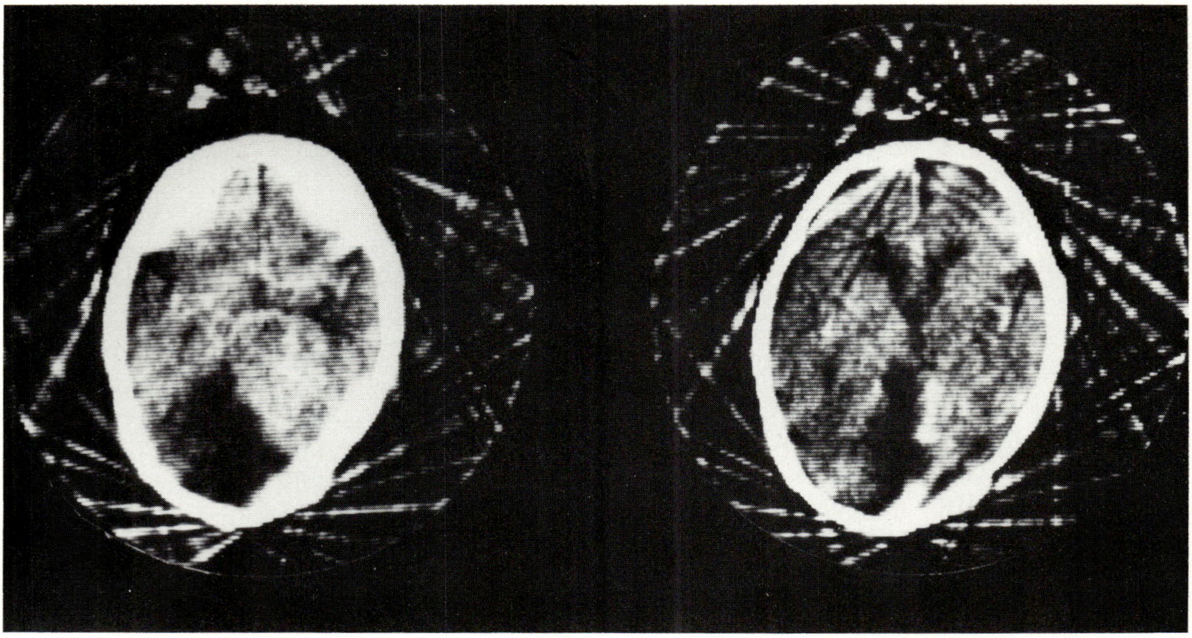

Figure 7–3b

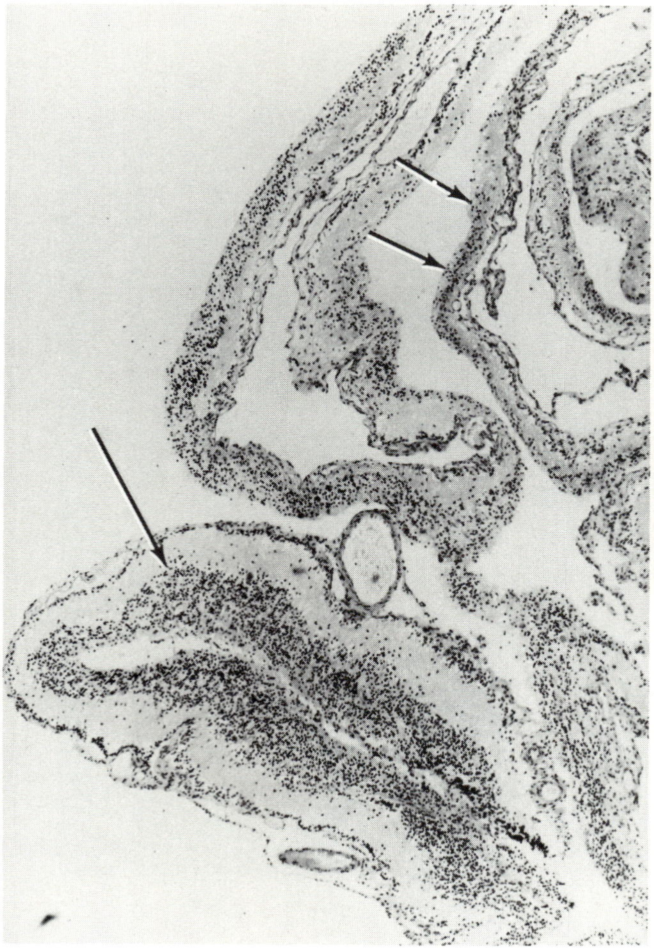

Figure 7–3c

1A

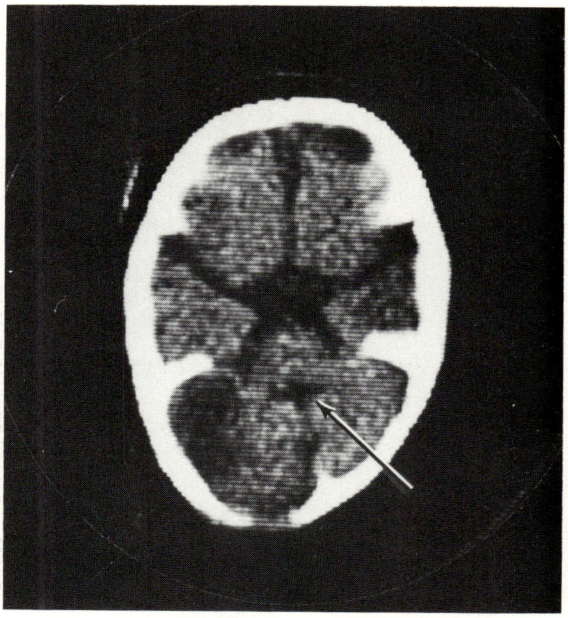

Figure 7–3d

d. The postsurgical CT scan shows that the fourth ventricle has returned to a more normal position and there now appears to be expansion of the left lobe of the previously compressed cerebellum.

LEFT FRONTAL PORENCEPHALIC CYST (Figure 7–4)

C. W. is a 21 year old male who had two grand mal seizures in the 2 months prior to admission. There was no history of birth trauma. He had had one episode of severe head trauma at age 8, associated with a questionable loss of consciousness.

a to d. The radionuclide scan appears essentially within normal limits.

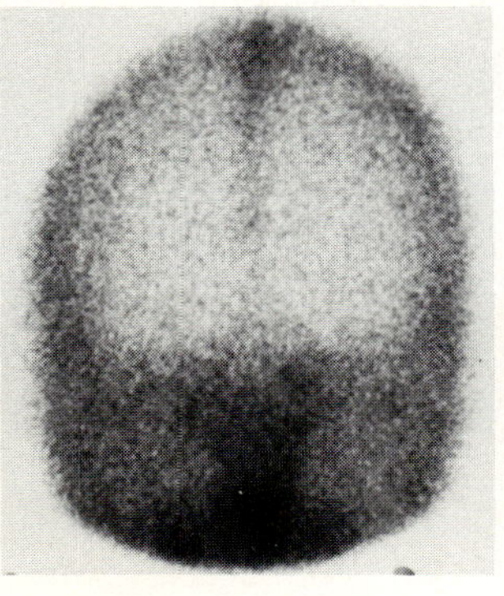

Figure 7–4a

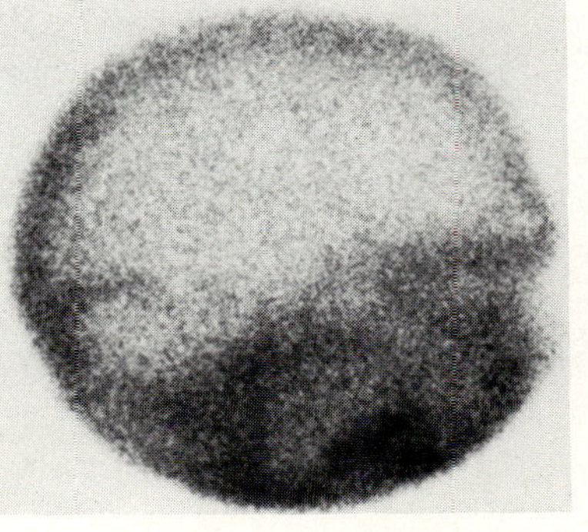

Figure 7–4b

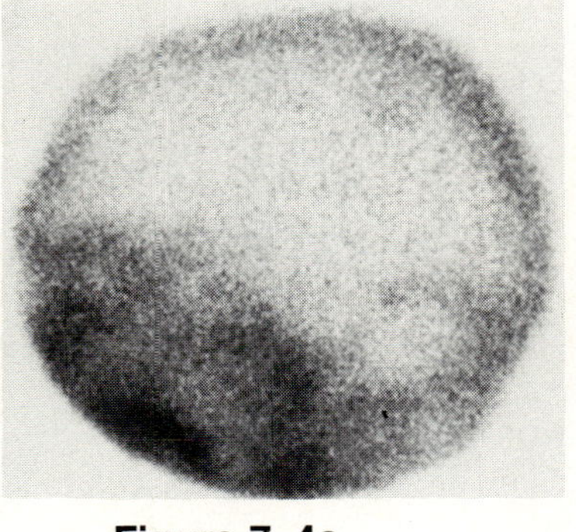

Figure 7–4c

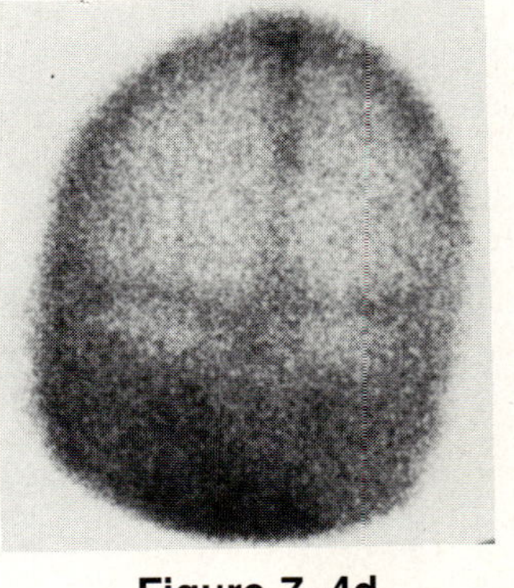

Figure 7–4d

e. The routine CT scan reveals a well-defined cystic area in the left frontal lobe with a density of cerebrospinal fluid. There was a slight shift of the frontal horns to the right best seen on cut 2A (arrow).

f. Following contrast infusion, no areas of enhancement are noted. This lesion is thought to be a benign porencephalic cyst with minimal mass effect.

1A 2A 3A

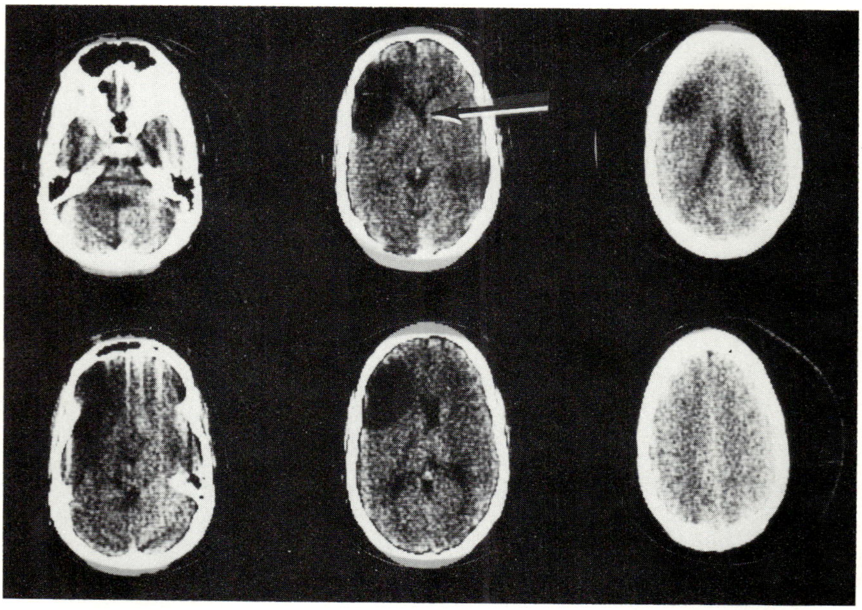

1B 2B 3B

Figure 7–4e

11A 12A 13A

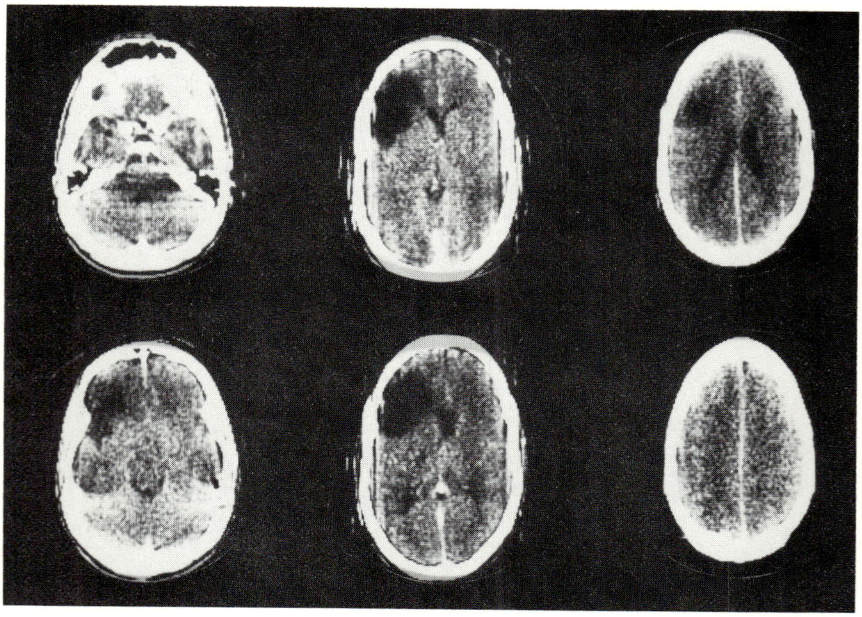

11B 12B 13B

Figure 7–4f

g to i. The arterial phase of the left carotid arteriogram (g) reveals slight posterior displacement of the anterior portion of the sylvian triangle (arrow), and mild stretching of the branches in the frontal region. The later phases show a large, relatively avascular area in the frontal lobe regions (arrows).

j. The anteroposterior arterial phase reveals mild bowing of the anterior cerebral artery across the midline (arrows). There is no shift of the internal cerebral vein.

The left frontal lesion was felt to be a benign porencephalic cyst, and it was elected not to perform surgery at this time.

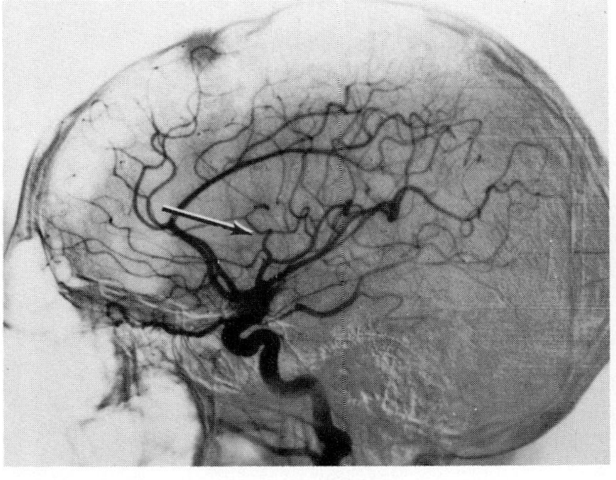

Figure 7–4g

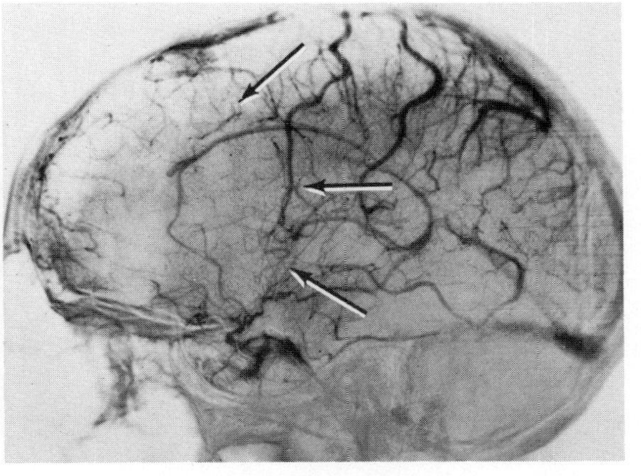

Figure 7–4h

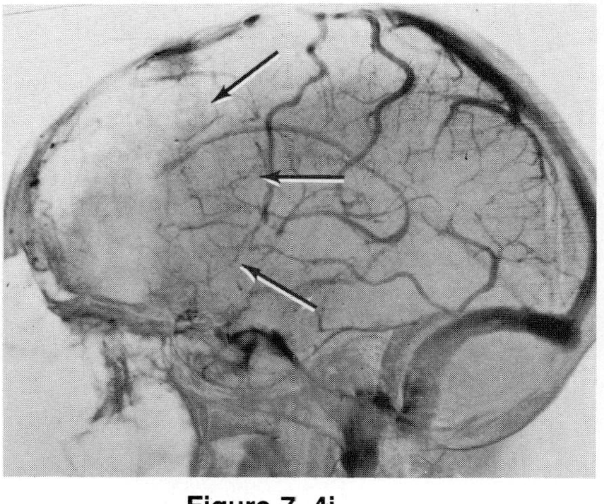

Figure 7–4i

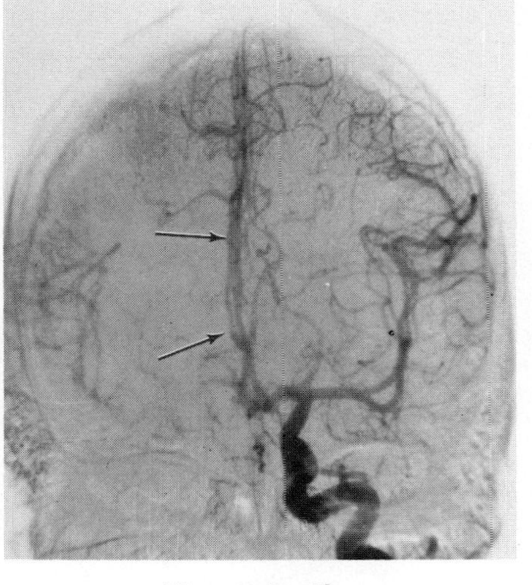

Figure 7–4j

Other Congenital Abnormalities

HEMIATROPHY (Figure 7–5)

D. V. is a 6 year old male.

The routine CT scan reveals a misshapen cranial vault which is smaller on the left than on the right side. The left lateral ventricle is enlarged, and there is a semilunar area of cerebrospinal fluid density adjacent to the atrophic left hemisphere.

There is shift of the midline toward the atrophic left hemisphere.

The findings here are quite typical of hemiatrophy on the left side; however, in less obvious cases care must be taken not to interpret the findings as a mass lesion—such as a subdural hematoma—on the right side causing shift toward the left.

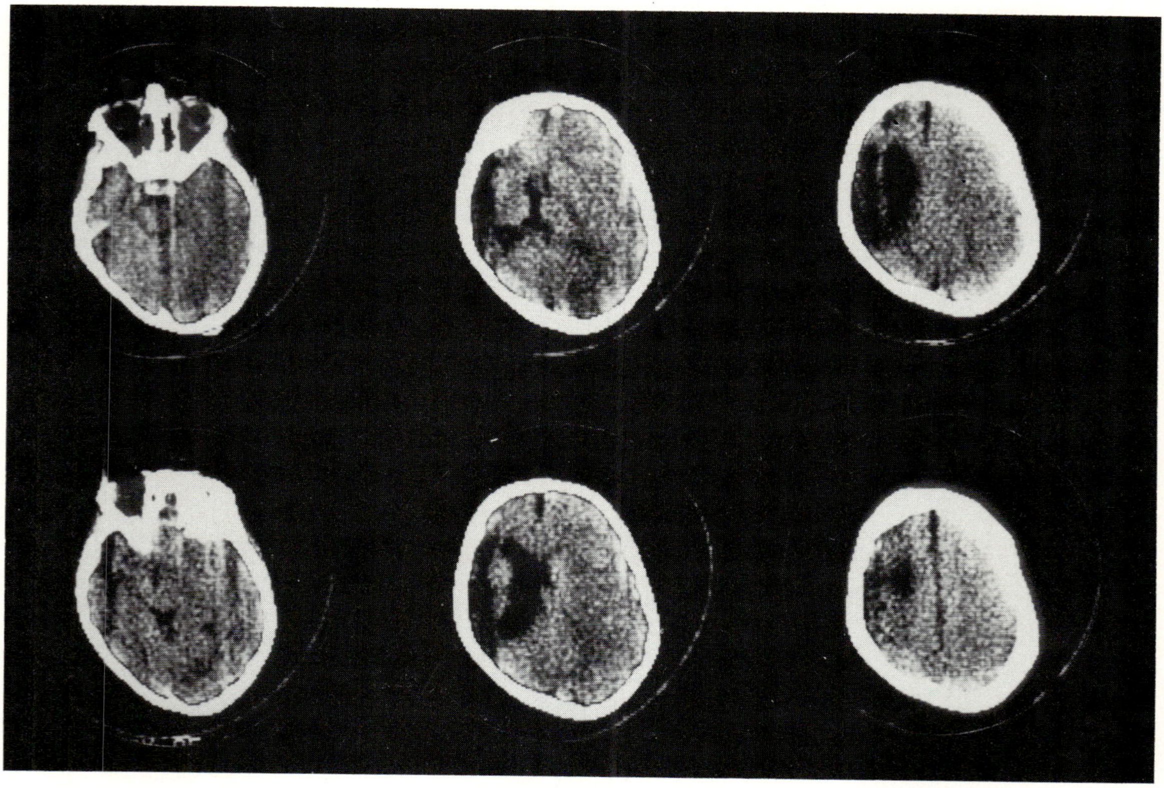

Figure 7–5

AGENESIS OF THE CORPUS CALLOSUM (Figure 7–6)

Agenesis of the corpus callosum may be partial or complete. In either case, there is a splaying apart of the lateral ventricles, which no longer meet in the midline as they would in a normal patient, and there is a resultant upward extension of the third ventricle between the lateral ventricles because of the absent corpus callosum (arrow).

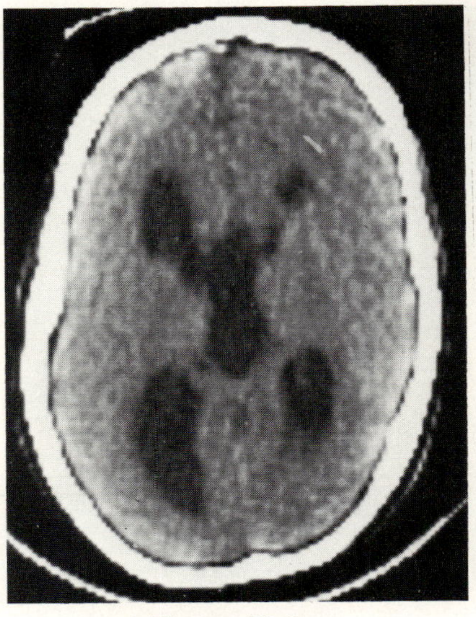

Figure 7–6a

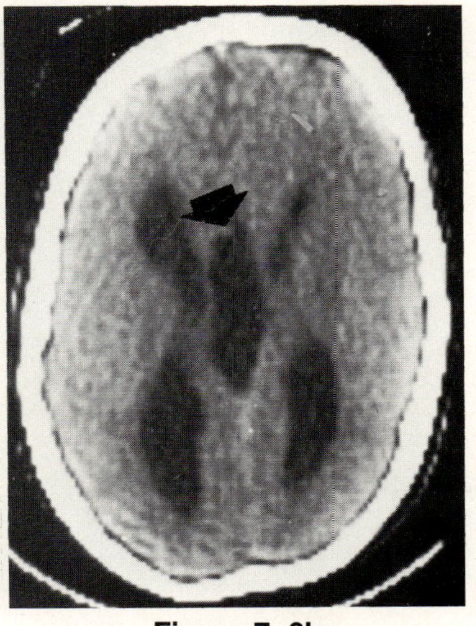

Figure 7–6b

STURGE-WEBER DISEASE (Figure 7–7)

a. The lateral view of the plain skull examination reveals the typical appearance of "tram tract" calcification in a gyral pattern in the occipital lobe of the brain. Occasionally this calcification may extend beyond the occipital lobes. This appearance is associated with the clinical presentation of seizures and a hemangioma of the face, usually in the ophthalmic distribution of the fifth cranial nerve and on the same side as the brain calcification. These children may be mentally retarded.

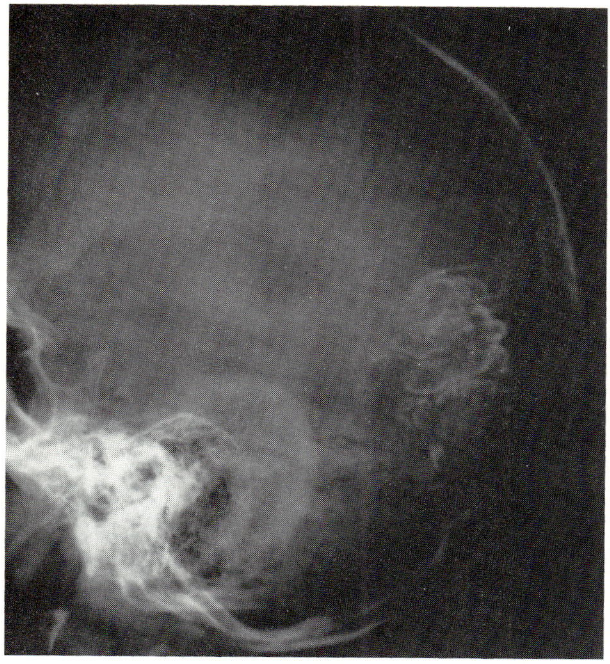

Figure 7–7a

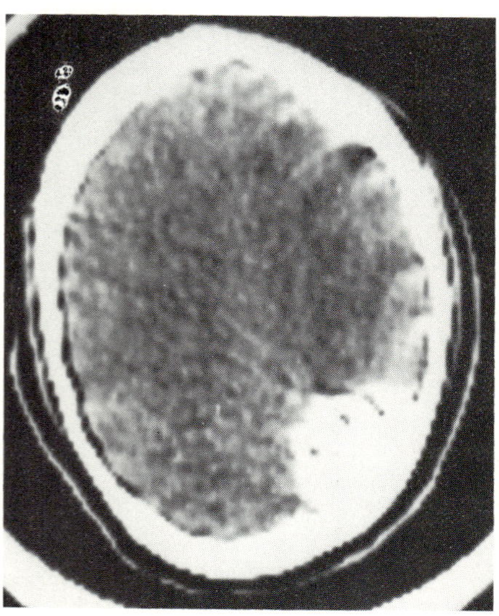

Figure 7–7b

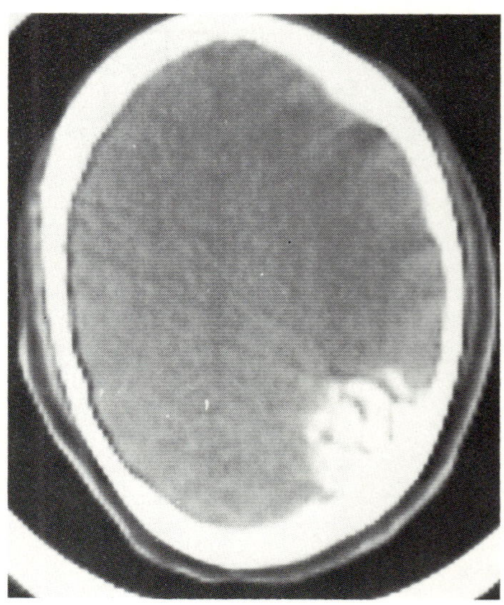

Figure 7–7c

b and c. The CT scan demonstrates the dense calcification seen on the skull film and the electronically enhanced scan (c) reveals the gyral pattern of the calcium distribution. Also note the shrunken right hemicalvarium secondary to hemiatrophy, a common finding, readily appreciated on CT.

TUBEROUS SCLEROSIS (Figure 7–8)

This 14 year old male had adenoma sebaceum in a butterfly distribution over the cheeks, convulsive seizures, and progressive mental deficiency.

a and b. The CT scan demonstrates multiple areas of calcification in a periventricular distribution. These calcifications are in giant glial tissue masses which are subependymal in distribution. These giant astrocytomas are malignant by location and may degenerate into glioblastomas in some cases.

The CT appearance is very typical for tuberous sclerosis, which is one of the neurocutaneous syndromes. This disease process is also associated with rhabdomyosarcomas of the heart as well as hamartomas of the liver and kidneys.

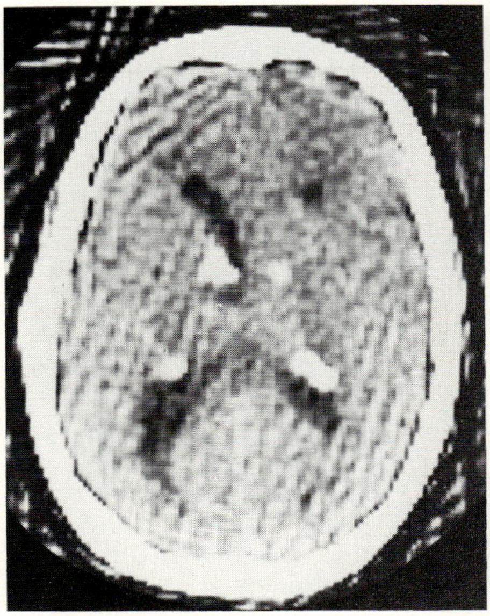

Figure 7–8a

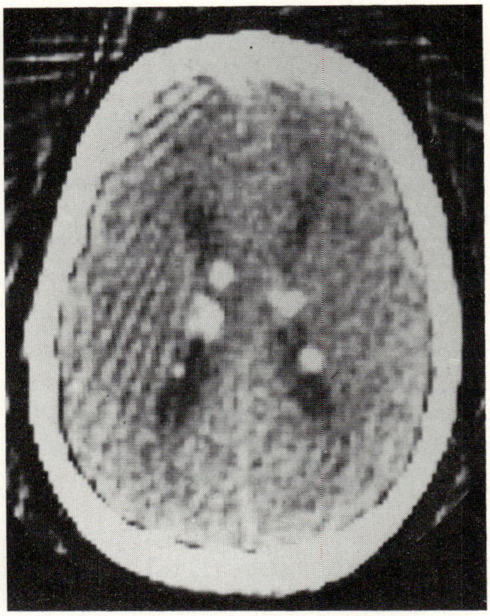

Figure 7–8b

LIPOMA OF THE CORPUS CALLOSUM (Figure 7–9)

a and b. The CT scan reveals the area of fat density in the region of the genu of the corpus callosum. The frontal horns of the lateral ventricles are splayed apart. There is typical peripheral calcification of the lipoma. There are also multiple "daughter" lipomas in this example (arrows). The appearance is pathognomonic and is confirmed by a density measurement in the negative number range.

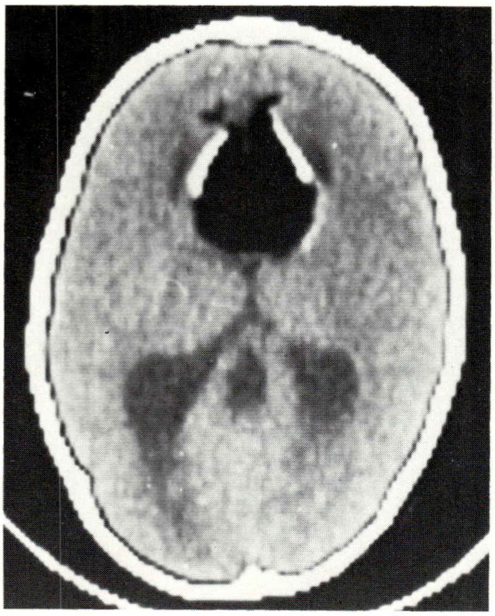

Figure 7–9a

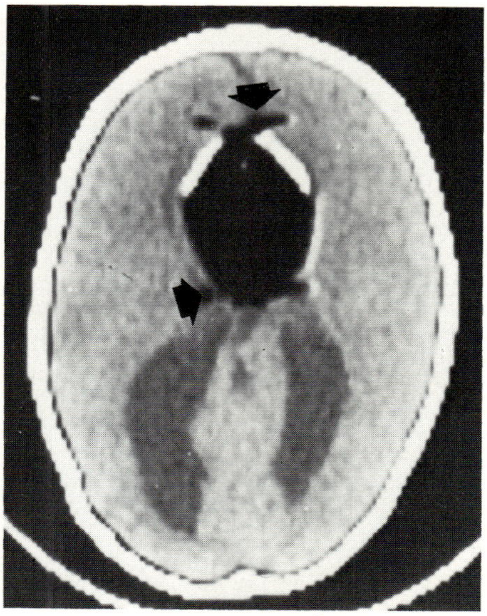

Figure 7–9b

HERPES SIMPLEX TYPE I ENCEPHALITIS (Figure 7–10)

Herpes encephalitis usually involves the temporal lobes of the brain.

a and b. A typical appearance includes a diffuse lucency of the temporal horns. In addition, there is a mass effect with compression of the lateral ventricles bilaterally, in this case slightly asymmetrically.

c and d. A follow-up examination 1½ weeks later reveals additional mass effect with further compression of the lateral ventricles. In addition, while there had been no enhancement on the postinfusion portion of the examination at the time of the initial scan, there is now bilateral diffuse enhancement of the involved temporal lobes.

These patients can now be successfully treated with vidaradine if treatment is started sufficiently early. Diagnosis is confirmed when a brain biopsy reveals intracellular virus particles.

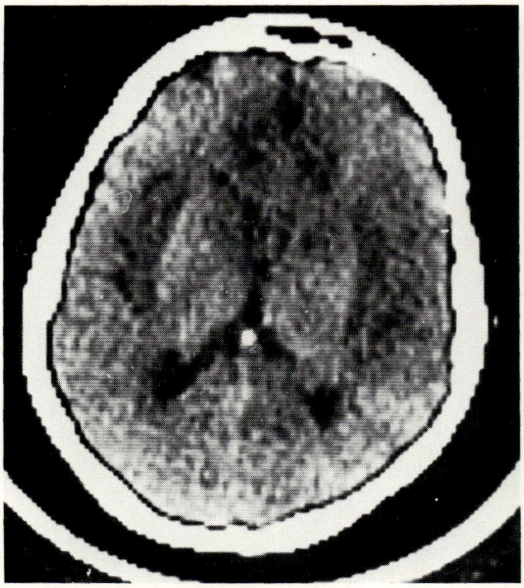

Figure 7–10a

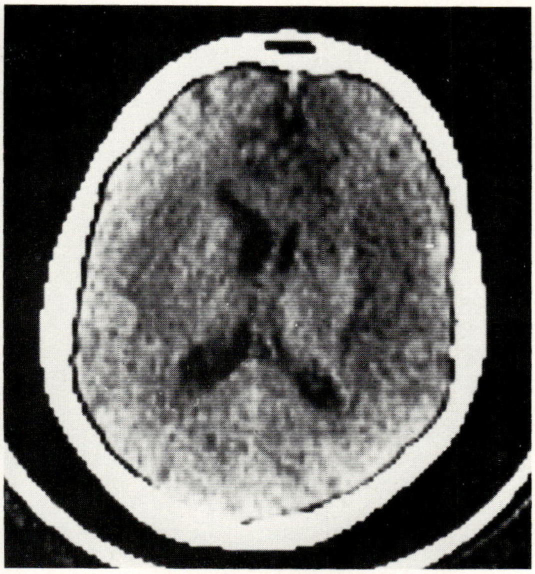

Figure 7–10b

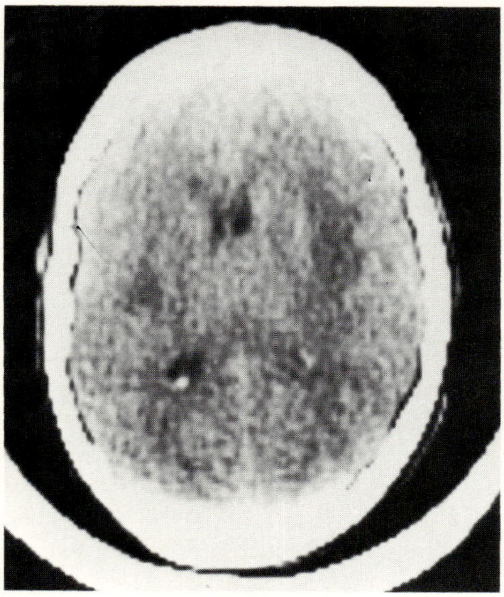

Figure 7–10c

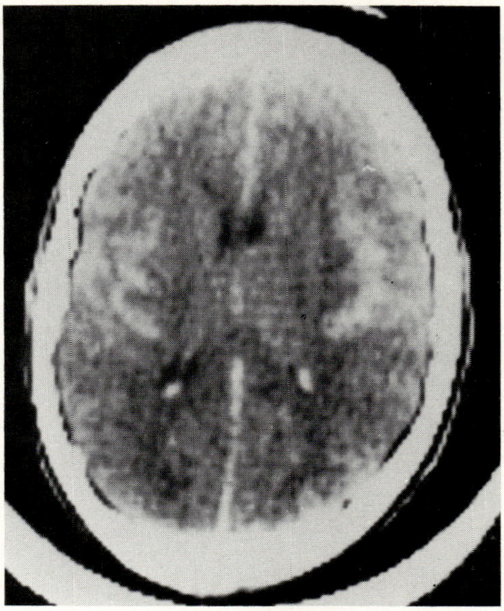

Figure 7–10d

CHAPTER 8

ORBITAL SCANNING

Orbital scanning is performed using cuts approximately one half the thickness used for a conventional scan. In addition there are new collimating devices that will allow 2 mm cuts to be obtained; this will further increase the resolution possible with orbital studies. One of the main advantages of orbital scanning is seen in the case of the patient with exophthalmos, either unilateral or bilateral, when one wants to rule out an orbital tumor. With the routine scan one can readily visualize the optic nerves bilaterally and, occasionally, outline the medial and lateral rectus muscles as well. The mass, if present, is identified on the initial scan and then better visualized after the infusion of contrast material.

In addition to identifying orbital masses, this method can also be used to locate foreign bodies in the globe. These are best localized in conjunction with routine radiographic techniques.

With exophthalmos due to hyperthyroidism no mass is visible but enlargement of the extraocular muscles can be detected.

NORMAL ORBITAL ANATOMY (Figure 8–1)

a. A normal view of the orbits. We photograph these at a window width of 100. The density is set at the level at which the optic nerves are best visualized. In day-to-day use we often take several photographs at different density settings. At least one photo is obtained on the measure mode. 1, This is a portion of the bolus bag that extends across to the other side. 2, Lateral wall of the orbit. 3, Globe. 4, Lens. 5, Medial wall of the orbit. 6, Ethmoid sinuses. 7, Optic nerve. 8, Lateral rectus muscle. 9, Region of the sella turcica.

b. The same picture as a, taken on the measure mode. Note that the optic nerves are quite distorted from the normal appearance.

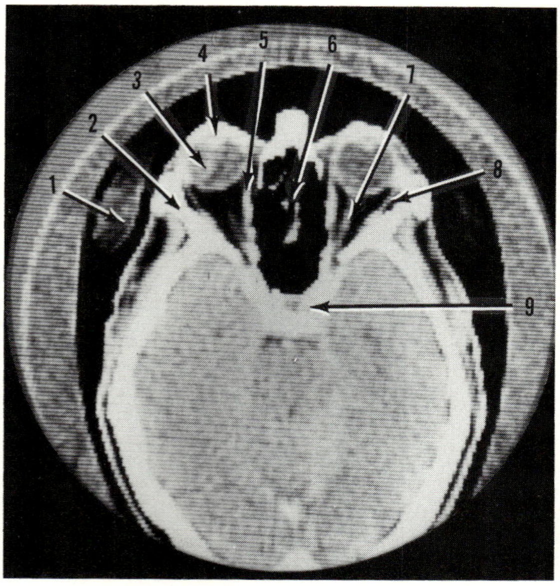

Figure 8–1a

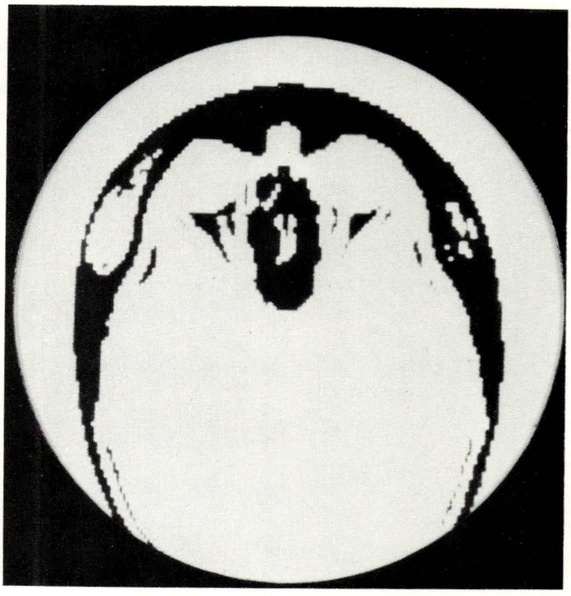

Figure 8–1b

NORMAL ORBIT (Figure 8–2)

The 4 mm axial cut of the orbit reveals the normal superior ophthalmic vein (SOV) as it crosses the optic nerve. The SOV crosses anteromedially to posterolaterally and then exits the orbit via the superior orbital fissure.

The ophthalmic artery (OA) is also demonstrated. The OA originates from the internal carotid artery and initially rests lateral to the ophthalmic artery; then the OA usually crosses superiorly over the optic nerve to be medial to it.

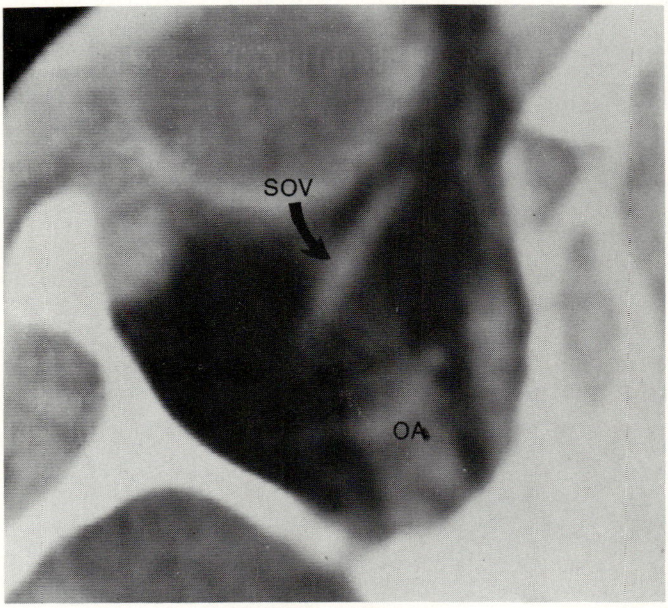

Figure 8–2

MEDIAL BLOW-OUT FRACTURE (Figure 8–3)

a. The break in the medial orbital wall–lateral wall of the ethmoid sinus is readily demonstrated. There is herniation of the orbital contents through the fracture into the ethmoid sinus (the medial rectus muscle and orbital fat).

b. Further posteriorly the fracture and herniated orbital contents are seen (arrow). The extraocular muscles are also nicely demonstrated bilaterally. The optic nerves are also seen: superior rectus muscle (S), lateral rectus

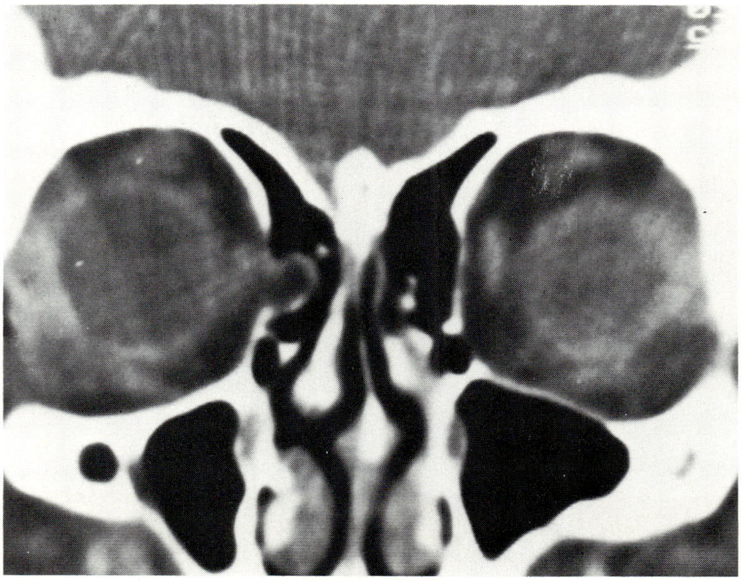

Figure 8–3a

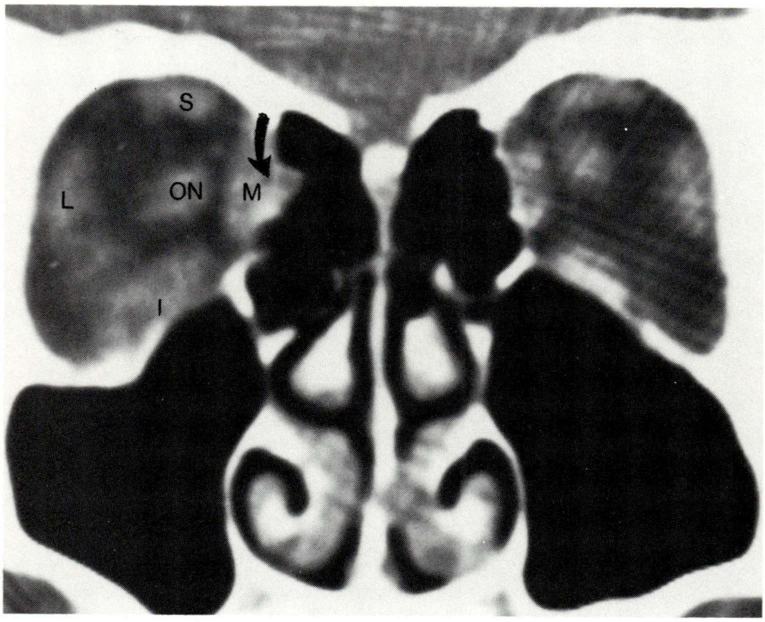

Figure 8–3b

muscle (L), inferior rectus muscle (I), medial rectus muscle (M), optic nerve (ON).

CT has been shown to be very helpful in the diagnosis of fractures of the facial bones and surrounding the orbits. As the availability of CT increases, it is possible that CT will replace radiographic tomography as the method of choice to study these problems.

FOREIGN BODY OF THE GLOBE (Figure 8–4)

This 19 year old male entered with a metallic foreign body in the left globe.

Cut 1A readily identifies the foreign body with its associated computer artifact (arrow). The higher cut no longer visualizes the metallic foreign body.

By determining the relationship with the optic nerve, one can arrive at an approximate level of the foreign body. Perhaps with the finer collimators and the subsequent thinner cuts we will ultimately increase our ability to localize foreign bodies; however, at present I feel these are best studied in conjunction with routine radiographic techniques.

1A 1B

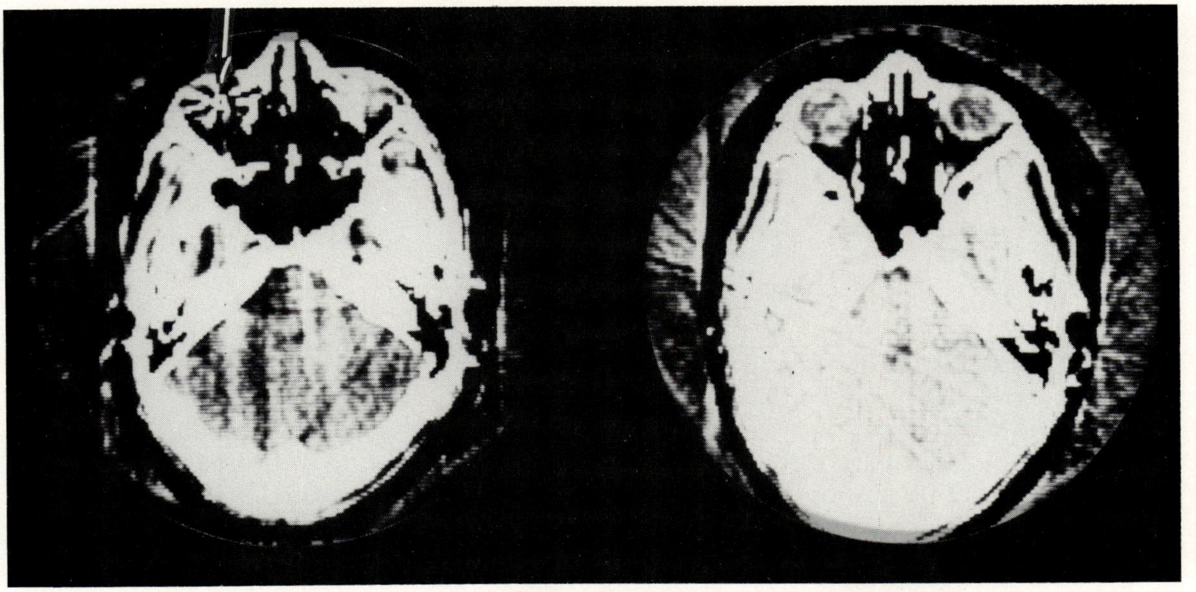

Figure 8–4

RETINOBLASTOMA (Figure 8–5)

This infant presented with visual loss and the typical amaurotic "cat's eye."

The CT scan demonstrates a calcified mass in the posterior aspect of the globe (arrow). This appearance is very typical of retinoblastoma. These tumors may also be bilateral.

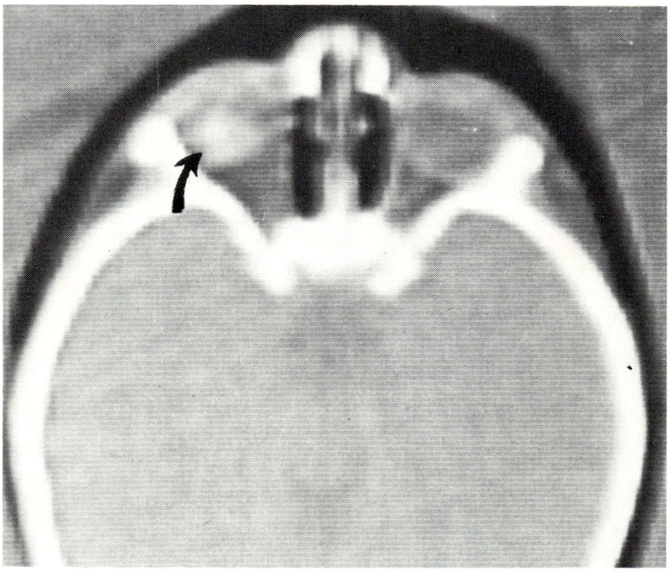

Figure 8–5

METASTASES TO ORBIT (Figure 8–6)

This 45 year old male presented with unilateral proptosis on the left side. Some 9 months earlier he had had a right lung tumor removed. Physical examination revealed that the left eye was displaced superiorly and laterally.

a. The lowest cut through the orbit reveals that the mass is visible in the lower, inner corner of the globe.

b. A slightly higher cut reveals that the mass is just larger than the globe itself, and displaces the globe foreward and laterally. The mass extends quite far forward to just below the level of the eyelid.

c. At a level through the optic nerve only a small portion of the mass is visible (M). In addition, the medial rectus muscle (MR) is infiltrated by tumor and is thicker than the normal muscle on the contralateral side.

Surgically this proved to be metastasis to the left orbit.

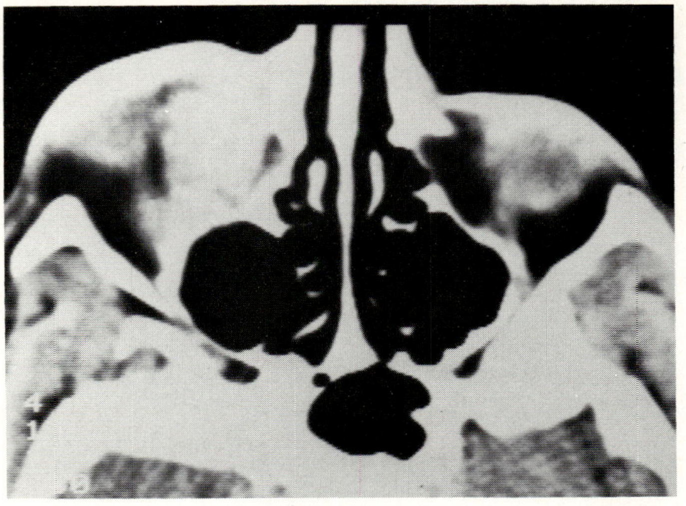

Figure 8–6a

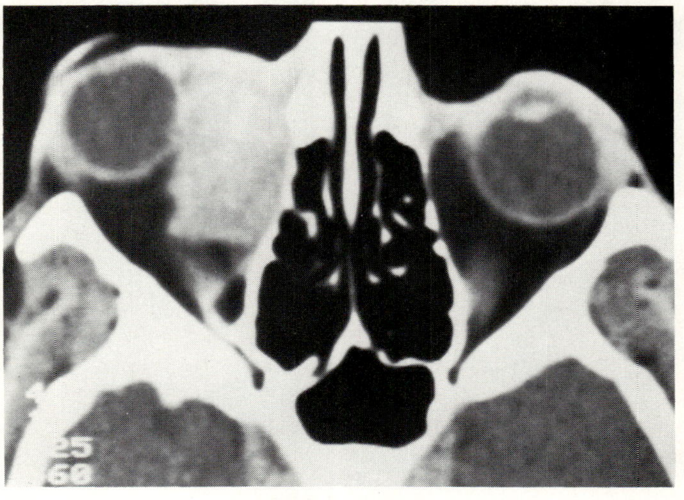

Figure 8–6b

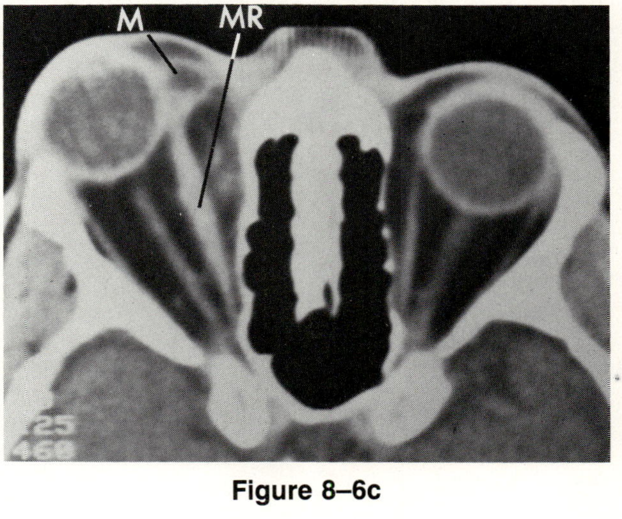

Figure 8–6c

HEMANGIOMA OF THE ORBIT (Figure 8–7)

The patient presented with progressive painless right proptosis.

a. The preinfusion scan demonstrates an oval, high density mass behind the globe on the right side. There is mild right proptosis.

b. The postinfusion scan demonstrates marked homogeneous enhancement of the mass.

This was a surgically proved hemangioma of the orbit. The CT appearance is quite typical. At times these hemangiomas may contain areas of calcification.

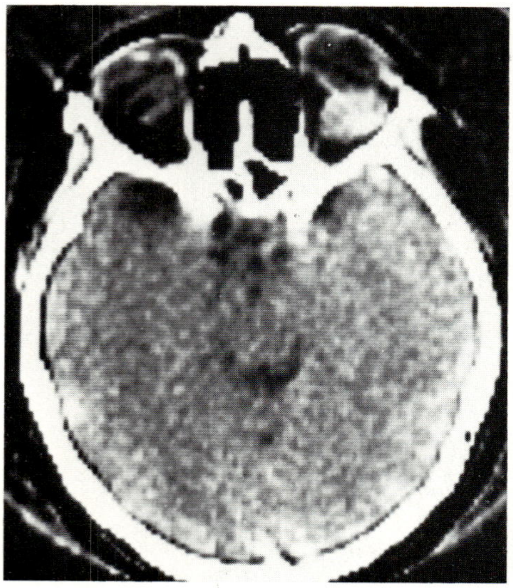

Figure 8–7a

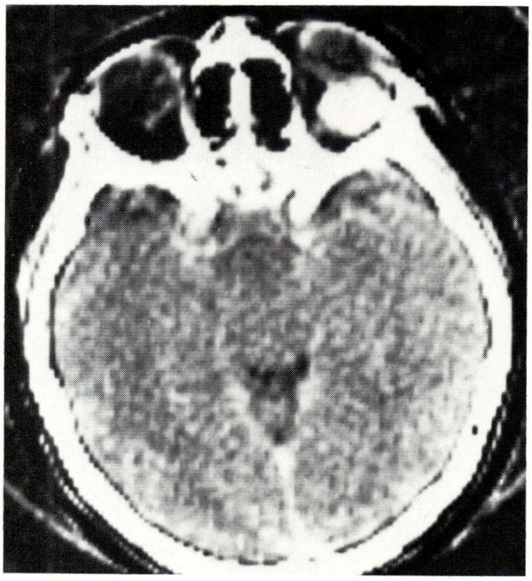

Figure 8–7b

HYPERTHYROID EXOPHTHALMOPATHY (Figure 8–8)

This 39 year old female had a 10-year history of Graves' disease with progressive exophthalmos.

The appearance is typical of Graves' disease. The CT appearance is usually diagnostic and is especially helpful in those patients with hyperthyroid Graves' disease who have unilateral exophthalmos.

a to c. The CT scan through the low (a) and mid (b) and upper (c) portions of the orbit demonstrates diffuse enlargement of the extraocular muscles. This increase in size results in exophthalmos.

Note the absence of a retro-orbital mass. The usefulness of CT is especially apparent in patients with unilateral exophthalmos when a mass lesion is easily ruled out.

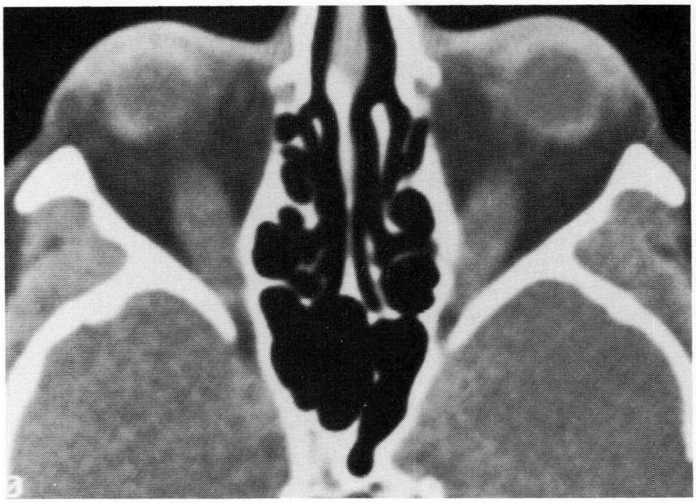

Figure 8–8a

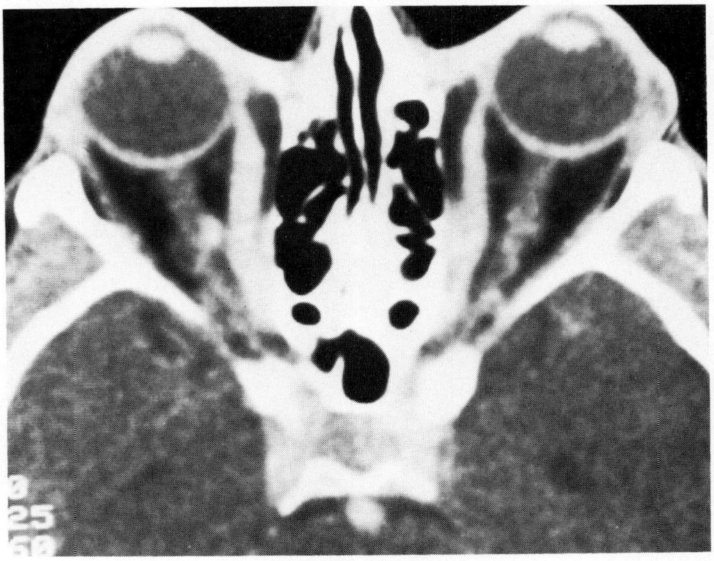

Figure 8–8b

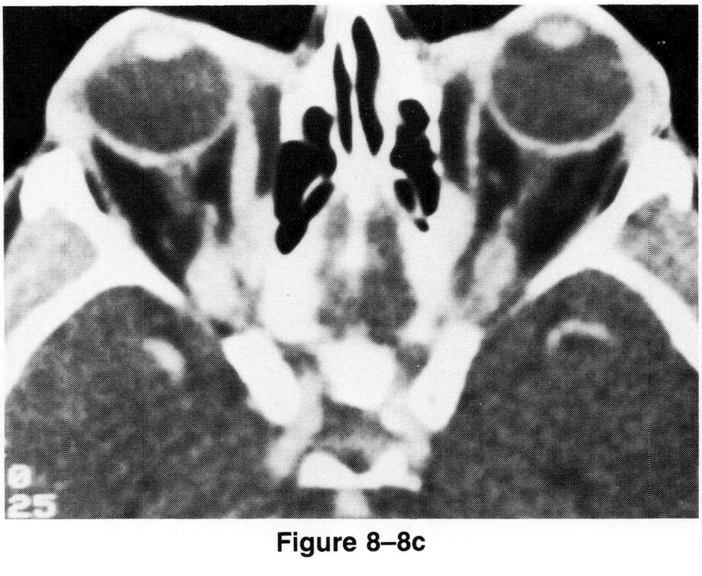

Figure 8–8c

ORBITAL PSEUDOTUMOR (GRANULOMA) (Figure 8–9)

This is a process of undetermined etiology that affects the globe of the eye. It is a nonspecific granulomatous process, usually associated with proptosis; it may be bilateral. This lesion responds well to steroids.

a. The preinfusion scan of the orbit reveals proptosis of the right eye and a diffuse thickening of the peripheral margin of the globe.

b. The postinfusion scan demonstrates that there is diffuse enhancement of the periphery of the globe, most marked posteriorly. The margin of the enhancing area is indistinct. This appearance is very typical of orbital pseudotumor.

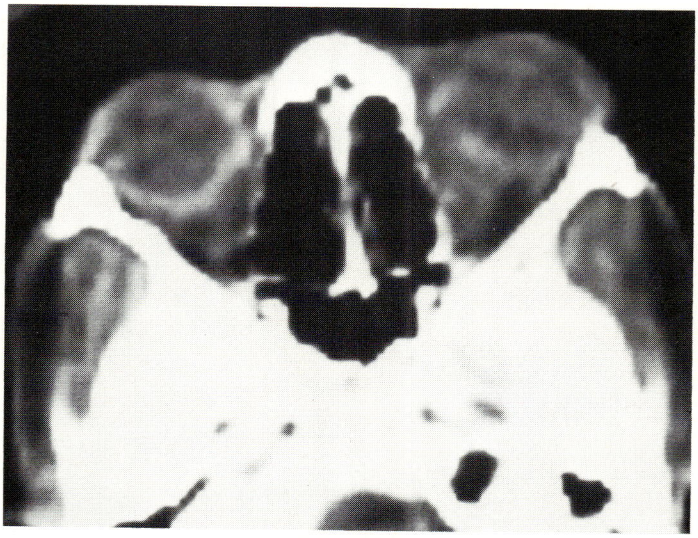

Figure 8–9a

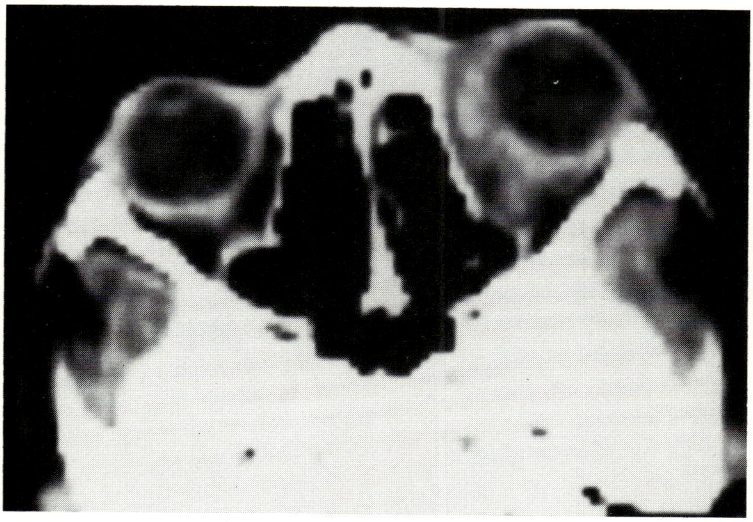

Figure 8–9b

CAROTID CAVERNOUS FISTULA (Figure 8–10)

This 69 year old female presented with the acute onset of left pulsating exophthalmos following a fall down the stairs.

a. The preinfusion scan demonstrates dilatation of the left superior ophthalmic vein (arrow).

b. The postinfusion cut demonstrates enlargement of the dilated superior ophthalmic vein (arrow) as it courses obliquely posteriorly in the upper portion of the orbit above the globe of the eye.

c. The postinfusion cuts through the cavernous sinus reveal fullness of the left cavernous sinus (large arrow) compared with the normal right side. This is secondary to excessive blood flow on the side of the fistula.

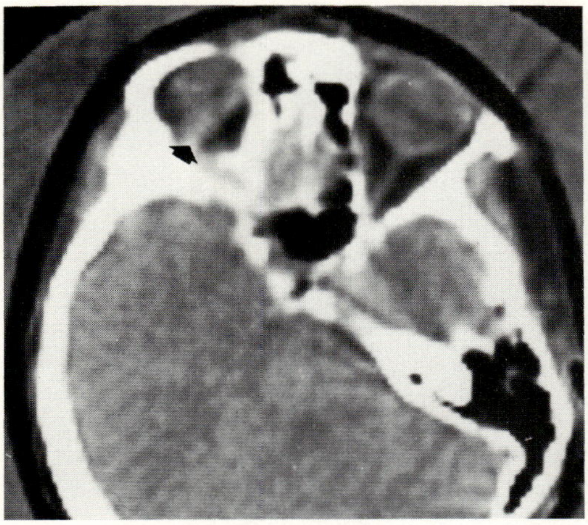

Figure 8–10a

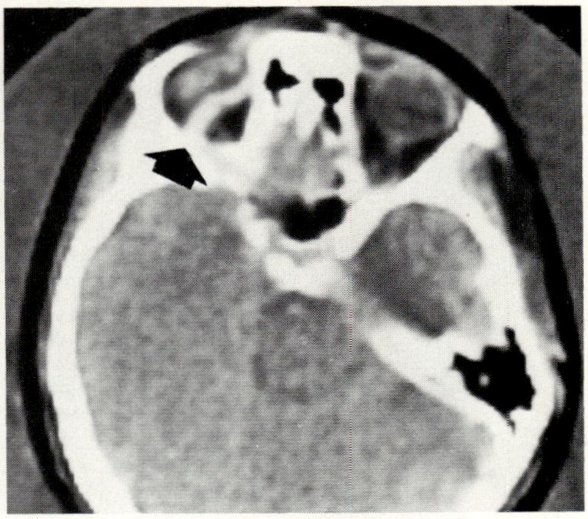

Figure 8–10b

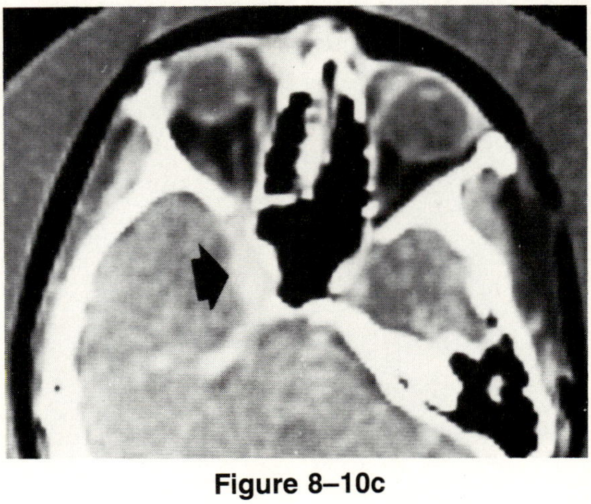

Figure 8–10c

d. The internal carotid angiogram reveals simultaneous filling of the intracranial circulation and the cavernous sinus (CS). There is retrograde flow through the greatly dilated superior ophthalmic vein (SOV).

This history and appearance are typical of a post-traumatic carotid cavernous fistula.

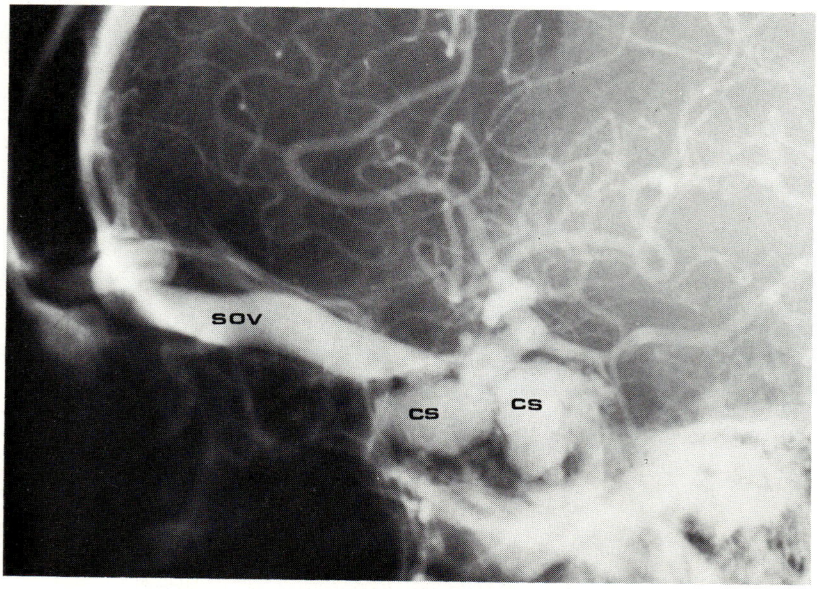

Figure 8–10d

HODGKIN'S DISEASE OF THE ORBIT (Figure 8–11)

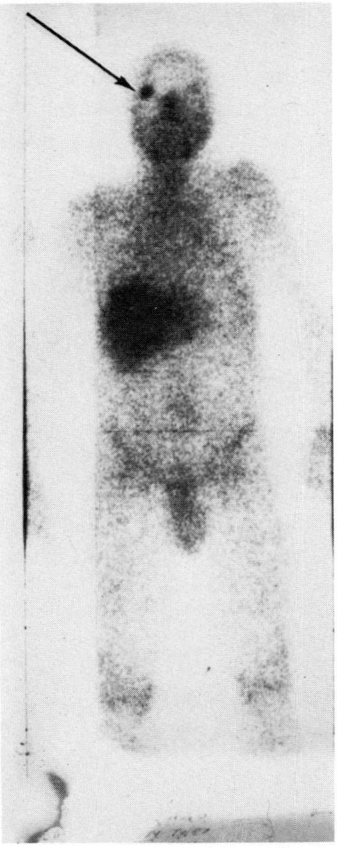

Figure 8–11a

T. P. is a 59 year old male who presented with a history of progressive exophthalmos on the right side over a period of several months. His past history was significant in that he had previously received total nodal treatment for Hodgkin's disease. There was no evidence of recurrent Hodgkin's disease.

a. The gallium scan reveals only the abnormal area of uptake in the region of the right eye.

b. The preinfusion scan discloses exophathalmos on the right side. A poorly defined mass can be seen behind the right globe, measuring from 20 to 36 u (arrow).

c. After infusion the mass can be better visualized and on this view with electronic enhancement can be seen to best advantage (arrow). The density has increased to 24 to 80 u.

Histologic diagnosis was recurrent nodular sclerosing Hodgkin's disease.

1A

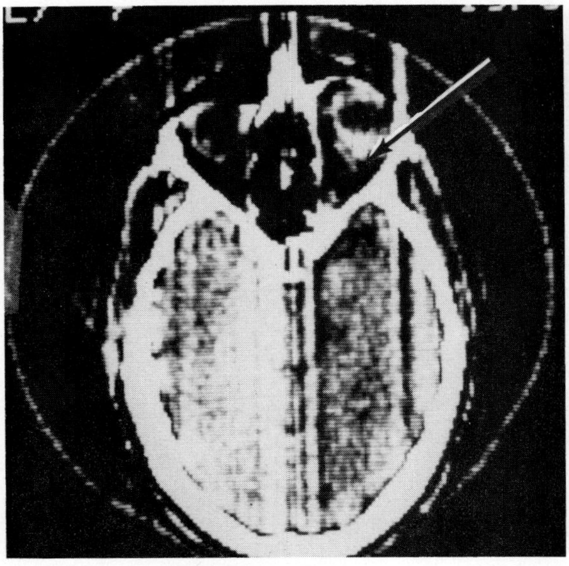

Figure 8–11b

11A

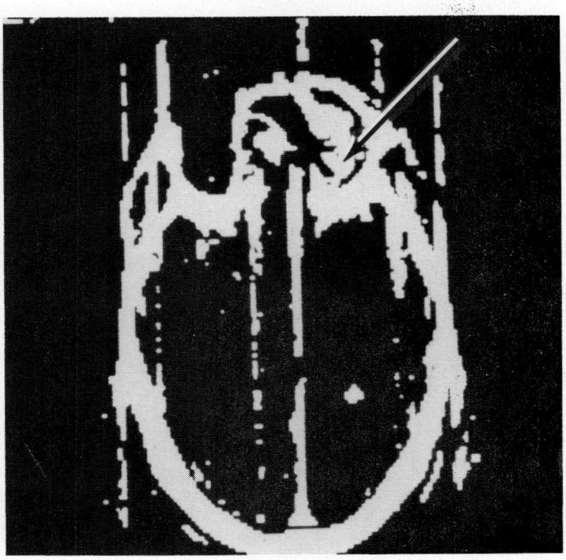

Figure 8–11c

OSTEOMA OF THE FRONTAL SINUS (Figure 8–12)

L. Y., an adolescent male, had a known large osteoma of the right frontal sinus. The CT scan was performed to rule out any intracranial extension of the tumor prior to attempted surgical removal.

a. The Caldwell view of the skull reveals a large osteoma occupying the right frontal sinus and extending over to the left side. The osteoma appears to extend into the ethmoid sinuses on the right side as well.

b. A lateral tomogram through the osteoma demonstrates a sizable mass lesion extending into both the frontal and ethmoid sinuses.

c. The low CT scan cut confirms the large osteoma extending into the ethmoid and frontal sinuses. There is no evidence of intracranial extension. The density ranges from 600 to 1000 u.

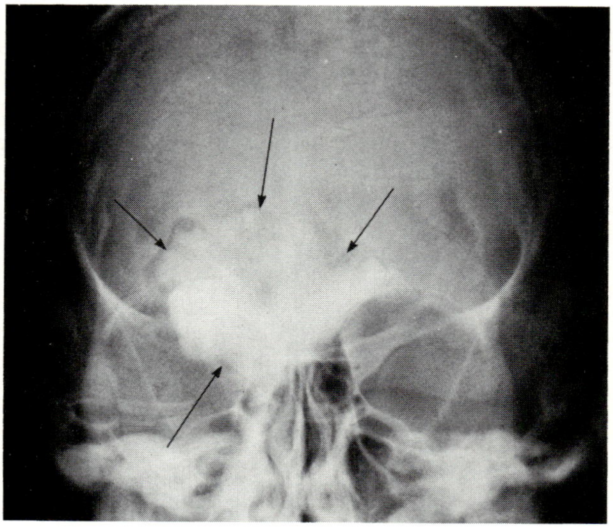

Figure 8–12a

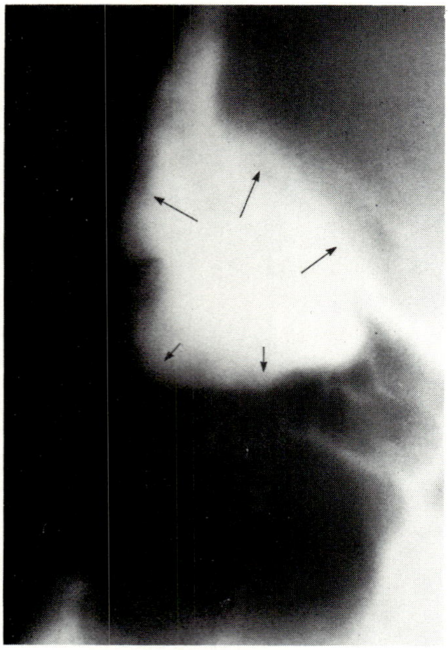

Figure 8–12b

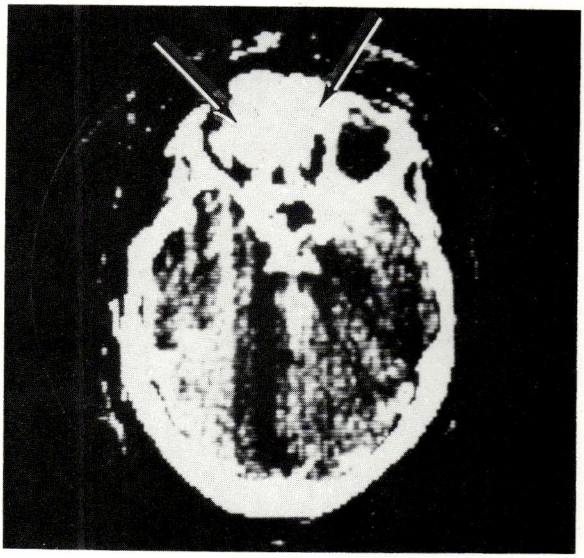

Figure 8–12c

CHAPTER 9

NEONATAL ULTRASOUND

The new ultrasound equipment with in-line transducers can be used to visualize the intracranial structures in newborn infants. The technique is particularly useful because the portable ultrasound units can be wheeled to the nursery for examination of infants (usually premature) rather than transporting the infants to the radiology department for a CT scan. Often these infants are quite fragile and maintained by life support systems; therefore the less they are transported the better.

Normal Examination and Method

The anterior fontanelle is used as an acoustic window and through it the lateral ventricles and other intracranial structures can be visualized. The infants are usually studied in several projections (see Figure 9–1). The most commonly used projections are the coronal, lateral, and sagittal. Careful perusal of the intracranial contents should be performed at the time of the first examination. The transducer should be applied gently to the anterior fontanelle and rocked back and forth until the lateral ventricles are demonstrated in various planes. There should be no midline shift and the ventricles should be slit-like. If the lateral fontanelle is used for the axial projection, the size of the ventricles can be evaluated and the alterations from normal appearance can be readily appreciated. Normally the choroid plexus of the lateral ventricle is more dense than the remainder of the brain structures, and therefore it stands out as an echodense area. This should not be mistaken for a hemorrhage, which also appears dense on ultrasound (see below). Of course, variations in positioning of the patient can be done in any projection desired, but a standard approach is best. There appears to be a range for the normal size of the lateral ventricles, but the usual appearance is slit-like and the corners of the ventricles should not be rounded.

Appropriate projections can also be used to visualize the posterior fossa structures, but that is somewhat more difficult and at this point evaluation is best left to the CT scan.

NORMAL NEWBORN ULTRASOUND (Figure 9–1)

a. The coronal projection reveals the normal-sized frontal horns of the lateral ventricles (outlined).

b. Coronal projection in another infant reveals that the frontal horns are generous in size. There is also a cavum septum pellicidum projecting between the frontal horns (arrow).

c. The parasagittal view reveals the slightly dilated lateral ventricle. The choroid plexus of the lateral ventricle projects as a high density area in the floor of the lateral ventricle.

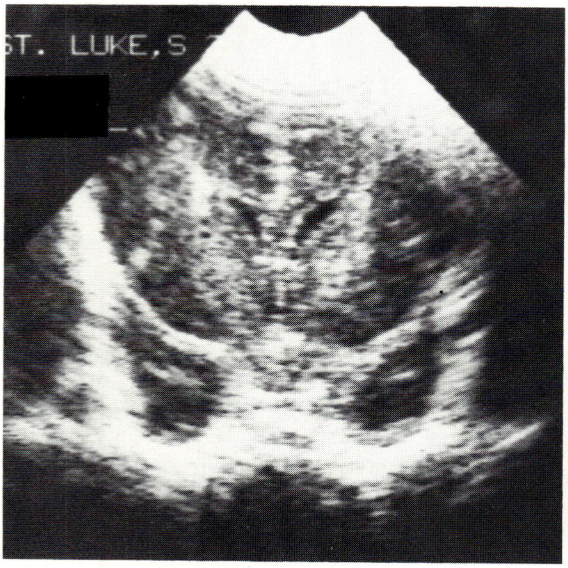

Figure 9–1a

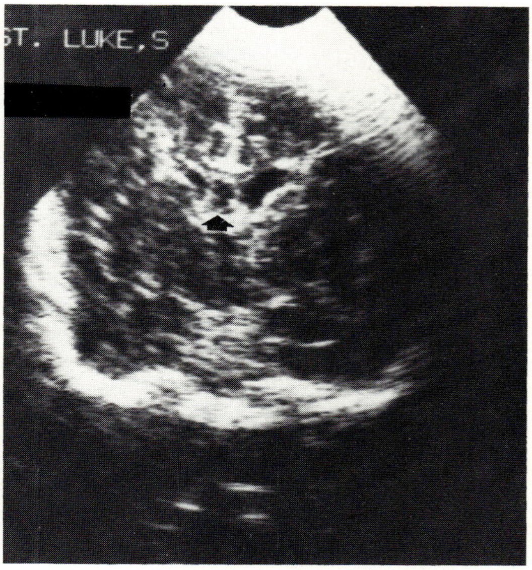

Figure 9–1b

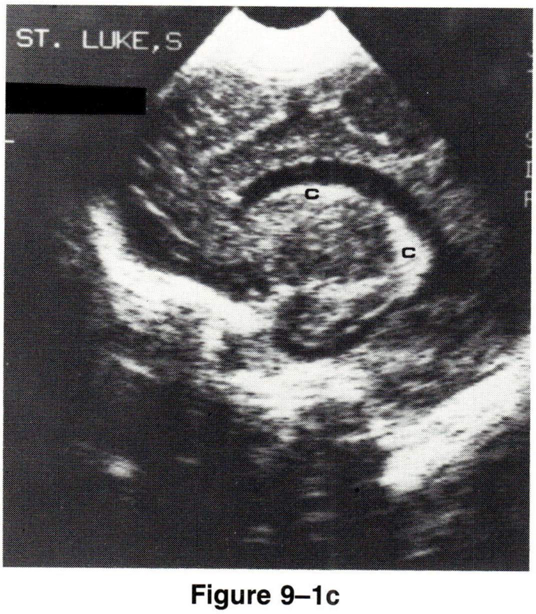

Figure 9–1c

Hemorrhage

There is normally a very vascular layer surrounding the lateral ventricles, called the *germinal plate*. This layer involutes and disappears in the full-term infant. It is this layer which hemorrhages at the time of birth. Hemorrhages are common in premature infants because a certain amount of trauma occurs when these tiny babies are born. The areas of hemorrhage can be variable in size from very tiny to much larger areas which rupture into the lateral ventricle and cause them to become greatly dilated. These areas of hemorrhage are readily apparent on ultrasound as areas of increased echogenicity. It should be mentioned that these areas of hemorrhage are not always apparent at the time of birth because delayed hemorrhages can occur. Therefore, it is appropriate and recommended that an initial study be performed at the time of birth and that regular follow-up examinations also be performed.

The increase or decrease in the size of these areas of hemorrhage can be readily appreciated and the change in ventricular size can also be evaluated on CT. In most cases one can predict with a fair degree of certainty whether the hemorrhage extends far into the cerebral substance and this may alter the prognosis in these infants. It can be readily appreciated if the hemorrhage has ruptured into the lateral ventricle. If the latter is the case, then the development of an obstructive or communicating hydrocephalus is a strong possibility.

GERMINAL PLATE HEMORRHAGE (Figure 9–2)

a. The parasagittal view reveals a long area of increased echogenicity along the wall of the lateral ventricle (arrows). This appearance is consistent with a germinal plate hemorrhage.

b. The follow-up examination obtained approximately 2 weeks later reveals that the lateral ventricle is enlarged and has a "corrugated" (arrows) upper margin secondary to the formation of multiple areas of porencephaly following destruction of the brain by the hemorrhage.

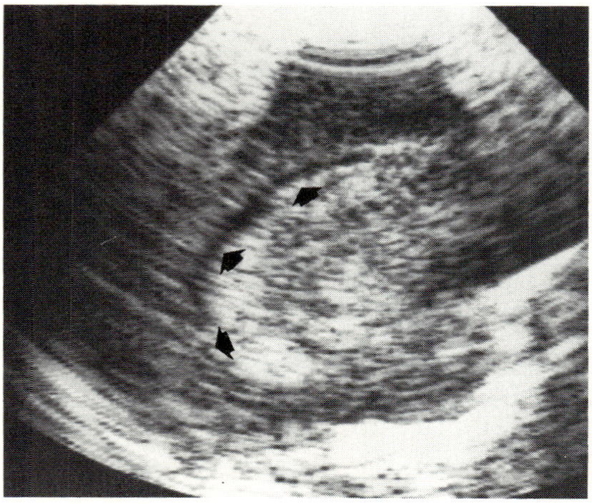

Figure 9–2a

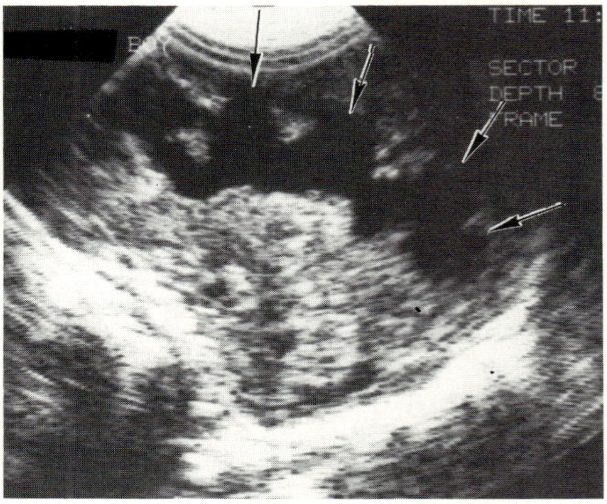

Figure 9–2b

GERMINAL PLATE HEMORRHAGE WITH RUPTURE INTO THE LATERAL VENTRICLE (Figure 9–3)

a and b. The coronal and transverse and parasagittal projections of the ultrasound reveal greatly dilated lateral ventricle filled with clotted (CL) blood. Note that the transverse projection (b) is obtained by using the lateral fontanelle as an acoustic window and correlates nicely with the CT scan appearance. The arrows outline the blood-filled lateral ventricles.

c to e. The follow-up examination approximately 3 weeks later was performed in the parasagittal (c and d) and coronal (e) projections and reveals that the large intraventricular clots have retracted while the lateral ventricles have dilated. This could be secondary to a communicating hydrocephalus, but it could also be related to an obstructive hydrocephalus secondary to a blood clot in the outlet of the third ventricle and in the fourth ventricle.

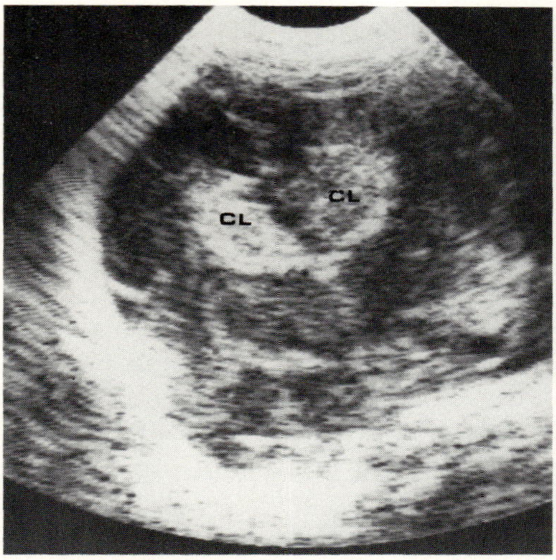

Figure 9–3a

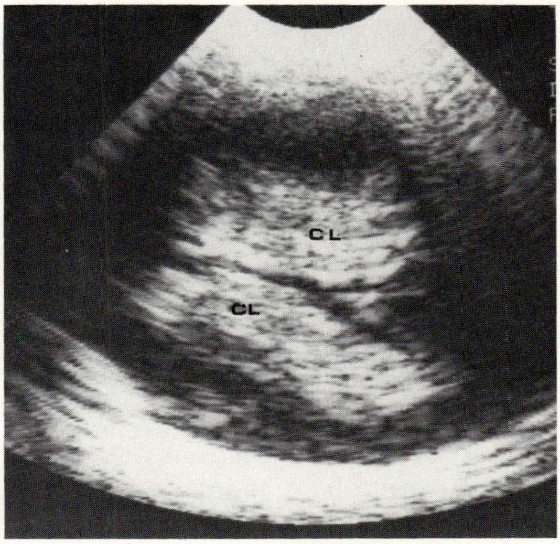

Figure 9–3b

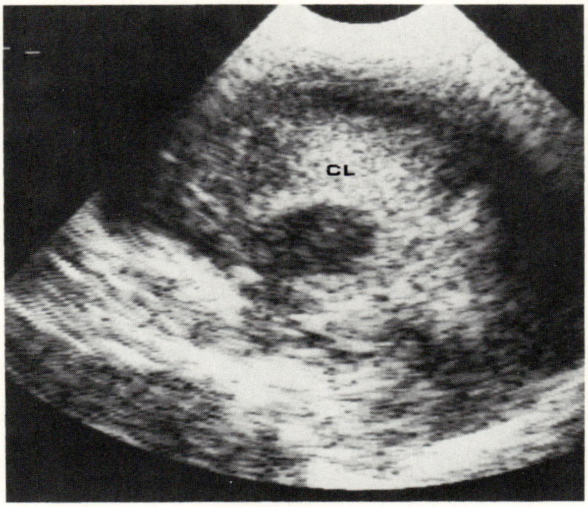

Figure 9–3c

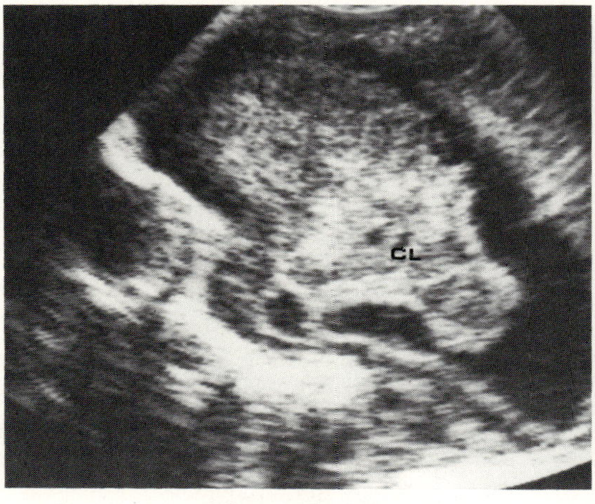

Figure 9–3d

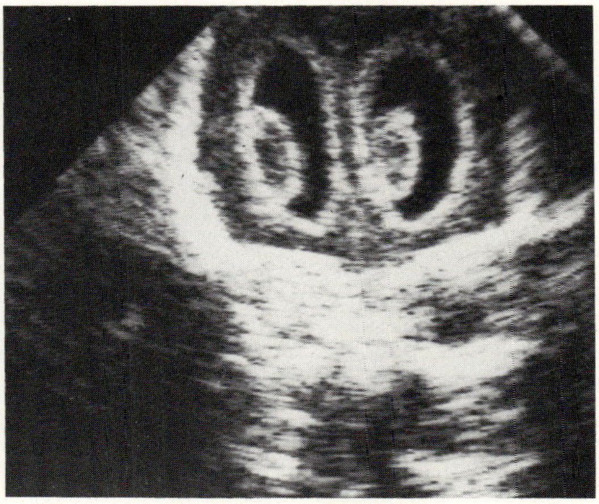

Figure 9–3e

Hydrocephalus

Hydrocephalus can be readily monitored by the use of ultrasound. The size and configuration can be demonstrated and any change in size can be determined by comparison with older examinations. Therefore, a standard magnification and technique should be used to facilitate comparison between examinations. In this way the ventricle size can be safely monitored noninvasively on a day to day basis and planning for shunt placement, if necessary, can be done.

In addition to the development of hydrocephalus, we have also observed the formation of areas of porencephaly secondary to areas of hemorrhage.

GERMINAL PLATE HEMORRHAGE WITH HYDROCEPHALUS AND PORENCEPHALY (Figure 9–4)

a and b. The initial scan was performed in the coronal (a) and parasagittal (b) projections and reveals a large germinal plate hemorrhage on the left side (XXX). The sonar-lucent ventricle projects above the clot.

c and d. A follow-up examination 1½ months later reveals that hydrocephalus has developed and the retracted clot can be identified resting in the frontal horn of the lateral ventricles (XXX in c). The lateral ventricles are dilated. In addition an area of low echogenicity can be seen projecting above the lateral ventricle (arrows in d). This is a porencephalic cyst.

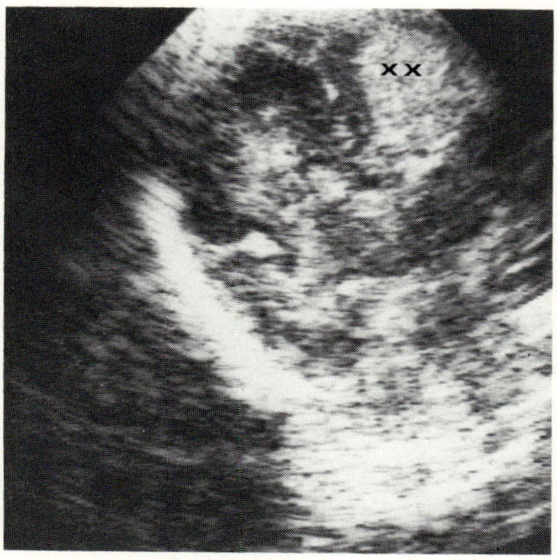

Figure 9–4a

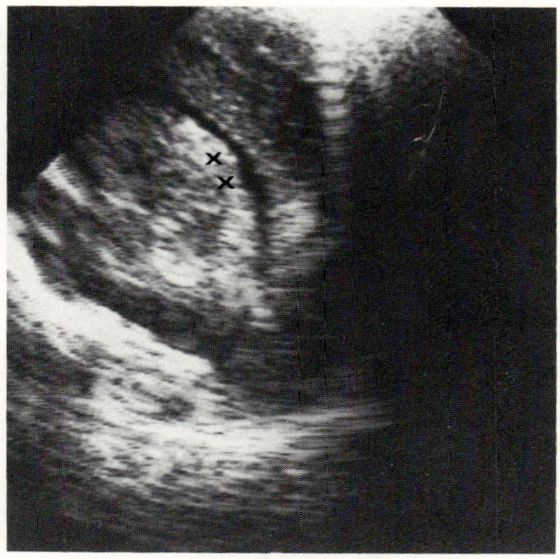

Figure 9–4b

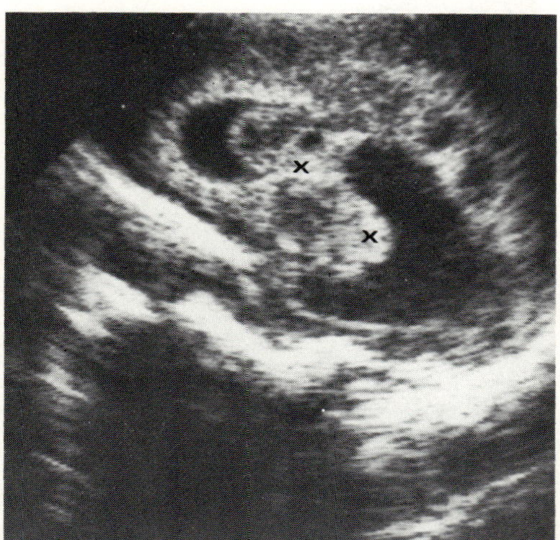

Figure 9–4c

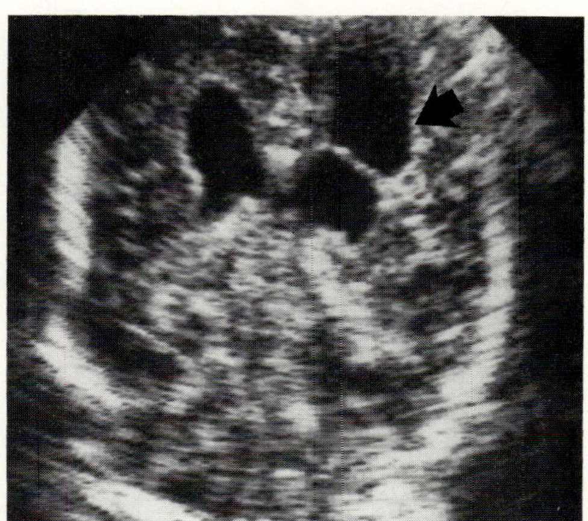

Figure 9–4d

e and f. Parasagittal views obtained at 3 months reveal the greatly dilated ventricle on the side without the hemorrhage (e) and the dilated ventricle with the multiple areas of porencephaly surrounding the roof of the lateral ventricle where the hemorrhage initially occurred (arrows).

g and h. The CT scan obtained at approximately the same time as the last ultrasound examination correlates nicely and demonstrates the enlarged lateral ventricles and the multiple areas of out-pouching of the lateral ventricles on the left side secondary to the formation of porencephalic cysts (arrows).

The excellent correlation between the CT and ultrasound findings has allowed us to eliminate the need for a CT scan in most cases. As mentioned previously, if a posterior fossa abnormality is suspected, then a CT scan is needed for evaluation.

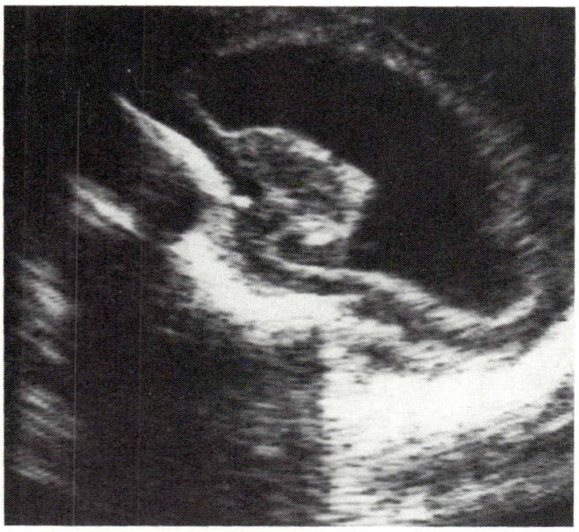

Figure 9–4e

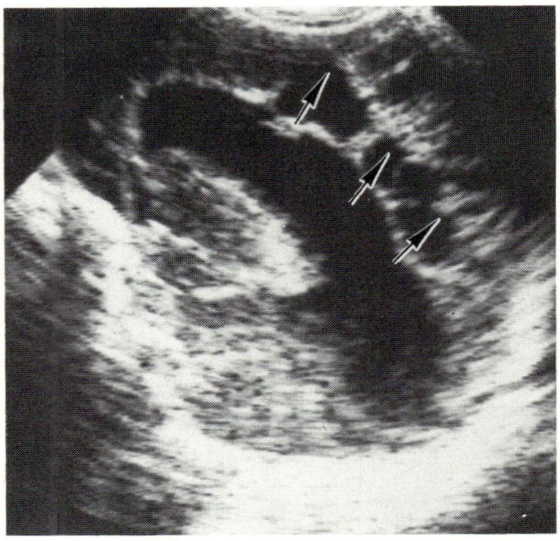

Figure 9–4f

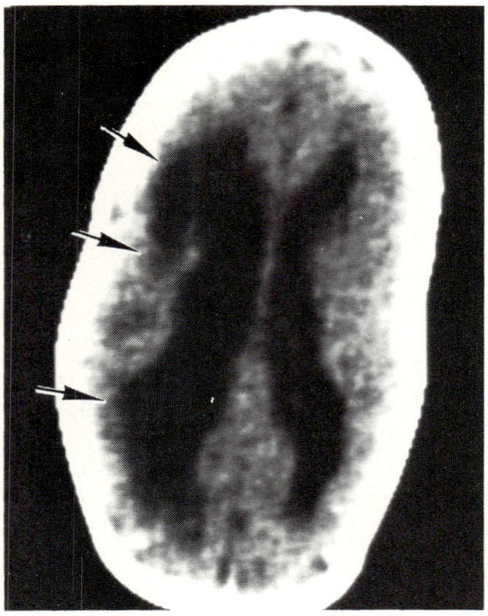

Figure 9–4g

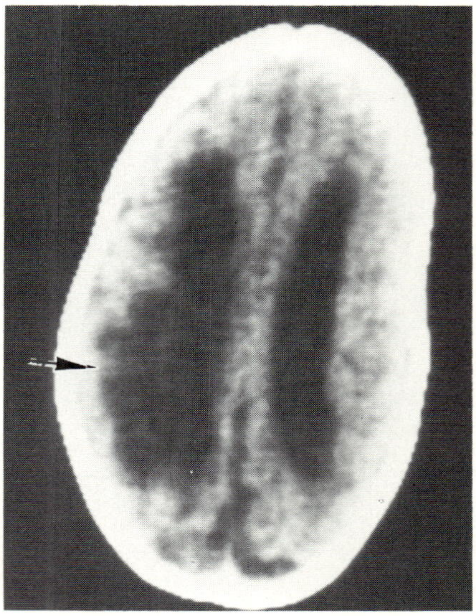

Figure 9–4h

Subdural Extracerebral Collections

Some observers have reported visualizing areas of extracerebral collections such as subdural hematomas, but I feel that these are best demonstrated and followed by the use of CT scanning.

Intraoperative Ultrasound

This is an area that shows great promise for the future. Intraoperative ultrasound is particularly helpful for shunt placement. It is possible to observe the shunt placement under direct vision and to make adjustments in the position of the shunt during the course of the operative procedure. The only drawback at this time is that this method requires two burr holes—one for the shunt tubing device and the other for the acoustic window for the ultrasound unit.

Ultrasound may also prove useful in the removal of brain tumors. In some cases the tumor has different ultrasonic characteristics than the remainder of the normal brain and therefore, while direct visualization of the tumor does not definitely identify the abnormal tissue, ultrasound may be helpful for better definition. This area is still open for future research.

CHAPTER 10

DIGITAL INTRAVENOUS SUBTRACTION ANGIOGRAPHY (DISA)

Digital intravenous subtraction angiography (DISA) is a new technique which allows visualization of the arterial system following the intravenous injection of contrast material. The technique is based upon the principle of manual film subtraction, in which a "mask" film is superimposed upon the contrast-filled film and a "subtracted" image is obtained. With modern equipment, this masking and subtraction process is performed electronically. Fluoroscopy, rather than cut film radiography, is the modality used. The images are stored temporarily on a disc which is then played back and reviewed. From the series of stored images appropriate views are chosen for subtraction and then recorded on x-ray film for viewing and permanent storage.

There are variations of this process from one manufacturer to another. The disc storage system can store the images in two ways: analog or digital. In the *analog* method the image is stored on the disc, as it is generated, as the fluoroscopic image without an assigned numerical density but in varying shades of gray. The *digital* storage method assigns numerical densities to the various shades of gray and stores these density numbers on the disc. Analog storage is faster and allows more fluoroscopic images per unit time. Digital data collection is more scientific, perhaps, but slower.

One advantage of the digital method is that it stores the images as a grid of number densities, which can be shifted side to side and up and down to compensate for patient motion during the study. With the analog storage method this compensatory image shifting is not possible. It can be seen that both analog and digital methods of storage have certain advantages and disadvantages which must be considered when purchasing equipment.

In addition, the size of the image intensifier, and therefore the field of view, also varies in size. A choice must be made concerning preference for a large or small field of view. Some systems allow a choice of two field sizes rather than only one.

DISA requires the injection of relatively large amount of contrast material, and therefore should not be used in patients with compromised renal function. Since this examination also requires a good cardiac output to carry a bolus of contrast material to the area of interest, the method is also contraindicated in patients with congestive heart failure.

Approximately 80 per cent of these studies are for examination of the extracranial carotid arteries. Other intracranial problems, such as large aneurysms or a tortuous vertebrobasilar system, are also studied. The method is also useful for evaluating renal artery stenosis and for examination of the peripheral vascular system (see Table 10–1).

Indications for the use of DISA are listed in Table 10–1. Since ulcerated plaques may not be visible using DISA, the clinical diagnosis of transient ischemic attacks (TIAs) is not an indication for this type of study.

The injection of contrast material can be made (1) via a 2½ inch needle in an antecubital vein, (2) via a 10 cm needle in an antecubital vein, or (3) via an end and multiple side hole catheter placed in the superior vena cava. In our opinion, the latter method is preferable. The catheter is placed using the Seldinger technique via an antecubital vein (preferable) or the femoral vein. It is technically easier to use a medial antecubital vein rather than a laterally placed vein.

We use 40 ml of Renographin 70 per cent with each injection. For extracranial carotid stenosis we use a minimum of 3 injections—in the right posterior oblique, left posterior oblique, and anteroposterior projections—and a maximum of 5 injections. For other studies and anatomic locations the patient position is varied accordingly.

There are certain dangers and technical difficulties involved with this method. Dangers include allergy to contrast material and extravasation of contrast material into the soft tissues of the arm with the short needle technique, or into the mediastinum or pericardium using the central injection. Technical difficulties are the inability to perform venipuncture because of small or fragile veins and the inability to advance the wire or catheter.

The benefits of DISA include the ease of performance, the fact that it is an outpatient procedure, a cost approximately one third that of angiography, the absence of risk of stroke secondary to the procedure itself, and ease of repetition.

Contraindications include known allergy to the contrast material, congestive heart failure, uncooperative patient, and the presence of renal failure.

TABLE 10–1. Indications for DISA in Neuroradiology

1. Preoperative patients for coronary by-pass
2. Preoperative patients for other major surgery such as total hip replacement in older patients
3. Asymptomatic carotid bruits
4. Follow-up carotid endarterectomy
5. ? Tortuous basilar artery
6. ? Superior sagittal sinus thrombosis
7. ? Large or moderate sized intracranial aneurysm
8. Follow-up intracranial arteriovenous malformations
9. Follow-up of superficial temporal to middle cerebral artery anastomosis

NORMAL VIEWS IN DISA (Figure 10–1)

a. The view of the arch in the RPO projection after injection into the superior vena cava (40 ml of 76 per cent Renographin) following right antecubital vein puncture. This reveals excellent visualization of the great vessels and ascending, transverse, and proximal descending aorta. Innominate artery (INN), right subclavian artery (RS), right common carotid artery (RCC), left common carotid artery (LCC), left subclavian artery (LS), left vertebral artery (LVA).

b. The view of the neck vessels in the RPO projection reveals the carotid bifurcations and both vertebral arteries. (1) Right common carotid artery, (2) right external carotid artery, (3) right internal carotid artery, (4) right vertebral artery, (5) left common carotid artery, (6) left internal carotid artery, (7) left external carotid artery, (8) left vertebral artery.

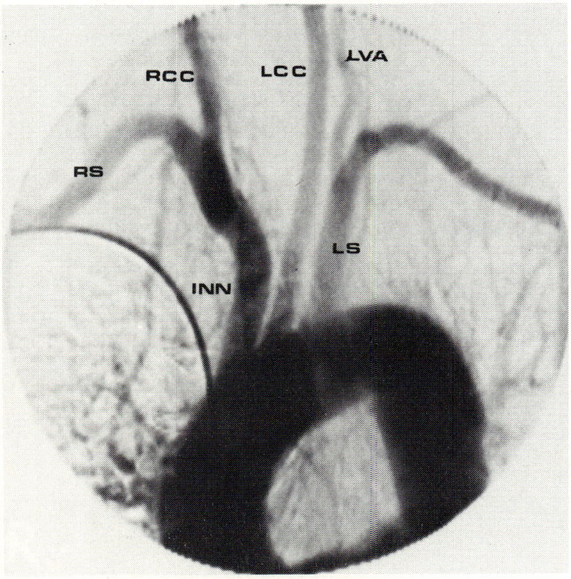

Figure 10–1a

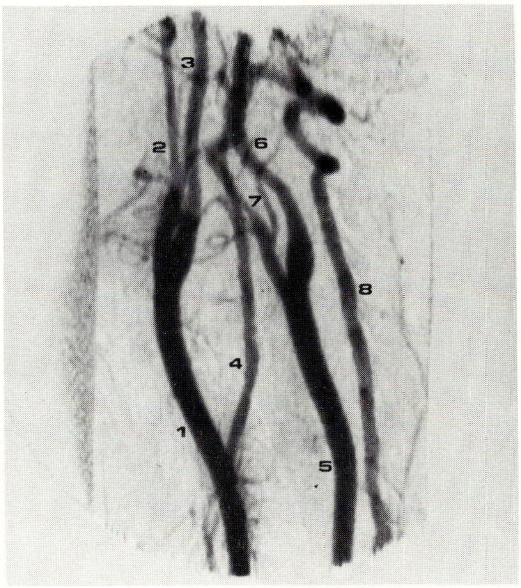

Figure 10–1b

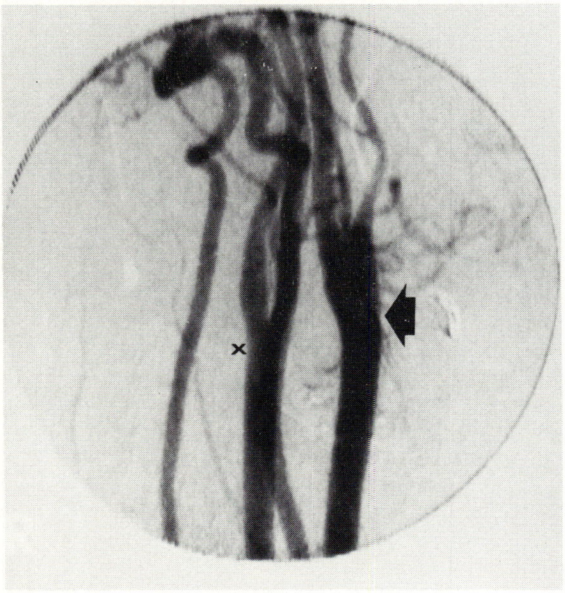

Figure 10–1c

c. The view of the neck vessels in the LPO projection reveals superimposition of the right external carotid artery over the left vertebral artery (X). The left internal and external carotid arteries are also superimposed in this projection (arrow).

OCCLUDED RIGHT INTERNAL CAROTID ARTERY AND WIDELY PATENT LEFT INTERNAL CAROTID ARTERY (Figure 10–2)

a. In this LPO projection the right internal carotid artery is shown to be occluded (right arrow) at this origin. The left internal carotid artery is widely patent at its origin (left arrow). The right vertebral artery appears normal (RVA). The left vertebral artery demonstrates areas of atherosclerosis in its proximal portion (arrowheads).

b. The intracranial series reveals that the right internal carotid distribution is filled by crossing over from the left side via the anterior communicating artery (arrow). No contrast is identified in the position of the right internal carotid artery.

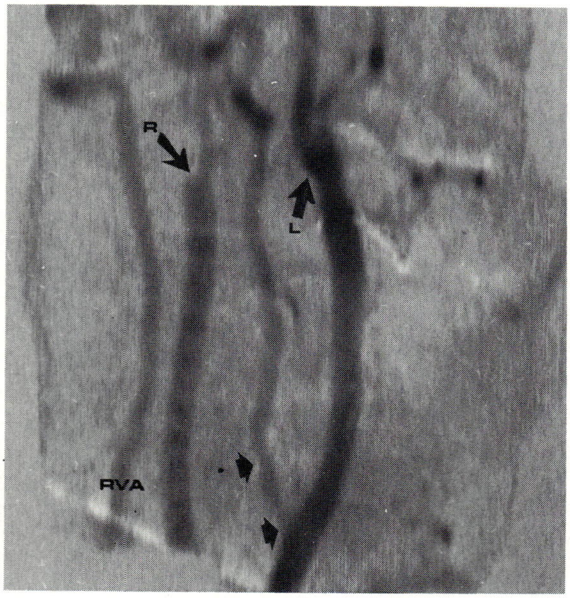

Figure 10–2a

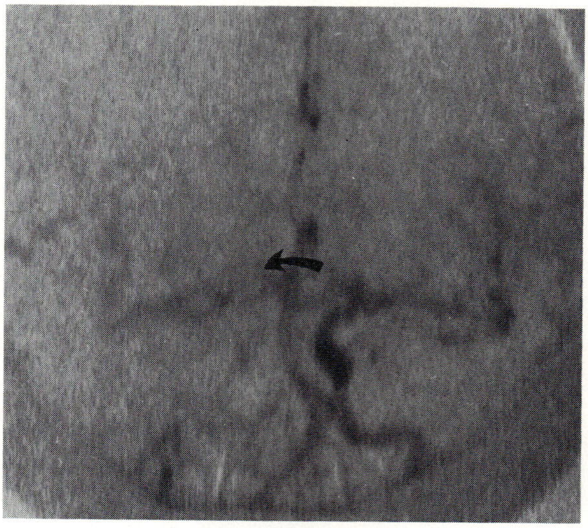

Figure 10–2b

NORMAL INTRACRANIAL CIRCULATION (Figure 10–3)

a. Normal subtraction image, with visualization in the AP projection. There is excellent visualization of the intracranial circulation. (1) Right internal carotid artery (RICA), (2) right vertebral artery (RVA), basilar artery (B), (4) left vertebral artery (LVA), (5) left carotid artery (LCA).

b. The same structures are now seen in an inverted image.

In an individual case, the normal or reversed image may give better visualization of the area of interest. Therefore, both images should be reviewed when necessary.

This technique of visualization of the intracranial vessels is particularly useful for evaluation of patients with pituitary tumors. The position of the vessels around the sella and their relationships to the tumor are readily appreciated.

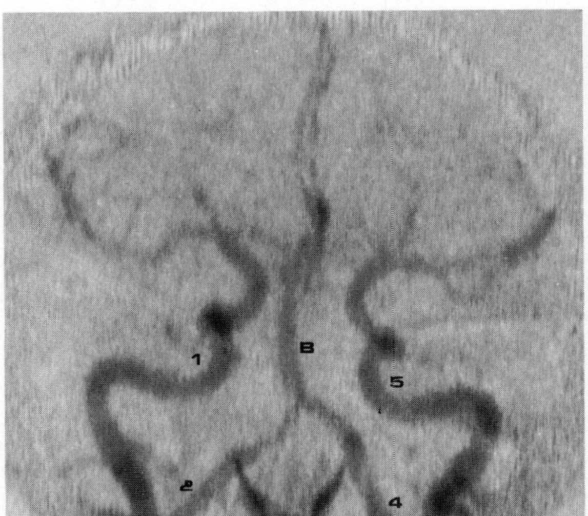

Figure 10–3a

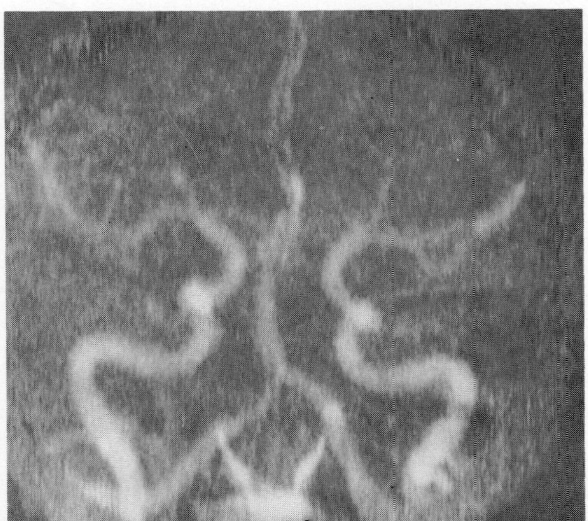
Figure 10–3b

NORMAL BUCKLING OF THE INTERNAL CAROTID ARTERY (Figure 10–4)

This 17 year old male had a pulsating mass below the angle of the jaw which had been present for many years.

a. The "white on black" (inverted) image in the AP projection demonstrates a large buckle of the left internal carotid artery (arrow) which projects laterally. This prominence of the left internal carotid artery corresponded to the clinically palpable mass.

b. The RPO image also demonstrates buckling of the right internal carotid artery which projects superiorly (arrow).

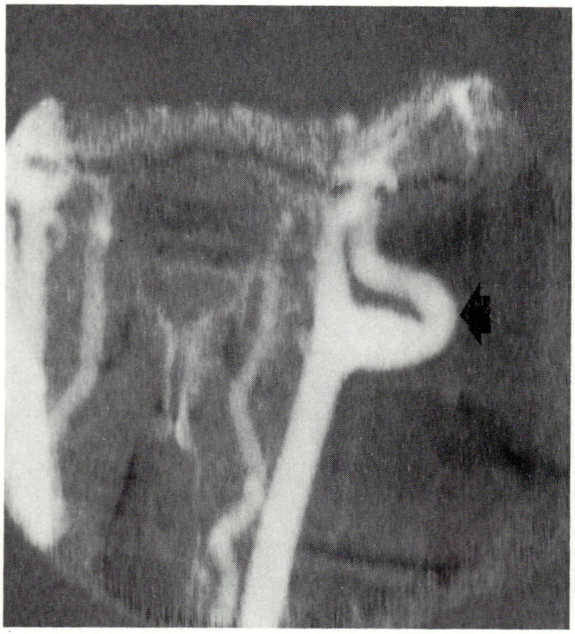

Figure 10–4a

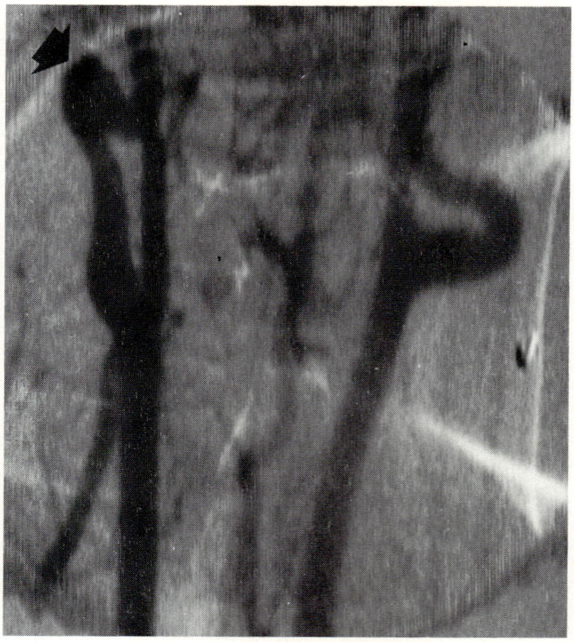

Figure 10–4b

ENLARGED THYROID GLAND (Figure 10–5)

This 59 year old female presented with a bruit in the left side of the neck.

a. The AP view of the neck reveals a very enlarged superior thyroid artery (large arrow) which supplies a very vascular enlarged left lobe of the thyroid gland (arrowheads). The left common carotid artery (LCCA) is displaced laterally by the enlarged thyroid.

b. The later phase demonstrates the dense blush of the enlarged left lobe of the thyroid gland.

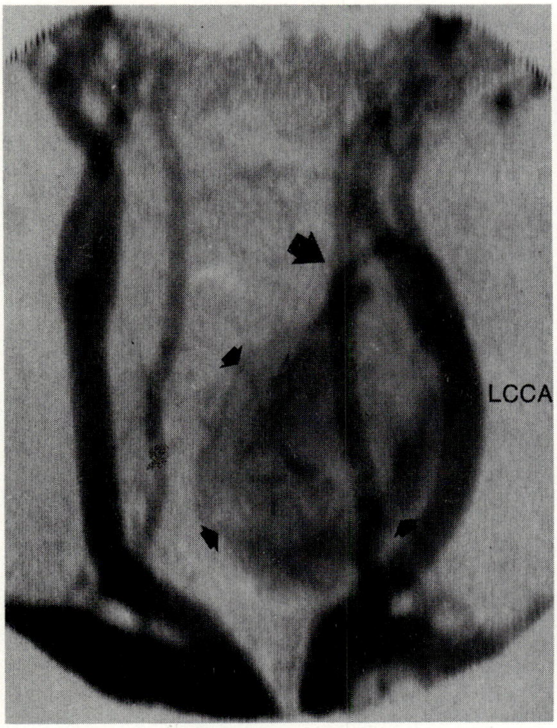

Figure 10–5a

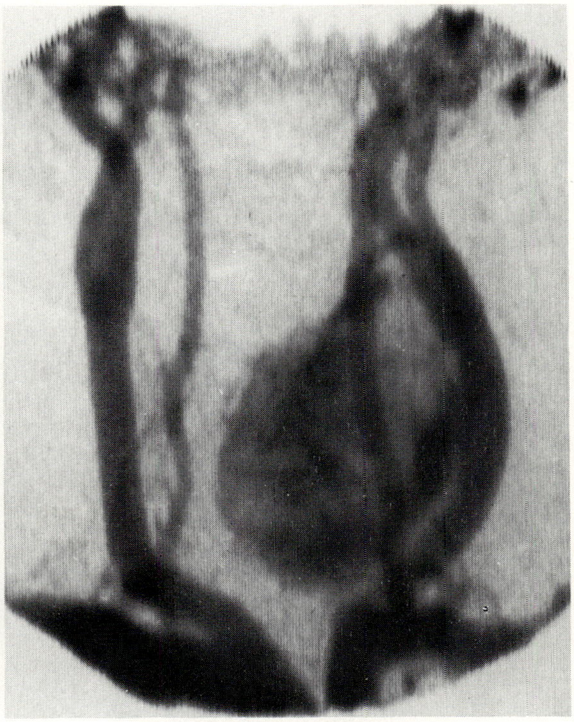

Figure 10–5b

PITFALLS IN THE USE OF DISA (Figure 10–6)

a. For technical reasons, the catheter could not be placed in the superior vena cava. Therefore, contrast was injected through a left antecubital vein with an 8-inch catheter. An arch view of the vein was attempted, but the entire area is obscured by the contrast flowing through the left subclavian vein and other venous tributaries from the left side. There is also retrograde flow into the left internal jugular vein (arrow). Additional artifact ("misregistration artifact") is caused by patient motion.

b. The later image faintly demonstrates the arch and left common carotid artery (arrow) but is otherwise nondiagnostic because of patient motion artifact.

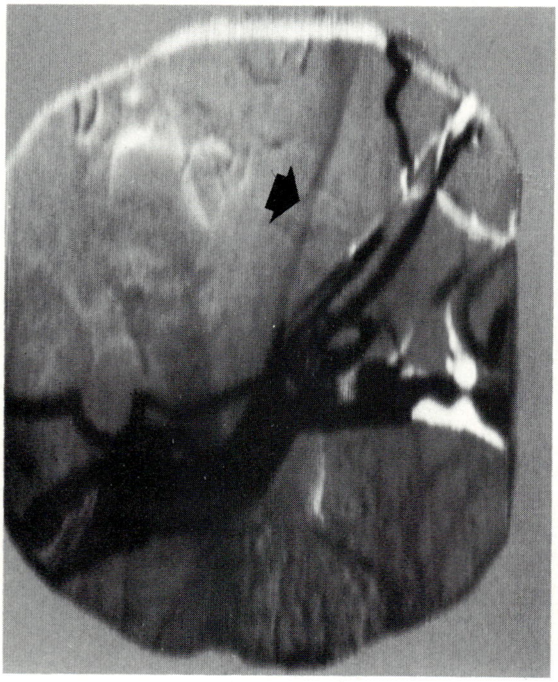

Figure 10–6a

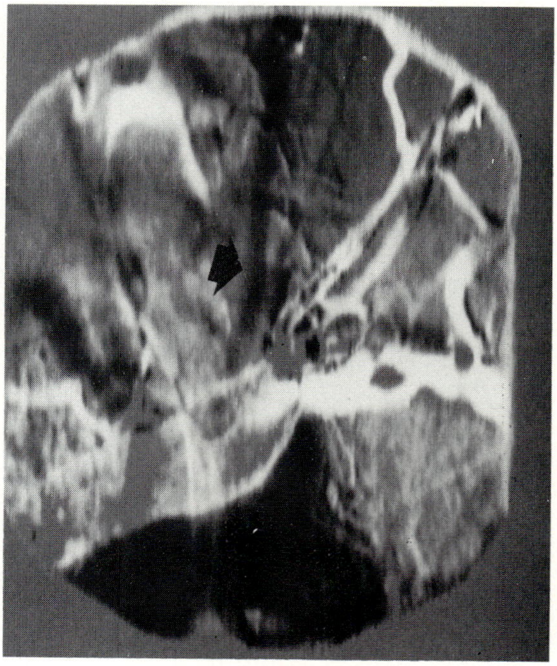

Figure 10–6b

CHAPTER 11

NUCLEAR MAGNETIC RESONANCE

Block and Purcell received the Nobel prize in physics for their work in chemical nuclear magnetic resonance (NMR) in 1952. In the last several years this technique has been applied to the study of biologic systems. The method is ingenious and does not require the use of ionizing radiation. Instead, it uses a magnetic field and the application of a radiofrequency pulse; no harmful biologic effects have yet been demonstrated.

The patient is placed in a large magnet (similar in appearance to the gantry of a CT scanner) to which a steady magnetic field with a gradient is applied. This causes the various protons (usually hydrogen is studied) to "line up" in the magnetic field. A pulsed radiofrequency wave is then applied to the system, causing some of the spinning nuclei to wobble and to give off a certain amount of energy. A measurement is made of this energy and the time required for the nuclei to return or "relax" to equilibrium. Two principal "relaxation" times are measured:

T_1, or the longitudinal relaxation time, is the characteristic time it takes for the system to "decay," or return to equilibrium with its surroundings ("lattice") after the excitation pulse ends.

T_2, or the dephasing relaxation process, is the time it takes for the energy of the system to cancel itself out.

T_1 and T_2 tend to measure whether matter is liquid or solid. In general, liquids tend to deaden the signals, and T_1 and T_2 are equal for water. Solids have short T_2 and long T_1 times. Fast-growing tissues, such as cancerous ones, tend to contain water and have short T_1 times.

Normal tissues tend to have characteristic decay times following the application of a certain radiofrequency pulse for a certain period of time. Unfortunately, there is some overlap in the decay times of various body tissues. In general, however, tumor cells contain a larger amount of water than normal tissues, so the T_1 of tumors appears to be longer than that of normal tissues. However, there continues to be an overlap among the various tissues and between normal and abnormal tissue measurements.

An additional drawback to the use of NMR is that bone and calcifications are poorly visualized or not demonstrated at all. The protons in these tissues are very closely bound in their crystal lattice and therefore are not free to rotate in response to the application of either the magnetic field or the radiofrequency pulse.

Further experimentation is necessary before we discover the best radiofrequency wave lengths to apply to each type of tissue and the length of the application times.

Images from the two types of magnets used in NMR, resistant and superconducting magnets, should be the same. The time needed to generate the images will probably be shorter with the superconducting magnets, however, and this will probably be advantageous.

NMR has some advantages over CT in addition to the fact that it does not require the use of ionizing radiation. One of the great advantages is that a large amount of information can be generated at the time of the scan because of the technique of "volume" imaging. When the patient is studied, the entire body part placed in the unit can be examinated and then viewed in the desired plane of imaging. Therefore, as seen in Figures 11–1 to 11–3, the body can be viewed in the plane most advantageous to the study of the body part being examined. This will obviously decrease the amount of time needed to examine an area, and various anatomic locations can be extracted from the data generated to suit the particular examination.

Many workers now using and studying NMR and its applications think that this new technique will eventually replace computed tomography. Time will tell if their hypothesis is correct.

5.0 KILOGAUSS SAGITTAL CRANIAL IMAGE (Figure 11–1)

This sagittal slice of cranial anatomy was acquired using a saturation recovery pulse technique at a 5.0 kilogauss magnetic field strength. Gauss (and kilogauss) is a measurement of magnetic field strength. The magnetic field of the earth is 0.6 G at Washington, D.C. (Reproduced courtesy of Technicare Corporation.)

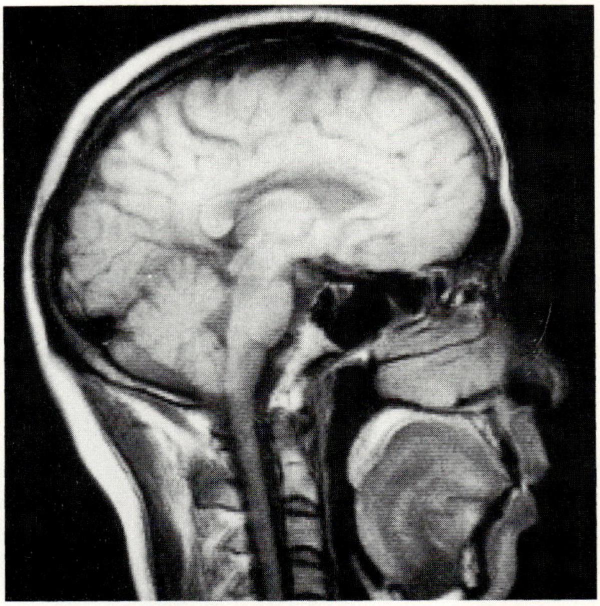

Figure 11–1

3.0 KILOGAUSS TRANSVERSE CRANIAL IMAGE (Figure 11–2)

Transverse slices of cranial anatomy were acquired using saturation recovery pulse technique at a 3.0 kilogauss magnetic field strength. (Reproduced courtesy of Technicare Corporation.)

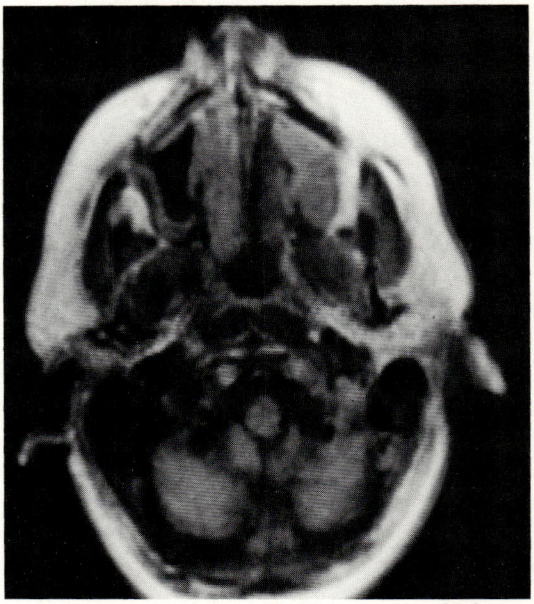

Figure 11–2

3.0 KILOGAUSS SAGITTAL SPINE IMAGE (Figure 11–3)

Sagittal slice of the dorsolumbar spine area. Image was obtained using two-dimensional acquisition and saturation recovery pulse technique. (Reproduced courtesy of Technicare Corporation.)

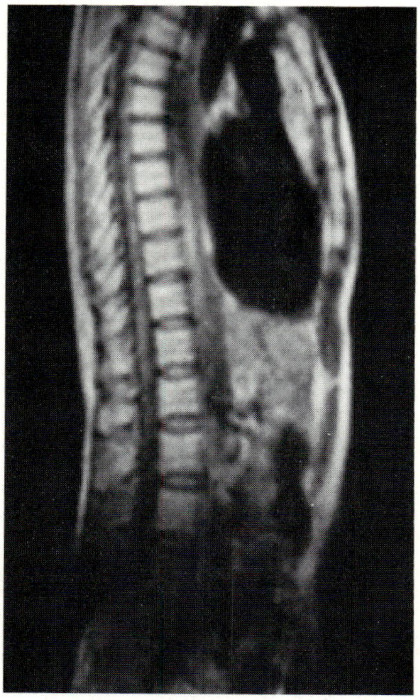

Figure 11–3

Selected References

Normal Anatomy

Berns, T. F., Daniels, D. L., Williams, A. L., et al.: Mesencephalic anatomy: Demonstration by computed tomography. AJNR (1981), 2(1):65.

Bolsen, B.: CT scanning of the brain: A revolution in only eight years (news). JAMA (1981), 246(23):2667.

Carmel, P. W., and Mawad, M.: CT scanning of the posterior fossa. Clin. Neurosurg. (1982), 29:51.

Daniels, D. L., Williams, A. L., and Haughton, V. M.: Computed tomographv of the medulla. Radiology (1982), 145(1):63.

Dutton, J. J., Klingele, T. G., Burde, R. M., et al.: Evaluation of the suprasellar cistern by computed tomography. Ophthalmologv (Rochester) (1982), 89(11):1220.

Gyldensted, C.: Measurements of the normal ventricular system and hemispheric sulci of 100 adults with computed tomography. Neuroradiology (1977), 14:183.

Kuulial, A. I.: The normal suprasellar subarachnoid space in computed tomography. Clin. Radiol. (1980), 31(2):155.

Lund, E., and Halaburt, H.: Irradiation dose to the lens of the eye during CT of the head. Neuroradiology (1982), 22(4):181.

Mawad, M. E., Silver, A. J., Hilal, S. K., et al.: Computed tomography of the brain stem with intrathecal metrizamide. Part I: The normal brain stem. AJR (1983), 140(3):553.

Mawad, M. E., Silver, A. J., Hilal, S. K., et al.: Computed tomography of the brain stem with intrathecal metrizamide. Part II: Lesions in and around the brain stem. AJR (1983), 140(3):565.

Taylor, S.: The petrous temporal bone (including the cerebellopontine angle). Radiol. Clin. North Am. (1982), 20(1):67.

Theerman, M. R., Shuster, A., and Fanale, J. E.: Nephrotoxic effects of computerized tomographic brain scan (letter). N. Engl. J. Med. (1979), 300(1):45.

Trefler, M., and Haughton, V. M.: Patient dose and image quality in computed tomography. AJR (1981), 137(1):25.

Yamamoto, Y., Satoh, T., Asari, S., et al.: Normal anatomy of cerebral vessels by computed angiotomography in the coronal, Towne, and semisagittal planes. J. Comput. Assist. Tomogr. (1982), 6(6):1049.

Brain Tumors

Ambrose, J., Gooding, M. B., and Richardson, A. E.: An assessment of the accuracy of computerized transverse axial scanning (EMI scanners) in the diagnosis of intracranial tumor. A review of 366 patients. Brain (1975), 98:569.

Bardfeld, P. A., Passalaqua, A. M., Braunstein, P., et al.: A comparison of radionuclide scanning and computed tomography in metastatic lesions of the brain. J. Comp. Assist. Tomogr. (1977), 1:315.

Butler, A. R., Horri, S. C., Kricheff, I. I., et al.: Computed tomography in astrocytomas: A statistical analysis of the parameters of malignancy and the positive contrast-enhanced CT scan. Radiology (1978), 129:433.

Crocker, E. F., Zimmerman, R. A., Phelps, M. F., et al.: The effect of steroids on the extravascular distribution of radiographic contrast material and technetium pertechnetate in brain tumors, as determined by computed tomography. Radiology (1976), 119:471.

Futrell, N. N., Osborn, A. G., and Cheson, B. D.: Pineal region tumors: Computed tomographic-pathologic spectrum. AJR (1981), 137(5):951.

Glanz, S., Geehr, R. B., Duncan, C. C., et al.: Metrizamide-enhanced CT for evaluation of brainstem tumors. AJR (1980), 134(4):821.

Maravilla, K. R., Kirks, D. R., Maravilla, A. M., et al.: Computed tomography in the evaluation of sellar and parasellar lesions: The value of sagittal and coronal reconstructions. Comput. Tomogr. (1978), 2(3):237.

Naidich, T. P., Pinto, R. S., Kushner, M. T., et al.: Evaluation of sellar and parasellar masses by computed tomography. Radiology (1976), 120:91.

Osborn, A. G., Williams, R. G., and Wing, S. D.: Low attenuation lesions in the midline posterior fossa: Differential diagnosis. CT (1978), 2(4):319.

Penley, M. W., and Pribram, H. F.: Diagnosis of cerebellopontine angle tumors with small quantities of air. Otolaryngol. Head Neck Surg. (1981), 89(3 Pt 1):457.

Segall, H. D., Zee, C. S., Naidich, T. P., et al.: Computed tomography in neoplasms of the posterior fossa in children. Radiol. Clin. North Am. (1982), 20(1):237.

Valavanis, A., Schubiger, D., Hayek, J., et al.: CT of meningiomas on the posterior surface of the petrous bone. Neuroradiology (1981), 22(3):111.

Vascular Diseases

Alcala, H., Gado, M., and Torack, RM: The effect of size, histologic elements and water content on the visualization of cerebral infarcts. Arch. Neurol. (1978), 35:1.

Araki-G., Mihara, H., Shizuka, M., et al.: CT and arteriographic comparison of patients with transient ischemic attacks—correlation with small infarction of basal ganglia. Stroke (1983), 14(2):276.

Campbell, J. K., Houser, O. W., Stevens, J. C., et al.: Computed tomography and radionuclide imaging in the evaulation of ischemic stroke. Radiology (1978), 126:695.

Davis, J. M., Davis, K. R., and Crowell, R. M.: Subarachnoid hemorrhage secondary to ruptured intracranial aneurysm: Prognostic significance of cranial CT. AJR (1980), 134(4):711.

Davis, K. R., Ackerman, R. H., Kistler, J. P., and Mohr, J. P.: Computed tomography of cerebral infarction: Hemorrhagic, contrast enhancement, and time of appearance. Comput. Tomogr. (1977), 1:71.

Davis, K. R., Taveras, J. M., New, P. F. J., et al.: Cerebral infarction diagnosis by computerized tomography. Am. J. Roentgenol. (1975), 124:643.

Golding, R., Peatfield, R. C., Shawdon, H. H., et al.: Computer tomographic features of giant intracranial aneurysms. Clin. Radiol. (1980), 31(1):41.

Inoue, Y., Takemoto, K., Miyamoto, T., et al.: Sequential computed tomography scans in acute cerebral infarction. Radiology (1980), 135(3): 655.

Kendall, B. E., and Pullicino, P.: Intravascular contrast injection in ischaemic lesions. II. Effect on prognosis. AJNR (1980), 19:241.

Kohlmeyer, K., and Graser, C.: Comparative study of computed tomography (CT) and carotid angiography (CAG) in stroke patients. Neuroradiology (1978), 16:162.

Manelfe, C., Clanet, M., Gigaud, M., et al.: Internal capsule: Normal anatomy and ischemic changes demonstrated by computed tomography. AJNR (1981), 2(2):149.

Martelli, A., Scotti, G., Harwood-Nash, D. C., et al.: Aneurysms of the vein of Galen in children: CT and angiographic correlations. Neuroradiology (1980), 20(3):123.

Norton, G. A., Kishore, P. R. S., and Lin, J.: CT contrast enhancement in cerebral infarction. Am. J. Roentgenol. (1978), 131:881.

O'Neill, M., Hope, T., and Thomson, G.: Giant intracranial aneurysms: Diagnosis with special reference to computerized tomography. Clin. Radiol. (1980), 31(1):27.

Pullicino, P., and Kendall, B. E., Contrast enhancement in ischaemic lesions, 1. Relationship to prognosis. Neuroradiology (1980), 19:235.

Shaw, C., Alvord, E. G., and Berry, R. G.: Swelling of the brain following ischemic infarction with arterial occlusion. Arch Neurol. (1959), 1:161.

Traupe, H., Heiss, W. D., Hoeffken, W., et al.: Hyperperfusion and enchancement in dynamic computed tomography of ischemic patients. J. Comput. Assist. Tomogr. (1979), 3(5):627.

Wing, S. D., Norman, D., Pollock, J. A., and Newton, T. H.: Contrast enhancement of cerebral infarcts in computed tomography. Radiology (1976), 121:89.

Yock, D. H., and Marshall, W. H.: Recent ischemic brain infarcts at computed tomography: Appearance pre- and post-contrast infusion. Radiology (1975), 117:599.

Trauma

Bergstrom, M., Ericson, K., Lavander, B., et al.: Computed tomography of cranial subdural and epidural hematomas: Variation of attenuation related to time and clinical events such as rebleeding. J. Comput. Assist. Tomogr. (1977), 1:449.

Davis, K. R., Taveras, J. M., Roberson, G. H., et al.: Computed tomography in head trauma. Semin. Roentgenol. (1977) 12:53.

Jeffries, B. F., Kishore, P. R., Singh, K. S., et al.: Contrast enhancement in the postoperative brain. Radiology (1981), 139(2):409.

Kim, K. S., Hemmati, M., and Weinberg, P. E.: Computed tomography in isodense subdural hematoma. Radiology (1978), 128:71.

Merino de Villasante, J., and Taveras, J. M.: Computerized tomography (CT) in acute head trauma. Am. J. Roentgenol. (1976), 126:765.

Tsai, F. Y., Teal, J. S., Quinn, M. F., et al.: CT of brainstem injury. AJR (1980), 134(4):717.

Zilkha, A., and Faegenburg, D.: Computed tomography of isodense subdural hematomas. Comput. Tomogr. (1979), 3(1):29.

Zimmerman, R. A., Bilaniuk, L. T., Gennarelli, T., et al.: Cranial computed tomography in diagnosis and management of acute head trauma. Am. J. Roentgenol. (1978), 131:27.

Acquired

Beck, R. W., Savino, P. J., Schatz, N. J., et al.: Plaque causing homonymous hemianopsia in multiple sclerosis identified by computed tomography. Am. J. Ophthalmol. (1982), 94(2):229.

Blaquiere, R. M.: The computed tomographic appearance of intra- and extracerebral abscesses. Br. J. Radiol. (1983), 56(663):171.

Enzmann, D. R., Ranson, B., Norman, D., et al.: Computed tomography of herpes simplex encephalitis. Radiology (1978), 129(2):419.

Fitz, C. R., and Harwood-Nash, D. C.: Computed tomography in hydrocephalus. CT (1978), 2(2):91.

Harwood-Nash, D. C.: Computed tomography and the abnormal brain in the neonate. J. Neuroradiol. (1981), 8(2):125.

Haughton, V. M., Ho, K. C., Williams, A. L., et al.: CT detection of demyelinated plaques in multiple sclerosis. AJR (1979), 132(2):213.

Heinz, E. R., Drayer, B. P., Haenggeli, C. A., et al.: Computed tomography in white-matter disease. Radiology (1979), 130:371.

Hughes, C. P., and Gado, M.: Computed tomography and aging of the brain. Radiology (1981), 139(2):391.

Ketonen, L., and Koskiniemi, M. L.: Computed tomography appearance of herpes simplex encephalitis. Clin. Radiol. (1980), 31(2):161.

Masdeu, J. C., Dobben, G. D., and Azar-Kia, B.: Dandy-Walker syndrome studied by computed tomography and pneumoencephalography. Radiology (1983), 147(1):109.

Nabawi, P., Dobben, G. D., Mafee, M., et al.: Diagnosis of lipoma of the corpus callosum by CT in five cases. Neuroradiology (1981), 21(3):159.

Naidich, T. P., Pudlowski, R. M., and Naidich, J. B.: Computed tomographic signs of chiari II malformation. II: Midbrain and cerebellum. Radiology (1980), 134(2):391.

Ramsey, R. G., and Huckman, M. S.: Computed tomography of porencephaly and other cerebrospinal fluid-containing lesions. Radiology (1977), 123:73.

Rosenblum, M. L., Hoff, J. T., Norman, D., et al.: Decreased mortality from brain abscesses since advent of computerized tomography. J. Neurosurg. (1978), 49(5):658.

Wang, A. M., Morris, J. H., Hickey, W. F., et al.: Unusual CT patterns of multiple sclerosis. AJNR (1983), 4(1):47.

Whelan, M. A., and Hilal, S. K.: Computed tomography as a guide in the diagnosis and follow-up of brain abscesses. Radiology (1980), 135(3):663.

Wu, S., Schenkenberg, T., Wing, S. D., et al.: Cognitive correlates of diffuse cerebral atrophy determined by computed tomography. Neurology (NY) (1981), 31(9):1180.

Orbit

Enzmann, D., Donaldson, S. S., Marshall, W. H., et al.: Computed tomography in orbital pseudotumor (idiopathic orbital inflammation). Radiology (1976), 120:597.

Gado, M. H., and Smith, M. E.: Computerized tomography of the orbit. Int. Ophthalmol. Clin. (1978), 18(1):151.

Hilal, S. K., and Trokel, S. L.: Computerized tomography of the orbit using thin sections. Semin. Roentgenol. (1977), 12(2):137.

Kadir, S., Aronow, S., and Davis, K. R.: The use of computerized tomography in the detection of intra-orbital foreign bodies. Comput. Tomogr. (1977), 1(2):151.

Tadmor, R., and New, P. F.: Computed tomography of the orbit with special emphasis on coronal sections. I. Normal anatomy. J. Comput. Assist. Tomogr. (1978), 2(1):24.

Wright, J. E., Lloyd, G. A. S., and Ambrose, J.: Computerized axial tomography in the detection of orbital space-occupying lesions. Am. J. Ophthalmol. (1975), 80:78.

DSA

Crummy, A. B., Strother, C. M., Sackett, J. F., et al.: Computerized fluoroscopy: Digital subtraction for intravenous angiocardiography and arteriography. AJR (1980), 135:1131.

Detmer, D. E., Fryback, D. G., and Strother, C. M.: Digital subtraction arteriography cost-effectiveness. *In* Mistretta, C. A., Crummy, A. B., Strother, D. M., et al.: (eds.): Digital Subtraction Arteriography. Chicago, Year Book Medical Publishers, Inc., 1982.

Meaney, T. F., Weinstein, M. A., Buonocore, E., et al.: Digital subtraction angiography of the human cardiovascular system. AJR (1980), 135:1153.

Roehrig, H., Nudelman, S., Capp, M. P., et al.: X-ray image intensifier video system for diagnostic radiology: Part I, design characteristics. SPIE 127 Optical Instrumentation in Medicine (1977), 6:216.

Strother, C. M., Sackett, J. E., Crummy, A. B., et al.: Clinical applications of computerized fluoroscopy: The extracranial carotid artery. Radiology (1980), 136:781.

Weinstein, M. A., Chilcote, W. A., Modic, M. E. T., et al.: Digital subtraction carotid angiography: A comparative study with conventional angiography in 100 patients. Radiological Society of North America, Dallas, 1980.

Weinstein, M. A., Modic, M. T., Buonocore, E., et al.: Digital subtraction angiography. Experience at the Cleveland Clinic Foundation. Appl. Radiol. (1981), 10:53.

NMR

Brant-Zawadski, M., Davis, P. L., et al.: NMR demonstration of cerebral abnormalities: Comparison with CT. AJR (1983), 140(5):847.

Doyle, F. H., Gore, J. C., Pennock, J. M., et al.: Imaging of the brain by nuclear magnetic resonance. Lancet (1981), 2(8237):53.

Huk, W., Heindel, W., Deimling, M., et al.: Nuclear magnetic resonance (NMR) tomography of the central nervous system: Comparison of two imaging sequences. J. Comput. Assist. Tomogr. (1983), 7(3):468.

Vermess, M., Bernstein, R. M., Bydder, G. M., et al.: Nuclear magnetic resonance (NMR) imaging of the brain in systemic lupus erythematosus. J. Comput. Assist. Tomogr. (1981), 7(3):461.

INDEX

Page numbers in *italics* refer to illustrations; (t) indicates tables.

Abnormalities, brain, acquired, 229–236
congenital, 237–251
Abscess, brain, 149–151, *149–151*
Absorption, coefficients of, in Hounsfield units, 5
Acoustic neurinoma, 98–107. See also *Neurinoma, acoustic.*
Adenocarcinoma, metastatic to brain, from unknown primary tumor, 126–127, *126, 127*
Adenoma, pituitary, 64–69, *64–69*
cystic, 70–71, *70, 71*
Agenesis, of corpus callosum, 247, *247*
Air cisternogram, 101, *101*
Aneurysm(s), 191–200
giant, of cavernous internal carotid artery, 72–73, *72, 73*
multiple, and tortuous basilar artery, 195–197, *195–197*
partially thrombosed, mimicking craniopharyngioma, 75–76, *75, 76*
posterior communicating artery, 200, *200*
suprasellar, large, 192–194, *192–194*
with intracerebral and intraventricular hemorrhage, 178, *178, 179*
Angiography, digital subtraction, 207. See also *Digital intravenous subtraction angiography.*
Aqueduct, cerebral, stenosis of, 74–75, *74*
Arteriovenous malformation, 201–206, *202–206*
Artery, basilar, tortuous, 199, *199*
and multiple aneurysms, 195–197, *195–197*
internal carotid, cavernous, giant aneurysm of, 72–73, *72, 73*
normal buckling of, 282, *282*
occluded, digital intravenous subtraction angiography for, 280, *280*
posterior communicating, aneurysm of, 200, *200*
Astrocytoma, cerebellar, 108–110, *108–110*, 121–122, *121, 122*
Grade II, 26–28, *26–28*, 38–45, *38–45*
Atrophy, of brain, 229–232, *230–232*
simulating subdural accumulations, 231–232, *231, 232*

Basal ganglion, hematoma of, 181, *181, 182*
moderate-sized, 189–190, *189*
Basal ganglion (*Continued*)
hematoma of, with intraventricular component, 183–184, *183, 184*
Basilar artery, tortuous, 199, *199*
and multiple aneurysms, 195–197, *195–197*
Battered child syndrome, 222–223, *222, 223*
Brain, abnormalities of, acquired, 229–236
congenital, 237–251
abscess of, 149–151, *149–151*
acute shearing injury to, 218–220, *218–220*
atrophy of, 229–232, *230–232*
simulating subdural accumulations, 231–232, *231, 232*
cavum septum pellucidum variation in, 13, *13*
CT scanning of, principles of, 1–3
hemiatrophy of, 246, *246*
normal anatomic variations of, 13, *13*
normal anatomy of, by CT, 1–4, *5–11*, 13–15, *13–15*
of child, 16, *16, 17*
postinfusion, 12, *12*, 18–20, *18–20*
preinfusion, 4, *6–11*
by nuclear magnetic resonance imaging, 287, *287*
normal intracranial circulation and, 281, *281*
nuclear magnetic resonance imaging for, 285–288
sagittal section on, 287, *287*
transverse section on, 287, *287*
postsurgical changes in, 20–23, *20–23*
post-traumatic abnormalities in, 211–227
spontaneous hematomas of, 172–190
tumors of, extracranial metastases with intracranial extension, 145–146, *145, 146*
metastatic, 125–151
pituitary, 63–76
primary, 24–123. See also names of specific types, such as *Glioma; Meningioma.*
vascular diseases of, 153–210. See also specific lesions, such as *Aneurysm; Infarct.*
Brain stem, hemorrhage of, 173, *173*
massive, 174, *174*
Breast, tumor of, metastatic to brain, 139–140, *139, 140*
at multiple sites, 143, *143–144*

Calcification, basal ganglion, 14, *14*
pineal gland, 14, *14*
Carcinoma, lung, metastatic to brain, 128–134, *128–134*, 138, *138*
at multiple sites, 143, *143–144*
splenic flexure, extracranial metastases of with intracranial extension, 145–146, *145, 146*
squamous cell, of face, without intracranial extension, 147–148, *147, 148*
Carotid artery, internal. See *Artery, internal carotid.*
Carotid–cavernous sinus fistula, 263–264, *263, 264*
Cavum septum pellucidum, 13, *13*
Cerebral hemorrhage. See *Hematoma, intracerebral; Hemorrhage, intracerebral.*
Cerebral infarct. See *Infarct.*
Chiari malformation, 239, *239*
with postoperative changes, 238–239, *238*
Child, battered, 222–223, *222, 223*
normal CT anatomy of brain in, 16, *16, 17*
sedation dosages for, in CT scanning, 16, 16(t)
Circulation, intracranial, normal, 281, *281*
Cisternogram, air, 101, *101*
Clivus, meningioma of, 123, *123*
Computed tomography, normal brain anatomy and, 12–19
orbital scanning and, 253–266. See also *Scanning, orbital.*
principles of, 1–3
printout sheet for, 3, *3, 4*
Computer artifacts on CT scan, following surgery, 20–23, *20–23*
Corpus callosum, agenesis of, 247, *247*
lipoma of, 250, *250*
Cyst(s), porencephalic, 240–245
cerebellar, 241–242, *241, 242*
following intracerebral hematoma, 227, *227*
left frontal, 243–245, *243–245*
Cystic pituitary adenoma, 70–71, *70, 71*

Digital intravenous subtraction angiography, 207, 277–284
enlarged thyroid on, 283, *283*
indications for in neuroradiology, 278(t)
normal buckling of internal carotid artery on, 282, *282*
normal intracranial circulation in, 281, *281*
normal views in, 279, *279*
pitfalls in use of, 284, *284*
DISA. See *Digital intravenous subtraction angiography.*

Encephalitis, herpes simplex type 1, 250, *251*
Exophthalmopathy, hyperthyroid, 260, *261*

Face, squamous cell carcinoma of, recurrent, without intracranial extension, 147–148, *147, 148*
Falx cerebri, meningioma of, 95–96, *95, 96*
Fistula, carotid–cavernous sinus, 263–264, *263, 264*
Foreign body, in eye, 257, *257*
Fossa, posterior, tumors of, 108–123
Fracture, blow-out, of medial orbital wall, 256–257, *256*
skull, depressed, 221, *221*
Frontal sinus, osteoma of, 266, *266*

Ganglion, basal, hematoma of, 181, *181, 182*
moderate-sized, 189–190, *189*
with intraventricular component, 183–184, *183, 184*
Ganglioneuroma, cerebellar, 108–110, *108–110*
Germinal plate, hemorrhage of in newborn, 269–274, *270, 271, 273, 274*
Glioblastoma multiforme, 29–31, *29–31*, 35–37, *35–37*, 46–47, *46*, 49–51, *49–51*, 53, *53*, 57–62, *57–62*
atypical, 52, *52*
hemorrhagic, 32–34, *32–34*
Glioma, 25–62. See also specific types, such as *Astrocytoma; Pinealoma.*
hypothalamic, 56–57, *56, 57*
pontine, 114–118, *114–118*
thalamic, 47–48, *47, 48*
Globe, foreign body in, 257, *257*
Granuloma, orbital, 262, *262*

Head trauma. See *Trauma.*
Hemangioma, of orbit, 260, *260*
Hematoma. See also *Hemorrhage.*
basal ganglionic, 181, *181–182*
moderate-sized, 189–190, *189*
with intraventricular component, 183–184, *183, 184*
epidural, acute, 217, *217*
left subfrontal, 225, *225*
intracerebral, and resulting porencephalic cyst, 227, *227*
postsurgical, 226, *226*
spontaneous, 172–190, 177, *177*, 180, *180*
in child, 175, *175*, 176, *176*
intraventricular, with basal ganglionic hematoma, 183–184, *183, 184*
subdural, acute left, 215, *215*
large left, 213, *213*
radionuclide scan of, 212, *212*
right, 214, *214*
subacute chronic, 216, *216*
ultrasound for, 275
Hemiatrophy, brain, 246, *246*
Hemorrhage. See also *Hematoma.*
brain stem, 173, *173*
massive, 174, *174*

Hemorrhage (*Continued*)
in germinal plate of newborn, ultrasound for, 269–274, *270, 271, 273, 274*
intracerebral, and aneurysm, 178, *178, 179*
spontaneous, in child, 175, *175*, 176, *176*
various CT appearances of, 185–188. *185–188*
intraventricular, and aneurysm, 178, *178, 179*
subarachnoid, acute, 198, *198*
Herpes simplex type 1 encephalitis, 250, *251*
Hodgkin's disease, of orbit, 265, *265*
Hydrocephalus, communicating, 232, *233*
low pressure, 232, *233*
ultrasound for, 272–274, *273, 274*
with germinal plate hemorrhage and porencephaly, 272–274, *273, 274*
Hyperthyroidism, exophthalmopathy in, 260, *261*
Hypothalamus, glioma of, 56–57, *56, 57*

Infarct(s), brain, 153–171
acute, 159, *159*
and small asymptomatic meningioma, 171, *171*
calcified, 160, *160*
cerebral, 161–162, *161, 162*
old, 156, *156*
large, with mass effect, 157, *157*
multiple small areas of, 158, *158*
secondary to sickle cell disease, 154–155, *154, 155*
with luxury perfusion, 163–169, *163–169*
with mass effect, 170, *170*
Injury. See *Trauma.*
Intracerebral hematoma, spontaneous. See *Hematoma, intracerebral.*

Lipoma, of corpus callosum, 250, *250*
Lung, carcinoma of, metastatic to brain, 128–134, *128–134*, 138, *138*
multiple brain metastases, 141–142, *141, 142*
Luxury perfusion, 153
in infarction, 163–169, *163–169*

Malformation, arteriovenous, 201–206, *202–206*
Chiari, 239, *239*
with postoperative changes, 238–239, *238*
Malignant melanoma, metastatic to brain, 135–137, *135–137*
Medulloblastoma, 111–113, *111–113*, 119–120, *119, 120*
Melanoma, malignant, metastatic to brain, 135–137, *135–137*
Meningioma, 77–97
anterior falx, 95, *95*
asymptomatic, infarct and, 171, *171*
cerebellopontine angle, 89–90, *89, 90*
clivus, 123, *123*
falx cerebri, 95–96, *95, 96*
and left acoustic neurinoma, 106, *106*
left frontal, 83–84, *83, 84*
parasagittal convexity, 97, *97*
right parasellar, 78–79, *78, 79*
right sphenoid wing, 93–94, *93, 94*
right-sided, 80–82, *80–82*
tentorial, 85–86, *85, 86*, 91–92, *91, 92*
with extracranial metastases, 87–89, *87, 88*
Metastases, extracranial, of meningioma, 87–89, *87, 88*
to brain, 125–151
to orbit, 258–259, *259*
Multiple sclerosis, 234–236, *235, 236*

Neonate, germinal plate hemorrhage in, 269–274, *270, 271, 273, 274*
ultrasound for, 267–275. See also *Ultrasound, neonatal.*
Neurinoma, acoustic, 98–107
bilateral, 105, *105*
left, 102–104, *102–104*
and falx meningioma, 106, *106*
right, 99–100, *99, 100*, 107, *107*
NMR imaging. See *Nuclear magnetic resonance imaging.*
Nuclear magnetic resonance imaging, 285–288
anatomy of brain on, 287, *287*
sagittal section of spine on, 288, *288*

Orbit, scanning of, 253–266
and metastases to, 258–259, *259*
hemangioma and, 260, *260*
Hodgkin's disease of, 265, *265*
in medial blow-out fracture, 256–257, *256*
normal anatomy on, 254–255, *254, 255*
pseudotumor of, 262, *262*
Osteoma, of frontal sinus, 266, *266*

Perfusion, luxury, 153
in infarction, 163–169, *163–169*
Pinealoma, 54–56, *54, 55*
Pituitary gland, adenoma of, 64–69, *64–69*
cystic, 70–71, *70, 71*
tumors of, 63–76
Plate, germinal. See *Germinal plate.*
Pons, glioma of, 114–118, *114–118*
Porencephaly. See *Cyst(s), porencephalic.*
Post-traumatic abnormalities, 211–227. See also *Trauma, abnormalities following.*
Printout sheet, for CT of brain, 3, *3*, 4
Pseudotumor, orbital, 262, *262*

Radionuclide scan, of subdural hematoma, 212, *212*
Resonance imaging, nuclear magnetic. See *Nuclear magnetic resonance imaging.*
Retinoblastoma, 258, *258*

Scanning, orbital, 253–266
in hemangioma, 260, *260*
in Hodgkin's disease of orbit, 265, *265*
in hyperthyroid exophthalmopathy, 260, *261*
in osteoma of frontal sinus, 266, *266*
normal orbital anatomy, 254–255, *254, 255*
of foreign body in globe, 257, *257*
of metastases to orbit, 258–259, *259*
of orbital pseudotumor, 262, *262*
of retinoblastoma, 258, *258*
Sclerosis, multiple, 234–236, *235, 236*
tuberous, 249, *249*
Sedation, dosage schedules of, for children, 16, 16(t)
Sickle cell disease, infarct secondary to, 154–155, *154, 155*
Sinus, frontal, osteoma of, 266, *266*
superior sagittal, thrombosis of, 207–210, *208–210*
Skull, fracture of, depressed, 221, *221*
Spine, sagittal section of, by nuclear magnetic resonance imaging, 288, *288*
Squamous cell carcinoma. See *Carcinoma, squamous cell.*
SSS. See *Sinus, superior sagittal.*
Stenosis, of adult cerebral aqueduct, 74–75, *74*
Sturge-Weber disease, 248–249, *248*
Subarachnoid hemorrhage, acute, 198, *198*
Subdural hematoma. See *Hematoma, subdural.*
Superior sagittal sinus. See *Sinus, superior sagittal.*
Suprasellar aneurysm, 192–194, *192–194*
Surgery, brain, changes in CT scan following, 20–23, *20–23*
ultrasound during, 275

Thalamus, glioma of, 47–48, *47, 48*
Thrombosis, superior sagittal sinus, 207–210, *208–210*
Thyroid, enlarged, on digital intravenous subtraction angiography, 283, *283*
Trauma, abnormalities following, 211–227
head, acute shearing injury to brain in, 218–220, *218–220*
tetrapolar, 224–225, *224*
Tuberous sclerosis, 249, *249*
Tumors, brain, metastatic, 125–151
pituitary, 63–76
posterior fossa, 108–123
primary, 25–123. See also names of specific types, such as *Glioma; Meningioma.*
breast, metastatic to brain, 139–140, *139, 140*
multiple brain metastases of, 143, *143, 144*

Ultrasound, intraoperative, 275
in germinal plate hemorrhage, 269–274, *270, 271, 273, 274*
in hydrocephalus, 272–274, *273, 274*
neonatal, 267–275
method of, 267
normal examination in, 267–268, *268*

Vascular diseases, of brain, 153–210. See also specific lesions, such as *Aneurysm; Infarct.*